THE SCIENCE OF
BEACH
LIFEGUARDING

THE SCIENCE OF
BEACH
LIFEGUARDING

Edited by

Mike Tipton
University of Portsmouth, UK

Adam Wooler
Rescue Marine Services, Cornwall, UK

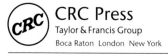
CRC Press
Taylor & Francis Group
Boca Raton London New York

CRC Press is an imprint of the
Taylor & Francis Group, an **informa** business

CRC Press
Taylor & Francis Group
6000 Broken Sound Parkway NW, Suite 300
Boca Raton, FL 33487-2742

First issued in paperback 2021

© 2016 by Taylor & Francis Group, LLC
CRC Press is an imprint of Taylor & Francis Group, an Informa business

No claim to original U.S. Government works

ISBN 13: 978-0-367-78769-1 (pbk)
ISBN 13: 978-1-4822-4597-4 (hbk)

**Visit the Taylor & Francis Web site at
http://www.taylorandfrancis.com**

**and the CRC Press Web site at
http://www.crcpress.com**

Dedication

This book is dedicated to Dr (Surg Rear Admiral) Frank Golden, Dr Mark ('Buster') Harries and Cdr Charles Thomson MBE, three legends who managed to scale the heights professionally but never lost sight of their Celtic roots. Respected by all, they did an enormous amount for both beach life-guarding and the editors of this book; we are proud to have had them as friends.

Contents

Foreword

The International Life Saving Federation (ILS) vision is a 'world free from drowning' and its mission is to lead, support and collaborate with national and international organisations engaged in drowning prevention, water safety, water rescue, lifesaving, lifeguarding and lifesaving sport.

The Science of Beach Lifeguarding provides an overview of current evidence in relation to beach lifeguarding. In particular, it supports the following objectives of ILS:

1. Recommend best practice in drowning prevention, aquatic lifesaving, resuscitation and emergency care
2. Encourage the conduct of training and development of standards available to the whole of the aquatic lifesaving world for drowning prevention and lifesaving
3. Promote uniformity concerning equipment, information, symbols and laws for control and regulation within the aquatic environment

The World Health Organization recently published its *Global Report on Drowning*, which found that drowning is the third leading cause of unintentional injury/death worldwide. The drowning chain recognises that appropriate surveillance is one of the intervention strategies that should be implemented to reduce death by drowning. Beach lifeguarding provides that level of supervision at beaches around the world and studies from both the United States and Australia indicate that many more people would have drowned if beach lifeguards were not present at our beaches.

This book will be of value to a wide range of individuals interested in beach lifeguarding, including local land managers who wish to set up a lifeguard service and those involved in the recruitment and training of lifeguards. The book will assist all those interested in beach lifeguarding and will support efforts to reduce the global burden of drowning.

While the book notes that much work still needs to be done in relation to researching the evidence that underpins current accepted beach lifeguard practices, it is pleasing to see the progress in this area. The book gives the information to improve both techniques and efficiency of lifeguarding and provides an evidence base for beach lifeguarding.

I highly recommend *The Science of Beach Lifeguarding* to not only all those involved in beach lifeguarding, but to all who are concerned with reducing the global burden of drowning.

Graham Ford
President, International Life Saving Federation

Acknowledgements

The following organizations have helped and supported the editors in the scientific journey that has led to this book: the University of Portsmouth, the Royal National Lifeboat Institution, Surf Life Saving GB, Surf Life Saving Australia and the United States Lifesaving Association.

The following authors contributed their time and expertise to the book:

Chris Brewster
Christine Branche
Julie Gilchrist
Ian Greatbatch
Michael Wright
Andrew Short
Adam Weir
Robert Brander
Tim Scott
Mike Tipton

Peter Wernicki
Kevin Moran
Christy Northfield
David Szpilman
Joost Bierens
Jenny Smith (nee Page)
Andrew Byatt
Justin Sempsrott
David Livingstone
David Anton
Polona Jaki
Tara Reilly
Norman Farmer
Thomas Mecrow

Finally, we thank Carole Tipton, whose expertise as a proofreader was invaluable, as well as the staff at CRC Press, who have been patient, enthusiastic and supportive along the way.

Editors

Mike Tipton was educated at the University of Keele (Staffordshire, UK) and the University of London, and joined the University of Surrey (Guidford, UK) in 1986. After 12 years at the Robens Institute (Guildford, UK) and European Institute of Health and Medical Science (Guildford, UK), he moved to the University of Portsmouth (UK) in 1998. In addition to his university positions, Professor Tipton was based at the Institute of Naval Medicine (INM; Gosport, UK) from 1983 to 2004 and was consultant head of the Environmental Medicine Division of the INM from 1996. He has spent over 30 years researching and advising the military, industry and elite sports people in the areas of thermoregulation, environmental and occupational physiology and survival in the sea. He has published over 500 scientific papers, reports, chapters and books in these areas.

Professor Tipton has been a consultant in survival and thermal medicine to the Royal Air Force and UK Sport. He sits on the Royal National Lifeboat Institution's Medical & Survival Committee and the Ectodermal Dysplasia Society's Medical Advisory Board. In 2004, Professor Tipton was made an honorary life member of the International Association for Safety & Survival Training in recognition of his work in sea survival. He chaired UK Sport's Research Advisory Group and now sits on the English Institute of Sports' Technical Advisory Group. Professor Tipton chairs the Energy Institute's Health Technical Committee and is a trustee of Surf Lifesaving GB and senior editor of the journal *Extreme Physiology and Medicine*. Professor Tipton is a Fellow of the Royal Society of Medicine and provides advice to a range of universities, government departments, industries, medical, search and rescue and media organisations.

Adam Wooler has considerable experience and expertise in lifeguarding, having instigated the establishment of the Royal National Lifeboat Institution (RNLI) Beach Lifeguard service. He also has a background in academic research. He earned an MPhil in arctic geophysics from the University of Plymouth (UK), Scott Polar Research Institute (Cambridge, UK), Cambridge University and Atlantic Geoscience Centre (Nova Scotia, Canada). The award of a Rotary scholarship allowed Adam to travel to the Antarctic and then to study at the University of Wellington (New Zealand) and the University of Western Australia (Perth).

On returning to the UK, Adam became the chief executive of Surf Life Saving GB and took up various committee positions with the International Life Saving Federation. Following a move to the RNLI in 2000, Adam instigated a partnership with the Universities of Portsmouth and Plymouth to conduct groundbreaking research into the field of beach lifeguarding.

Following a further 3-year secondment as CEO of Surf Life Saving GB, Adam returned to the RNLI as head of Coastal Safety and Research, establishing the Operations Research Unit. Although Adam left the RNLI in 2012, he continues to act as an external supervisor for PhD students and has co-authored several papers on lifeguard-related research.

Introduction

Progress is driven, in part, by the evaluation and re-evaluation of that which has gone before. Each time this occurs, current thinking and expectations are used as the tools by which to gauge the value of that which exists. So it is that as we have moved into an era of 'evidence-based' decision making, much of what has gone before, in numerous disciplines, appears largely based on opinion, albeit expert opinion or experience. That is not to say that this is an invalid approach; it is simply less defensible than hard data. At a time when everything exists to be challenged, the more valid the basis of decisions, the more supporting evidence, the greater the ability to defend the consequences, whether those consequences be the exclusion of someone from employment, adoption of a medical procedure or introduction of a beach safety campaign.

The idea for this book came about when the editors undertook a series of studies on behalf of the Royal National Lifeboat Institution (RNLI). Having been asked to become involved in beach lifeguarding and being confronted with the currently accepted pre-employment fitness test, they asked the question 'why?' to which the answer was invariably, 'because we've always done it this way'. The initial groundbreaking research by a team from the University of Portsmouth (UK), including Dr Tara J. Reilly, therefore quantified the scientific rationale behind a new RNLI-specific fitness standard. This research was then expanded to cover a fairly broad range of topics, from strength standards for the operation of inshore rescue boats and rescue watercraft, to visual acuity, to surveillance techniques, to surf swimming. Two things became apparent during these studies. Firstly, in many areas not much work had been undertaken on the specific topic of the occupational, as opposed to sporting, aspects of beach lifeguarding. Secondly, many of the current practices in beach lifeguarding were consequently not well evidence-based or had simply been imported from other areas with little attempt to check the validity of such a transfer.

We have therefore attempted to assemble a book focused on the scientific evidence that underpins what is taught and practised in beach lifeguarding. We believe it is the first book to try and pull together all the different areas involved in beach lifeguarding and to evaluate their evidence base. Each chapter is written by an expert or experts in the respective field, with the brief of including, as far as possible, the evidence base for existing practice and recommendations. Where areas are not covered or only mentioned (e.g. the choice of specific pieces of lifeguard equipment), it is generally because they lack any data-driven evidence base. The process of identifying these gaps in our scientific knowledge and proposals for further research are therefore addressed in the concluding chapters.

It is hoped that this book will be of value to a wide range of individuals interested in the topics surrounding beach lifeguarding, from those studying areas from drowning to employment standards, to those responsible for the management, recruitment and training of beach lifeguards. The World Health Organisation recently published its *Global Report on Drowning*, which found that drowning is the third leading cause of unintentional injury death worldwide. In light of this publication, this book has become even more relevant and important as part of the global effort to reduce this considerable public, but often hidden, health risk.

This book would not have been possible without the cooperation of the excellent organizations acknowledged as well as a large cohort of young (and slightly less young) beach lifeguards who volunteered both information and themselves for research studies. They are a credit to their generation; we thank them and applaud what they do. We hope this book is of some use to them in achieving their laudable aim of saving lives and that it gives the profession of beach lifeguarding greater recognition within the emergency services community.

Mike Tipton
University of Portsmouth, Portsmouth, UK

Adam Wooler
Rescue Marine Services, Cornwall, UK

Contributors

David Anton MSc (Occ Med), MBBS, DAvMed FFOM (Retd)
Formerly Consultant Occupational Physician,
Royal National Lifeboat Institution, Poole, UK

Joost Bierens MD, PhD, MCPM
Maatschappij tot Redding van Drenkelingen,
Amsterdam, The Netherlands

Christine Branche PhD
National Institute for Occupational Safety and
Health, Centers for Disease Control and
Prevention, Washington, DC

Robert Brander MSc, PhD
School of Biological, Earth and Environmental
Sciences, University of New South Wales, Sydney,
New South Wales, Australia

Chris Brewster BS
International Life Saving Federation – Americas
Region, United States Lifesaving Association,
San Diego, California

Andrew Byatt BSc (Hons), PGDip
Surf Life Saving GB, Exeter, UK

Norman Farmer ESM
Surf Life Saving Australia, Sydney, Australia

Julie Gilchrist MD
Division of Unintentional Injury Prevention,
National Center for Injury Prevention and
Control, Centers for Disease Control and
Prevention, Atlanta, Georgia

Ian Greatbatch MPhil, PhD
Department of Geography and Geology
School of the Natural and Built Environment
Faculty of Science, Engineering and Computing
Kingston University, London, UK

Polona Jaki MD, PhD
Eye Hospital, University Medical Centre,
Ljubljana, Slovenia

David Livingstone MSc
Department of Geography and Geology
School of the Natural and Built Environment,
Faculty of Science, Engineering and Computing
Kingston University, London, UK

Thomas Mecrow MPH
Royal National Lifeboat Institution, Poole, UK

Kevin Moran MEd, PhD
Faculty of Education, University of Auckland,
Auckland, New Zealand

Christy Northfield BA, MA
Morgan Stanley, Vero Beach, Florida

Tara Reilly PhD
Human Performance Research and Development
DFIT, Canadian Armed Forces, Ottawa, ON,
Canada

Tim Scott PhD
School of Marine Science and Engineering,
Plymouth University, Plymouth, UK

Justin Sempsrott MD, FAAEM
Lifeguards Without Borders
Emergency Medicine and EMS Faculty,
Wake Forest University, Winston-Salem,
North Carolina, USA

Andrew Short MA, PhD
School of Geosciences, University of Sydney,
New South Wales, Australia

Jenny Smith (nee Page) MSc, PhD
Department of Sport and Exercise Science,
University of Chichester, Chichester, UK

David Szpilman MD
Drowning Resuscitation Centre, CBMERJ,
Research and Teaching Center, Miguel Couto
Hospital, Rio de Janeiro, Brazil

Mike Tipton MSc, PhD
Extreme Environments Laboratory,
Department of Sport and Exercise Science,
University of Portsmouth, Portsmouth, UK

Adam Weir BSc, MAppSc
Surf Life Saving NSW, Belrose, Australia

Peter Wernicki MD, FAAOS
Department of Orthopedic Surgery,
Florida State College of Medicine,
Tallahassee, Florida

Michael Wright BSc, MSc, CPsychol, AfBPsS
Greenstreet Berman Ltd., London, UK

Adam Wooler BSc, MPhil
Rescue Marine Services, Cornwall, UK

PART 1

History and Context

History of beach lifeguarding

CHRIS BREWSTER

LIFESAVER/LIFEGUARD

This chapter uses the terms *lifesaver* and *lifeguard*. The term *lifesaver* is used to refer to all people who rescue others in peril in the water, whether acting as volunteers or as compensated employees, under the premise that lifesaving is an act which they both perform. The term *lifeguard* is used to refer to people compensated for that role. This chapter also uses the term *professional* to refer to those who practise lifesaving as a profession. Volunteers can, of course, perform at a highly professional level as well.

INTRODUCTION

Beaches have not always been a popular destination. They were once shunned by most people. That has changed, of course, but the intense popularity of beaches we know today is something very new in an historical sense. It has developed over just the past 100 years or so. With that popularity has come a new role – the beach lifesaver.

In the 1800s, the beach wasn't seen as an attraction, but a dangerous place. The population of many countries was mostly spread out in rural areas [1]. There were no cars or paved roads. Water was important to the founders of cities like London, New York and Sydney as a medium for moving people and goods aboard ships. Such cities were understandably positioned around harbours, with protected anchorage and docks. For most of the population, a trip to the beach was a journey, an adventure few chose and perhaps fewer could consider with the limited time available for recreation. That changed over a surprisingly short period of time, with beachfront property going from being undesirable to being prized, and beach recreation went from being an oddity to a passion. This current reality will not come as a surprise to the reader.

The dynamics that brought about such rapid change in the perceived desirability of the beach varied somewhat from place to place. The manner in which those visiting the beaches and swimming in their waters came to be protected also varied. Here are some stories of that evolution of the beach into a highly sought destination and domicile, and why lifesavers have come to be so essential.

BATHING AND SWIMMING

Lifesavers are not needed if few people choose to enter the water, and for much of human history few did so intentionally. Open-water bathing came first. Bathing (the recreational sort) might be described as passive enjoyment of the water – sitting or wading in it, for example. Without the skill to propel oneself through water (swimming), bathing was the way one might enjoy a pond or lake. Of course, the threat of drowning was ever present, particularly at an ocean beach with waves and currents.

One of the most interesting inventions that helped popularize ocean bathing was the bathing machine. Scarborough, on the Yorkshire coast of England, has a record of the earliest bathing machines in 1735 [2]. These machines were actually cabins on wheels which could be pulled by horses or men to the water's edge. The bather would then descend some steps straight into the sea in something resembling a private ocean pool. Women often enjoyed total privacy thanks to a refinement which allowed a canvas hood to cover the area of sea around the steps [3]. Obviously this was not ocean bathing for the masses, but dunking for the elite.

Some of the fisher folk of Brighton, a town which was transformed in the 1700s from a small village into a thriving resort through the popularity of sea bathing, found new and profitable employment as 'dippers' and 'bathers'. Dippers were for the ladies and bathers for the gentlemen, but their task was the same: to plunge their subject vigorously into and out of the water. By 1790, there were some 20 locals offering this strenuous service to the rich, titled and even royal visitors who flocked to the town [4]. These were not lifeguards per se, but attendants.

George, Prince of Wales, started to frequent his beloved Brighton in 1783 and his father, King George III, adopted Weymouth in Dorset as his pet resort after his first of many visits and dips in the sea there in 1789. Sea bathing had now received the royal seal of approval and had become, if not compulsory, at least very difficult to resist among the fashionable of the age. In Australia, there were no bathing machines, but as early as 1850 there were plenty of bathhouses in Sydney harbour, which were quite popular [5].

Over time, some people naturally became interested in swimming as a distinct skill that allowed the practitioner to move forward in the water and, in fact, prevent drowning [5]. This text, though, is not a history of bathing or swimming. It is a history of beach lifesaving, by volunteers and professionals. We now turn our attention to the reasons that lifesavers were needed, which of course meant that more than just the elite would need to favour the water.

THE FIRST LIFESAVERS

The beaches of the East Coast of the United States were lightly inhabited in the early 1800s. Those who lived near the shore were well aware of its hazards, though. Shipwrecks were common. Volunteer efforts to mount shore-based rescues of imperilled sailors were first initiated by the Massachusetts Humane Society in 1807. In 1848, the US Congress approved $10,000 to pay for 'surfboats, rockets, carronades (line throwing mortars), and other necessary apparatus for the better preservation of life and property from shipwrecks along the coast of New Jersey' [6]. They were positioned in eight stations, to be staffed by volunteers in case of shipwrecks. In 1850 for example, using this gear, at least 201 shipwrecked people were saved by beach-based rescuers, but many still died [6].

In Great Britain, similar efforts took place. The Royal National Lifeboat Institution (RNLI) was founded in 1824 as the National Institution for the Preservation of Life from Shipwreck [7]. The first RNLI Gold Medal was awarded to Charles Fremantle of the Lymington Coastguard in 1824 for swimming with a line from a beach to rescue the crew of the Swedish brigantine *Carl Jean*, which was in difficulty close to the shore near Christchurch [7].

In the United States, the volume of problems related to shipwrecks along the shoreline brought about the creation of the US Life-Saving Service in 1878 (which would later, in 1915, merge with the

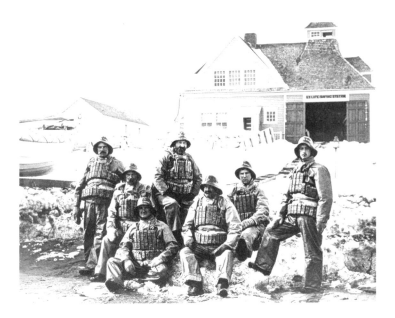

Figure 1.1 US Life-Saving Service crew (Wallis Sands station) beside their surfboat wearing storm suits with cork life vests. (U.S. Coast Guard; http://www.uscg.mil/history/CG)

Revenue Cutter Service to become the US Coast Guard) [6]. It appears to be the first in the world to use the term *life-saving* to apply to the effort to rescue people from drowning [5]. They used tools such as double-ended surfboats, launched from shore with six rowers and a man at a tiller oar, and lines fired from shore to vessels in distress, along with a variety of other devices to bring people to safety (Figures 1.1 and 1.2). There ultimately came to be 279 lifesaving stations, whose lifesavers had rescued over 150,000 from drowning by 1915 [6].

This is not a history of the beach-based rescue of mariners, which took place in other countries as well, but a history of beach lifesaving would be incomplete without mention of those first beach-based rescuers who were engaged in the rescue of shipwrecked people. Their work, methods and equipment set the stage for, and perhaps inspired, what came later.

THE FIRST BEACH LIFESAVERS TO PROTECT SWIMMERS

United States bathing resorts and lifeguards

Philadelphia, Pennsylvania is known as the birthplace of democracy in the United States. It is where the first US Congress met, and it also offered

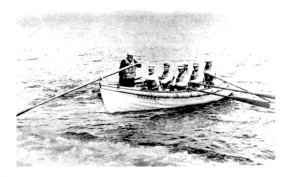

Figure 1.2 US Life-Saving Service surfboat drill (Orleans station), with crew wearing summer working suits and keeper in the standard uniform, with cork vests, 1908. (U.S. Coast Guard; http://www.uscg.mil/history/CG)

inspiration that eventually brought about creation of the first professional beach lifeguard corps – ironic, since Philadelphia is some 50 miles from the Atlantic coast and from any ocean beaches.

In summer, Philadelphia can swelter in heat and humidity. Before air conditioning, it was a hot summertime stew of humanity. Some entrepreneurs had an idea. What if we were to build a railroad to the coast, where the cool sea breezes would temper the heat of summer, and a dip in the ocean all the more so? What if we were to build a resort by the sea? They attracted investors, convinced the Camden and Amboy Railroad to build a line to Abescon Island and constructed the United States Hotel on a 'deserted pile of sand' [8]. The name of the 'resort': Atlantic City.

Atlantic City opened for business with 600 guests taking the train there on 1 June 1854. The entrepreneurs were the first in the United States by 10 years to establish direct train service to an ocean resort, but many were to duplicate their concept elsewhere [8]. The ocean resort, accessible by train, had arrived. It was 'the first planned city by the sea' [8]. They promoted the resort as beneficial to health, much as had the promoters of bathing machines in England. The author Gay Talese relates their exaggerated claims, bolstered by doctors, that the cool breezes, 'had a salubrious effect upon those suffering from asthma, consumption, laryngitis, pneumonia, diabetes, digestive disorders and other maladies, including insanity' [9]. They also promoted the healthiness of the salt water, but there was a particular problem unmentioned in that regard – drowning.

Atlantic City soon became popular. As the volume of visitors grew there and at other resorts that came to be built elsewhere along the Jersey Shore, it was inevitable that drowning would be a problem that could not be ignored. There were 13 drowning deaths in Atlantic City in 1865, for example, which brought about the installation of ropes extending out into the water attached to poles. The theory was that people could use them to steady themselves or (hopefully) pull themselves to safety, although they were largely ineffective at stemming the tide of drowning [8].

Volunteer lifesavers had begun offering their services in Atlantic City early on, walking the beaches and rescuing people with a ring buoy [10]. They offered assistance at no cost, but asked for a donation in return. Indeed some were even listed in the Atlantic City directory and compensated to some extent by the railroad or a hotel [10]. The drowning deaths also caused the larger hotels (there were now many) to employ lifeguards [9] to watch over the bathers, and in 1855 the Atlantic City council appointed two men whom they called 'Constables of the Surf' [10].

Most of the lifesavers, though, were quite unofficial. Talese relates, 'The lifeguard brigade of the mid-1800s was composed of a few petty brigands who received no municipal salary and therefore supported themselves in summer by unsubtly soliciting donations from the proprietors and patrons of bathhouses and the largess of anyone they rescued from drowning. When their funds ran low, they would fake rescues' [9]. Indeed, he reports, one of their fake victims was a young W.C. Fields, who was paid $10 a week to swim out and feign rescue, sometimes 12 times a day [11]. In his later life as a famous comic actor he reflected upon those days, saying that he'd quit swimming and drinking water because he'd ingested enough [11].

Since the blended approach of volunteers and a few paid constables wasn't working well, in 1875 the city hired more Constables of the Surf. By 1884, there were 25 in the city's employ [10]. They were city policemen with specialized responsibilities, who would return to land-based police duties after bathing hours were over. They were perhaps more effective than the volunteers, but police were needed ashore in a seaside resort with the many law enforcement issues that arose.

On 12 June 1892, the Atlantic City Beach Patrol was created as a municipal service with two lifeguards [10]. Hotels, bathhouses and associations had paid lifeguards before this, but this service was organized by the city [10]. By 1900, there were 55 members of the Atlantic City Beach Patrol (Figure 1.3), and by 1910 there were 64. It has continually operated since that time, saving lives each year as the fortunes of Atlantic City itself have risen and fallen repeatedly. These US efforts to protect bathers and swimmers along the Jersey Shore appear to have been the first in the world [5].

Volunteer lifesavers were to precede paid lifeguards in other areas of the United States as well. An organization called the US Volunteer Life Saving Corps was created in 1892 [5]. Loosely organized, it reported rescues in various parts of the country. In 1908, off Venice Beach, California, a member named George Freeth, who had been brought from Hawaii as a performer to attract people to seaside bathhouses and billed as 'the man who walks on water' (on a surfboard), rescued

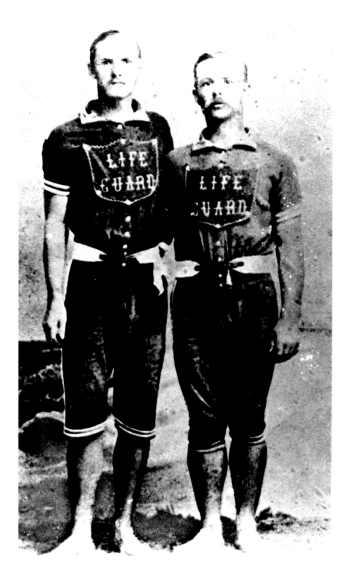

Figure 1.3 On 12 June 1892, the Atlantic City Beach Patrol was added to the city payroll with two paid lifeguards: Dan Headley and Nick Jefferies. The white belts had a loop at the back, which they would fasten to their rescue device. (Courtesy of Michael 'Spike' Fowler. With permission.)

seven men from drowning in a storm that cap-sized their fishing boats [12]. He was one of many citizen rescuers awarded the Gold Lifesaving Medal by the US Life-Saving Service [13], and he is also credited with introducing surfing to the US mainland [14].

On the West Coast of the United States, the city of Long Beach, California, hired its first municipal lifeguard in 1908, and the city of San Diego began a municipal beach lifeguard operation overseen by the police department in 1914 [14,15]. In each instance, bathhouses or hotels built beside the ocean, fed by regular train service, drew large numbers of people to the beach and the water. In 1918, 13 people died in one day in rip currents off San Diego's Ocean Beach, which caused the city to realize it needed to further bolster its lifeguard staffing levels [15]. Other lifeguard agencies were formed on the West Coast in later years, just as happened on the East Coast and Gulf Coast.

The American Red Cross (ARC) became involved as well, at the urging of Wilbert E. Longfellow,

Commodore-in-Chief of New York City's US Volunteer Life Saving Corps. The ARC created a standardized lifesaving training programme and issued certificates [16]. In the absence of any other source of standardized national training, some beach lifeguard agencies came to use elements of the ARC programme in their training or as a prerequisite, while others eschewed the ARC programme entirely.

As the volume of rescues rose, the volunteer approach faded away. Beach lifeguards in the United States came to be viewed as an essential municipal service, expected just as were police and fire departments, needed to ensure the safety of tourists and locals alike and to protect economies based on beach tourism. Today many of these beach lifeguard organizations are major municipal services, with annual budgets in millions of dollars.

Australian bathing clubs and lifesavers

In Australia, things evolved differently. There was a ban on daylight ocean bathing imposed by many local and state governments, including Sydney. It was perhaps reluctantly enforced by the police, but served to discourage more responsible Australians from venturing into the surf. Even so, there were drowning deaths, which raised concern. In 1899, a Life Saving Brigade was formed at Manly Beach, but it was reactive, with a bell to be rung if volunteers from the community were needed to respond to a person in distress, and it existed for only a few years [5].

In New South Wales, the law against daylight bathing was not lifted until 1903 and only then because of protests by a growing number of people. The most public of protests was conducted by the editor of the *Manly and North Sydney News*, William Gocher, who, sensing the support of his readers, marched into the waves in a comically oversized costume on three occasions at midday until the Sydney police ultimately arrested him [5,17]. Things changed rather rapidly thereafter, and thousands took up the pastime within a few years [5].

The need to rescue people in distress became quickly apparent, but how to organize lifesaving services was another matter. Unlike the beach resorts that had been built in the United States, which were commercial operations created to attract tourists and generate income, Sydney's ocean beaches were bordered by small communities, and the beach patrons were mostly daytrippers or locals. The heavy commercial aspect was lacking, along with the financial support it lent and the imperative to minimize drowning deaths to protect the income of resort owners. The local council of Manly paid for a 'surf attendant', but others were not willing or able to accept such an expense [5].

In 1907, a club was formed at Bondi Beach, which Surf Life Saving Australia (SLSA) now recognizes, with some controversy, as its first surf club [5]. Others formed in neighbouring communities in short order. Australian disputes as to which club came first aside, a key was that volunteer clubs allowed for protection of bathers without substantial costs to the local councils to hire lifeguards. In turn, the councils provided land for clubhouses and various benefits to the members. These surf clubs were essentially swimming clubs that agreed to protect others. This solution was to be followed throughout Australia.

Oddly enough, the clubs did not initially choose to collaborate for reasons related to surf lifesaving. Instead they united over an objection to local ordinances requiring very modest bathing costumes, which were uncomfortable for swimming [5]. When the clubs came together to form the Surf Bathing Association of New South Wales in 1907, their overriding interest was to fight the rules. Freedom versus modesty was the biggest issue to occupy them at its inception: should men be forced to wear an additional skirt over their neck-to-knee costumes? The association said definitely not [18].

More and more, however, the clubs became involved in protecting swimmers. It was what their members had to offer councils in return for permission to build clubhouses and occupy exclusive areas of the beach. By 1910, the association had instituted the basic qualification required for volunteer lifesaving – the Bronze Medallion [5].

The clubs initially enjoyed a positive relationship with the Royal Life Saving Society (RLSS), but they were also frustrated that the rescue methods it taught were not designed for the surf. Over the years, the relationship became strained. When the surf clubs renamed themselves the 'Surf Life Saving Association of New South Wales', the end was near.

In 1924, a key agreement was reached. The RLSS would confine its activities to inland waters and enclosed baths. The SLSA would confine itself to coastal beaches [5].

Calling themselves 'SLSA Australia' did not mean they represented the entire country – far from it. Over time, though, surf lifesaving clubs that developed in other states decided to become affiliated with the single body and every state was included with a state organization by the early 1950s (Figure 1.4) [5].

The US Volunteer Life Saving Corps had preceded SLSA as a volunteer movement, having been founded in 1890. It is reported to have saved over 17,000 people from drowning by 1938 [19]. It gradually faded from existence, however, as professional lifeguards were employed in accordance with local custom, albeit without the benefit of the standards offered by a national organization. (There was no Bronze Medallion equivalent in the United States, as there was no national association overseeing all surf lifesaving to create it.)

Over time, Australia's beach safety approach would gradually come to rely, in substantial part, on professional lifeguards. It was perhaps inevitable that, as tourism and beach attendance grew, volunteers alone (being mostly available on holidays and weekends) would be inadequate to ensure the daily need for beach safety. Thus local councils employed 'beach inspectors', now typically referred to as *lifeguards*.

Independent associations of Australian beach lifeguards began in 1937, and in 1980 the Australian Professional Surf Lifeguards Association united with SLSA, which provided funding [20]. This lasted only until 1984, when an acrimonious split took place, and the organization, now known as the Australian Professional Ocean Lifeguard Association, is decidedly independent with its own standards [20]. SLSA, though, had begun to contract with local councils to provide professional beach lifeguards in 1970 and is now the largest contract provider of professional lifeguards in Australia [20].

It can seem strange for a professional lifeguard from the United States, for example, to learn that Australia's professionals work mostly weekdays, leaving beach safety responsibilities to volunteer lifesavers on weekends, when attendance is presumably much higher and challenges greater, but the ethos of Australian lifesaving is founded in that reality.

More lifesaving origins

There are more than 120 countries with lifesaving organizations today. The following were kind enough to respond to an invitation to share their histories.

NEW ZEALAND

Surf Life Saving New Zealand (SLSNZ) declares that 'Surf Life Saving is one of the best

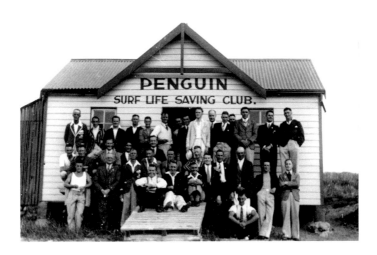

Figure 1.4 Surf lifesaving clubs came to exist in every state in Australia. This one, the Penguin Surf Life Saving Club, was founded in 1931 at Preservation Bay, Tasmania. (Courtesy of Surf Life Saving Australia; http://sls.com.au/)

imports we've ever had from Australia' [21]. In New Zealand, lifesaving began at Lyall Bay and New Brighton in 1910, but there were four more clubs by year end [21]. SLSNZ clubs were much like those in Australia, depending primarily upon the reel, line and belt. From the beginning, the camaraderie and democracy the clubs offered were a hallmark. 'All clubbies were treated equally – lawyers, plumbers and farmhands worked together to save lives. Their only qualification was an ability to move through the surf' [21]. Women were accepted as full club members from the early years.

SOUTH AFRICA

In South Africa, the RLSS formed its first South African Branches for teaching and certifying its lifesaving techniques at swimming pools and inland waterways in 1913 [22]. SLSA representatives visited in 1927, 'paraded along the beachfront of Durban, demonstrated lifesaving techniques and encouraged the formation in Durban of the first two clubs, the Durban Surf Life Saving Club and the Pirates Lifesaving Club' [22]. Lifesaving South Africa maintains its ties to this day with the RLSS, but also with SLSA.

BRAZIL

Brazil's history of beach lifesaving started in the city of Rio de Janeiro, which abuts beautiful beaches in a tropical climate. As in other areas of the world, the attractiveness of the ocean also holds great hazards. These characteristics are what have turned Rio de Janeiro into one of the leading regions of Brazil for drowning deaths. Hearing of these conditions, Commodore Wilbert E. Longfellow of the United States visited Rio de Janeiro (then the capital of Brazil) in 1914 and began teaching the lifesaving programmes of the ARC. At first, the goal was to organize and train lifeguard volunteers who would stand guard on all the beaches of Brazil. Realizing the challenge of fully accomplishing this goal, a campaign at a national level was implemented in hopes of educating and alerting everyone to the potential dangers on all beaches nationwide. Longfellow's slogan was 'Every person a swimmer, every swimmer a lifesaver'. Today the paid lifeguard service in Rio is responsible for beach safety along a 60-mile stretch, with 1200 lifeguards on

staff year-round (David Szpilman, MD, Sobrasa, personal communication via e-mail, 9 March 2015).

GERMANY

Germany's lifesaving organization, *Deutshe Lebens-Rettungs-Gesellschafte* (DLRG), was founded in 1913. It was initially focused on harnessing volunteers to educate the public with swimming and lifesaving instruction. In 1922, the DLRG resolved to add lifeguard service to its field of responsibilities, and water rescue service (*Wasserrettungsdienst*) became one of the tasks set out in its new constitution. Mobile (and also later fixed) lifeguard stations were established at dangerous bathing places along the coasts and at inland waters. At the beginning of the 1920s, an estimated 8000 people drowned in Germany per year. By the mid-1930s, the intensified instruction of lifeguards and the establishment of additional lifeguard stations, along with improved swimming instruction for the population by the DLRG and public schools, had reduced this number to about 3500.

In 1950, the number of deaths by drowning in German waters was still quite high at 2105, but today those numbers are down to about 400. Water rescue service is presently the only state responsibility in Germany that is still taken on by volunteers. It extends beyond beaches to flood rescue and disaster response. Each year between 40,000 and 60,000 DLRG lifesavers volunteer 2.2 million hours of voluntary service (Frauke Schroeder, Deutsche Lebens-Rettungs-Gesellschaft e.V., personal communication on 23 March 2015, via e-mail).

UNITED KINGDOM

In the United Kingdom, as had been the case in Australia before the existence of the SLSA, the only recognized qualification for a beach lifesaver was that given by the RLSS, which after its formation in 1891 was influential in saving lives in lakes and rivers as well as municipal baths. Their test, carried out in still water, came to be considered inadequate for the demands of lifesaving in the sea and, thus, it was an Australian lifesaver who introduced the country to surf lifesaving as he knew it [23]. Allan Kennedy had served as a lifesaver and as state superintendent for Queensland from 1941 to 1946 [24]. During World War II, he instructed Australian and US troops sent to recuperate on the Gold Coast in the techniques of surf lifesaving, awarding the Bronze Medallion to those who passed the test.

In 1951, Kennedy's job sent him to England. To ease symptoms of withdrawal from his beloved world of lifesaving, in May 1952 he made his way to Bude in Cornwall. Kennedy soon discovered that those concerned with beach safety in Bude could and should be much better equipped to deal with emergencies in the surf and wrote to see if the SLSA might provide a reel, line, belt and surf ski to get things started in Cornwall. In August 1953, the equipment eventually arrived, courtesy of HM The Queen, who had agreed to bring the equipment back on the Royal Yacht *Britannia* following her tour of Australia. Kennedy began an intensive week of instruction with members of the Bude Youth Club and others. By the end, 22 volunteers had qualified for the coveted Australian Bronze Medallion and the first British surf lifesaving club was founded (the 'Royal Reel' is now displayed in Bude SLSC's clubroom) [23].

Drowning deaths in other parts of the United Kingdom inspired the spread of surf lifesaving. New clubs were formed with the guidance of the Bude lifesavers. In the spring of 1955, a meeting was held and the Surf Lifesaving Association of Great Britain (SLSGB) was born. As a mark of proud parental approval, the high commissioner of Australia invited a deputation from St. Agnes to Australia House in London in May 1955 to be presented with a belt, line and reel, a gift from the North Bondi Surf Lifesaving Club [23].

Over the years, continued rivalry between the SLSGB and RLSS UK had arguably led to a decreasing emphasis on volunteer lifesaving. Although initially there was a corresponding increase in the provision of paid lifeguards by local authorities, eventual financial cutbacks due to the lack of clarity over where the statutory responsibility lay resulted in a highly variable standard of beach lifeguard provision across the United Kingdom. This situation finally resulted in the RNLI, probably the best known and funded lifeboat charity worldwide, being asked to take an active role in beach lifeguarding by both the SLSGB and RLSS UK. Since its inception in 2000, the RNLI beach lifeguard service has proven quite successful and has offered a seamless link between the lifeboat and lifeguard services.

IRAN

Beach lifesaving began in Iran in 1959 on northern beaches under the leadership of Davoud Nasiri. It was officially established in 1961. Lifesavers initially used inner tubes from truck tires and small fishing boats for their rescues. Tourism brought US and European lifesavers to Iran, which allowed for an exchange of information, leading to adoption of newer techniques and equipment. Nowadays, some of the lifesavers are paid by the Red Crescent Society and some are volunteers (Behrooz Esfandiari, Iran Lifesaving and Diving Federation, personal communication via e-mail, 30 March 2015).

TAIWAN

Taiwan is one of many lifesaving organizations that was established because of the influence of SLSA. SLSA sent an educational team of 15 to Taiwan in 1971, at which point surf lifesaving began. Taiwan's lifesavers are both volunteer and paid (Simon Hsu, Director of International Affairs, Chinese Taipei Water Life Saving Association, personal communication via e-mail, 13 March 2015).

JAPAN

In Japan, beach lifeguarding commenced in 1963 in Kanagawa Prefecture. It is composed of both paid and volunteer lifesavers. Today more than 50% of the Japan Lifesaving Association's members are university students, and one-third of its clubs are university clubs. This advantage is also a disadvantage, since upon graduating many of these students leave lifesaving (Shusaku Miyabe, Japan Lifesaving Association, personal communication via e-mail, 28 March 2015).

THE EVOLUTION OF BEACH LIFESAVING EQUIPMENT

Lifesaving equipment has been a major aspect of the evolution of lifesaving. Innovated over time, lifesaving organizations have learned from each other's advances and gradually, although not completely, gravitated towards international standardization.

Rescue lines

The reel, line and belt (also called the *landline* and other names in different places) involves a lifesaver swimming a line out to a victim in distress

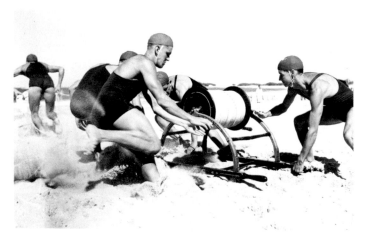

Figure 1.5 The reel, line and belt achieved an iconic status in Australia, surviving as a primary method of lifesaving for decades. (Courtesy of Surf Life Saving Australia; http://sls.com.au/)

and lifesavers (or others) ashore pulling them back (Figure 1.5). It was being used as early as 1902 in the United States [5]. It was used both on the East and West Coasts. In Australia, it was first placed in service at Bondi Beach in 1907 [5]. Atlantic City ceased using it early on after one of their lifeguards was pulled ashore dead, having become entangled in the line. That tragedy was repeated in Australia where in 1924 a lifesaver died on the line, then two more in 1950, and a fourth in 1967 at Coledale Beach [23,25].

Hazards aside, use of the line was considered a reliable method of rescue, despite some notable disadvantages. There is the drag on the swimmer making way towards the victim, for example, and the need for multiple lifesavers for the rescue of a single person.

The reel, line and belt achieved an iconic status in Australia, surviving as a primary method of lifesaving for decades. SLSA's extended reluctance to give up the line in favour of more modern lifesaving tools (e.g. rescue floatation devices) drew some derision. In correspondence between themselves in 1977 and 1978, the secretary of World Life Saving (WLS) (a New Zealander) joked that if Australia ran out of nylon line everyone would drown, while the WLS president referred to it as 'a lifesaving method so archaic I can't even believe it' [26]. (Considering that the WLS president at the time was American, he was either unaware of or equally dismissive of the line's widespread use in his own country by lifeguards on the New Jersey Shore.)

Today the line is used almost exclusively in competition, not in lifesaving, although the New Jersey Bathing Code maintains the following requirement: 'A 600 foot ¼ inch poly rope shall be provided at each lifeguard station at ocean bathing beaches' (8:26-5.12 Lifesaving equipment for bathing beaches).

Rescue floatation devices

Rescue floatation devices (RFDs) have become the most fundamental rescue implement of lifesavers today. Their utility is manifold. They can be carried and towed easily behind a single lifesaver with minimal drag; can be pushed to a victim in distress, thus eliminating direct contact with a panicked victim; and, with the leash and harness, allow the lifesaver to swim normally when returning to the beach. The first RFDs were life rings towed by a lifeguard with a sling over the shoulder, but they created quite a drag and a better solution was needed [10].

The first rescue buoy is reported to have been developed by Captain Henry Sheffield, an American who was touring Durban, South Africa, in 1897. It was four feet long, made of sheet metal, sharply pointed at both ends and quite heavy [14]. The design was modified in a myriad of ways in the United States. The heavy sheet metal was replaced with copper, balsa wood, aluminium (rounded on both ends), or fibreglass. A version made of copper was being used by Atlantic City lifeguards as early as 1901 [10].

Walter Biddell of the Bronte Surf Club in Australia introduced a 'torpedo buoy' of canvas and kapok in 1907 to be used in conjunction with the reel and line, or independently. However, no device of this sort would be officially adopted by SLSA for more than 60 years [25]. Conversely, the US lifeguard organizations, which were all independent of each other, used what they wanted, and they wanted rescue buoys.

An advantage of the early rescue buoy designs was that they moved fairly smoothly through the water, producing less drag than a life ring. A disadvantage was that they sometimes caused injuries, both to rescuers and those being rescued.

In 1935, in Santa Monica, California, lifeguard Pete Peterson came up with a different approach. He wanted something to secure a victim in the surf, not just something the victim could hold onto. He produced an inflatable, bright yellow rescue tube with a snap hook moulded onto one end and a 14-inch strap on the other, based on a design by Reggie Burton and Captain George Watkins. A line and harness were then attached. This highly visible RFD was used by many lifeguard services into the early 1960s [27].

In response to the buoyancy problems related to punctures and climatic conditions, Peterson redesigned the tube, constructing it of flexible foam rubber with an orange skin to keep water out of the interior. While this was an improvement, the skin was still subject to piercing and the underlying open cell foam would then act like a sponge, becoming waterlogged. In the late 1960s, however, closed-cell foam rubber was invented, and the tube was manufactured with this material so that punctures to the skin no longer resulted in water absorption. This device is still known to some as the *Peterson tube*, but it is more commonly known as the *rescue tube* [27]. Ironically, this tool to help secure victims in the turbulence of the surf is now widely used in the calm environment of pools, often to support lifeguards rather than victims.

The modern plastic rescue buoy was developed as a result of concerns by Los Angeles County lifeguard Lieutenant Bob Burnside (the founding president of the United States Lifesaving Association) about injuries to lifeguards struck by aluminium rescue buoys. He noticed a plastic pliable statuette sitting on his desk and wondered if the buoy could be constructed of similar material. He consulted with Professor Ron Rezek, an industrial design expert at the University of California at Los Angeles. They sketched different designs until they arrived at one that seemed to work and, using a new method called *rotational moulding*, the plastic rescue buoy was born in 1968. Known to many as the *Burnside buoy* or *can* (a terminology throwback to the original metal design) and used by lifesavers throughout the world, it was made iconic by the 1980s television show *Baywatch*, whose lifeguards seemed to use it exclusively [27] (Bob Burnside, personal communication via e-mail, 12 April 2015).

There is much discussion among lifesavers about the relative merits of the tube and buoy. The buoy is highly buoyant and, particularly in its larger size, can facilitate the rescues of numerous victims simultaneously, although they must be conscious and able to maintain their grips on the handles. The tube, while less useful for multiple victim rescues, is particularly secure for a single victim, around which it can be wrapped and secured. Thus the buoy tends to be used on beaches with high rescue volumes [27].

Rescue boards

One man seems to have been a primary factor in introducing the surfboard to lifesavers: the swimming and surfing legend Duke Kahanamoku. Charles Paterson, a member of an Australian club, brought a surfboard from Hawaii in 1912 that was, typical of the time, solid redwood and 45 kilos. However, the effort to use it for surfing by club members was a failure, apparently due to the lack of any board riding experience, and it was quickly retired [25]. Several years later, in 1915, Kahanamoku visited Australia and demonstrated to the lifesavers how to surf on these boards. Thus began the surfing culture in Australia. Lifesavers did endeavour to use these boards for rescue, but found them so unwieldy and dangerous that they were banned for that practice [5]. Amazingly, the design of surfboards in Australia went largely unchanged until 1956.

Kahanamoku also visited the US West Coast in 1913 and struck up a friendship with Roy 'Dutch' Miller of the Long Beach, California, lifeguards. Realizing the utility for rescue, the Long Beach lifeguards arranged to have modified surfboards made by the city's maintenance shop and used them for rescue thereafter [28]. Other lifeguard agencies in California used them for rescue as well.

Although he was not a trained lifesaver, Kahanamoku was involved in at least one extraordinary rescue. He and fellow surfers were credited with using their boards to save the lives of 13 people when a gas launch overturned off Laguna Beach, California, in June 1925 [29].

Australians and Americans exchange concepts to their betterment

A dramatic evolution in Australian and US lifesaving, as well as Australian surfing, took place in 1956 (Figure 1.6). Upon the occasion of Australia's hosting of the Olympic Games, SLSA decided to organize a concurrent event, the Australian Olympic International Surf Championships at Torquay, not far from Melbourne, the centre for the Olympic Games. Teams of lifesavers from other countries including South Africa, Great Britain, Ceylon (now Sri Lanka), New Zealand and the United States were invited. In the absence of a national US lifesaving organization, some California lifeguards created one on the fly, calling themselves the Surf Life Saving Association of America. In fact, it would barely have qualified as a club in Australia, although it was composed of professional lifeguards from several organizations [27].

The Americans brought with them three lifesaving tools: the rescue buoy, the rescue tube and the short and light Malibu balsa surfboard.

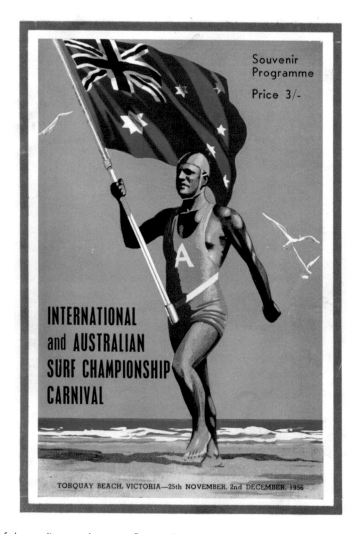

Figure 1.6 One of the earliest and most influential international exchanges of lifesaving knowledge took place in 1956 at an event hosted at Torquay Beach, Australia, by Surf Life Saving Australia. (Courtesy of Surf Life Saving Australia; http://sls.com.au/)

Up until then, Australian lifesavers had been relying on the reel, line and belt, and surfing was limited to the massive plank design that Duke Kahanamoku (who was in attendance) had introduced. A movie made at the time entitled *Service in the Sun* details the outcome [30,31].

In one instance, lifeguard Tad Devine, the son of movie star Andy Devine (who had also been a beach lifeguard), demonstrated the rescue tubes and buoys to the Australian lifesavers. The US team captain noted that each US lifeguard was assigned one and they needed just one lifeguard for a rescue of up to five people, instead of the five or six lifesavers needed to rescue a single person with the reel, line and belt [25,31].

A sponsor, Ampol Petroleum, offered to donate rescue tubes for use on all of Australia's beaches if SLSA agreed to adopt them [25]. Sadly, it was not to be, explains Alleyn Best: 'Despite favourable results from testing the tube in July 1957 by two Collaroy club members in difficult conditions at Bilgola Beach inaction by the various gear committees of state and national Boards of Examiners led to a lack of interest for many years. So entrenched was the reel, line and belt in the Australian surf lifesaving movement's traditions and culture that 30 years elapsed before the flexible rescue tube was adopted nationally' [25].

It was a different story with respect to surfboards. Several of the California and Hawaiian lifeguards, notably Greg Noll, Mike Bright and Tom Zahn, were also expert surfers and attracted huge attention with their surf riding skills, which had never before been seen in Australia. Their boards were lighter, shorter and much more manoeuvrable. Several minutes of *Service in the Sun* are devoted simply to showing the Americans surfing. According to *Australian Beach Cultures: The History of Sun, Sand and Surf*, by Douglas Booth, 'Australian surfing at the time was, in Zahn's words, "like nowhere". They were still going straight off on 16-foot paddleboards' [18].

The Americans left their boards behind and surfing in Australia changed forever, but so did lifesaving. The lifesavers came to use them in rescues and added handles. They were eventually made of fibreglass and shortened to the present 2.8 metres to lighten them [25]. They would still not replace the reel, line and belt though.

Why might Australians have preferred the rescue board, but rejected the rescue buoy and tube? Tradition, it seems. It was not until an

international conference was hosted in Australia in 1976 that word was passed, to the horror of many, that the reel, line and belt would eventually be retired in favour of rescue tubes, boards and other devices [32]. In fact, the SLSA standard for rescue tubes was not published until 1986 [25]. SLSNZ notes their move a bit differently, stating, 'A major shift of thinking was needed to free lifesaving [from the reel, line and belt] to take to the water with fins and neoprene rescue tubes ... in the 1970s' [21].

The value of the trip to the Americans was easily equal, but in a very different way. Their local lifeguard employers all worked independently. There was no national association and there were no national standards for beach lifesaving. Inspired by what they had seen, the Americans went on to found what is now the US Lifesaving Association (USLA), in 1964. One of them was Bob Burnside, who drove the creation of the USLA and became its founding president. One of its primary founding goals was national standards for beach lifeguarding, a goal that was ultimately achieved [27].

Several years after the Americans introduced Malibu surfboards to Australia, a similar impact was made on surfing in Great Britain by surf lifesavers from Australia. John Fuller, Ian Tiley, John Campbell and Warren Mitchell headed to the United Kingdom in 1961, bringing along two fibreglass Malibu surfboards and attaining jobs as beach lifeguards. Surfing in the United Kingdom was then what Tom Zahn thought of it in Australia when he visited, but the Australians changed it entirely. They were asked to give surfing demonstrations, and people were fascinated. The boards began to be copied and surfing in Great Britain was changed, as it had been in Australia, by lifesavers [23].

Rescue boats

SURFBOATS

Boats launched from the beach and rowed to people in distress were in use by the US Life-Saving Service and by Constables of the Surf long before the first beach lifeguards [6]. The standard New Jersey lifeguard surfboat has changed little from the early days. They are about 16 feet long, 4 feet wide, with a pointed bow and a gunwale at the stern, with two seats for two rowers and two sets of oarlocks [8]. They are iconic, although rarely used in rescue today. On the US West Coast the lifeguards used somewhat different surf dories. A modified, double-ended version of some of the original boats is used in US competitions sanctioned by the USLA. To this day, California law declares, 'No person shall own or conduct a resort unless it is equipped with at least one lifeboat [and 200 feet of line]' (Health and Safety Code 115980). No California beach resort is presently known to be in compliance.

In Australia, rowed boats developed differently. Beginning in 1907, various types of rowed surfboats were employed. A standardized design was approved in 1920 that was 18–20 feet long, double-ended, with buoyancy tanks to keep the vessel afloat if it capsized [25]. It was rowed by four lifesavers and guided by a fifth on a sweep oar. Similarly designed boats had been used in whaling and by the US Life-Saving Service since the 1700s [33]. The Australian surfboats evolved over the years. In the 1940s and 1950s, the design became narrower and a square transom appeared at the stern (a 'tuck stern' in Australian parlance). Why a crew of five for the SLSA boats, versus the one or two for the American lifesaver's boats? Smaller vessels initially developed in Australia proved inadequate to deal with the surf [25].

SURF SKIS

In the realm of rowed vessels used by lifesavers, the surf ski bears mentioning. It was invented around 1913 in Australia and was made an official piece of lifesaving equipment by SLSA in 1937 [25]. Modern versions are used exclusively in competition, having evolved to a highly streamlined design lacking any apparent utility for rescue. Early versions, which were broader and more stable, were also used for recreation and competition, although the SLSA manual included instructions for their use in rescue until 2002 [34]. Beginning in the 1970s, South Africa and Great Britain began using a modified design with a broader deck for rescue. It appears to have originated in the United States for rescue, although it is unclear if US lifesavers ever used it for that purpose. As was the case for surf skis, it was eventually replaced by rescue boards.

THE FIRST MOTORIZED BOATS

Motorized rescue boats were the next advance. Long Beach, California, lifeguards put their first one in service on 1 July 1924 [28]. Based in Long Beach harbour, lifeguards navigated it offshore where they could pick up victims (and lifeguards) at the heads of rips. Los Angeles County lifeguards first acquired motorized rescue vessels in the 1930s [35]. The current fleet of 13, 32-foot (9.75-metre) Baywatch vessels patrol Santa Monica Bay and Catalina Island, some with firefighting capability and paramedic lifeguards aboard [36]. (The *Baywatch* television show borrowed the name of the Los Angeles County rescue boat fleet, although it featured boats of a decidedly different design.) Several other US lifeguard agencies have long had boats of similar size and capabilities, as well as smaller hard-hull rescue boats, both inboard and outboard (Figure 1.7).

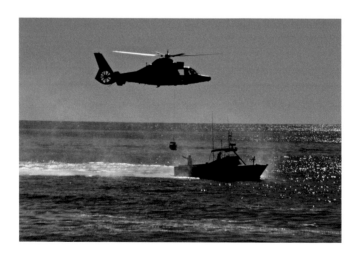

Figure 1.7 A Los Angeles County Baywatch boat crew delivers a patient to a US Coast Guard MH-65 Dolphin helicopter. There are thirteen, 32-foot Baywatch boats that patrol the coastline of Los Angeles County. (Courtesy of Joel Gittelson. With author's permission.)

JET RESCUE BOATS

SLSA began experimenting with motorized rescue boats in the 1950s and 1960s, with some limited success [25]. A unique advance was the 1960s creation of jet-powered surfboats. These originally 5-metre, fibreglass, inboard motor vessels used a Jacuzzi jet unit [25]. They were later built at 17 feet [23]. Still in use today with some modifications, their very shallow draft and wave-deflecting forward superstructure allows the jet rescue boat to be used very near shore and to navigate through the surfline, even punching through breaking surf if need be. The San Diego Lifeguard Service later successfully copied parts of the design of this boat, albeit with a stock hull and outboard engine.

INFLATABLE RESCUE BOATS

With the inflatable rescue boat (IRB), SLSA offered another unique solution to motorizing lifesaving boats. Warren Mitchell had helped introduce Malibu surfboards to Great Britain and while there observed the initial deployment of inflatable boats by the RNLI. In 1969, he proposed the use of small inflatables that could be launched from the beach. His first demonstration of the concept to SLSA officials came in eight-foot surf off Avalon Beach, NSW using a retired army inflatable with a 25 horsepower engine and his brother as crew. It was dramatic and successful, although a nasty cut to his brother's chin from the fuel tank bouncing in his face may have inspired the use of fuel bladders, rather than cans [23].

The IRB took some time to be accepted by SLSA. It was competing with the jet rescue boat and perhaps seen as one more challenge to the traditional methods of lifesaving so prized by SLSA (Figure 1.8). By 1976 though, SLSA had drawn up their own specifications for manufacturers to follow [23]. Use of the IRB was not without incident. A swimmer's foot was severed by an IRB propeller at Bondi Beach in 1977, underlining the need for effective propeller guards [23].

By the 1981–1982 season, 22% of SLSA rescues were attributed to the IRB. Moreover, the idea had been exported. Sergeant Bill Owen of the San Diego Lifeguard Service (who trained this chapter's author as an IRB operator) had toured Australia and convinced his superiors to acquire one in 1980. After a critical rescue using the IRB, he wrote SLSA Executive Director Gus Staunton, 'And so, Gus, a man here in America is alive today because of the work, dedication and humanitarian ideas of the Australian Surf Lifesaving Association [sic]' [23].

The IRB solved many problems. Unlike other motorized boats, a nearby harbour was not needed. It could be stored and launched directly from the beach like a rowed surfboat, but it was faster than any rowed boat, more nimble in the surf and able to handle the largest waves. Moreover, it was relatively inexpensive and easy to repair. The IRB made the motorized rescue boat affordable and practical for beach lifesaving. Its use was adopted not only in the United States, but in New Zealand, Great Britain,

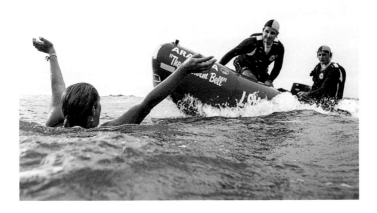

Figure 1.8 Australian surf lifesavers demonstrate the use of the IRB. (Courtesy of Surf Life Saving Australia; http://sls.com.au/)

South Africa and many other countries. Specialized designs for rescue and in-surf use greatly added to their utility [23].

PERSONAL WATERCRAFT

Personal watercraft (often referred to by the trade name Jet Ski®) has been used in beach lifeguarding since the 1990s. The original model required the operator to stand and balance on the device, but subsequent sit-astride, jet-drive variations by several manufacturers facilitated their use in rescue. Moreover, the addition of specially designed sleds towed behind allowed for an operator and crewmember to rapidly rescue those in distress without the need to bring them aboard the vessel. Many lifeguard organizations that once used IRBs have moved to these jet-drive vessels, while others that never had IRBs have acquired them. In 2004, the USLA issued their *Training and Equipment Guidelines for Rescuers Using Personal Watercraft as a Rescue Tool*, but they are by no means alone in promoting operations standards.

The attractiveness of the personal watercraft (PWC), also referred to by many lifesaving organisations as the rescue watercraft (RWC), in comparison to the IRB includes ready commercial availability, the safety of jet drives versus propellers, their speed, their ability to sustain a rollover and their ability to be used by a single operator. They lack the deck, albeit small, of an IRB, the ability for operator and crewmember to remain out of the water, and the simple hull repairs of an inflatable. Whether both of these rescue boats will continue to be used or one will win out remains to be seen, but the fact that IRBs are used in competition by several lifesaving organizations may ensure a substantial longevity for them.

Motor vehicles

TRUCKS AND AUTOMOBILES

The use of motorized lifesaving vehicles appears to have begun in the 1920s in Southern California. One photo depicts a Ford Model T lifeguard vehicle in San Diego [37]. The need was no doubt partly attributable to the expanse of beaches covered in some areas and the distance between beaches. Vehicles could rapidly respond with personnel and equipment to reports of emergencies and requests for backup. The California Vehicle Code

was amended in 1959 in part to make clear that lifeguard vehicles were authorized to respond on highways as emergency vehicles: 'An authorized emergency vehicle is: (a) Any publicly owned and operated ambulance, lifeguard, or lifesaving equipment …' (Section 165).

In the early years, lifeguards deflated the tires to allow them to drive on the beach. Later, as four-wheel drive Jeeps became available, they were used, and ultimately with the wide commercial availability of four-wheel drive vehicles the options broadened significantly. In Wildwood, New Jersey, the lifeguards at one time used motorcycles with sidecars, in addition to regular vehicles [10]. The typical lifesaving response and patrol vehicle is now four-wheel drive, with a rack above for a rescue board and stretcher.

In some areas, lifeguard vehicles are of unusual size and capability. The San Diego Lifeguard Service added a crane to one of its vehicles to help facilitate coastal cliff rescues in the 1930s. The vehicle has been repeatedly replaced, most recently in 2015 with a mechanical crane and winch system. Los Angeles County has long maintained 'call cars', which can be used for paramedic lifeguard response. Today, some US lifeguard agencies have fleets of more than 25 emergency response vehicles.

The benefits of lifeguard vehicles also bring with them a hazard. Unnoticed beach visitors have been run over and injured, or even killed. This danger has prompted extensive policies and training at many lifesaving organizations in an effort to ensure that accidents of this nature are avoided.

ALL-TERRAIN VEHICLES

The introduction of all-terrain vehicles (ATVs), especially as they expanded to have four wheels and substantial carrying capacity, offered an option to smaller lifesaving organizations with more limited budgets. They offer another benefit in that there are less serious consequences in accidents involving beach visitors (Figure 1.9). ATVs, however, do not allow for high-speed emergency responses via regular roads.

Helicopters

Australia pioneered the use of helicopters for lifesaving beginning in 1966 (Figure 1.10) [25]. They were viewed as a tool both for rescue and shark spotting. Cost was, of course, an issue. Thus a sponsorship with a prominent bank was

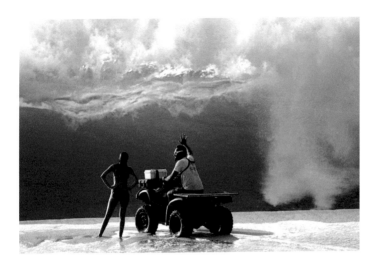

Figure 1.9 City and County of Honolulu Lifeguard Kainoa McGee warns a beach visitor at Ke Iki Beach, North Shore of Oahu. (Courtesy of Vince Cavataio. With author's permission.)

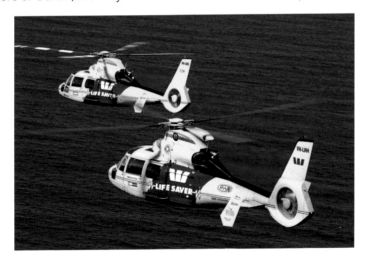

Figure 1.10 Australia pioneered the use of helicopters for lifesaving beginning in 1966. (Courtesy of Surf Life Saving Australia; http://sls.com.au/)

key to funding the service on an ongoing basis, in 1973 in Sydney, 1976 at the Gold Coast, 1979 in Victoria and 1983 in Western Australia. The programme has not been without challenge. Victoria's service had to be terminated in 1987 for financial reasons and was not funded again until 2002 [25].

In New Zealand, the Auckland Surf Life Saving Association launched a helicopter ocean rescue service in 1970. It was used primarily for rescues from the surf on Auckland's west coast beaches. This oversight continued until 1990, when a charitable trust was formed to oversee the service, with trustees selected from the community and business sectors of the greater Auckland region.

It offers emergency air ambulance and search and rescue [38].

Rio de Janeiro, Brazil, initiated a helicopter service in 1974. This involves utilizing existing government helicopters and assigning them to water rescue when needed. In water rescue cases, the helicopters typically include a lifeguard on board who exits the helicopter into the water to come to the aid of a victim, and both are then retrieved using a 'fish basket' type device that is hung from the helicopter on a static line [39].

The United States has used a variety of approaches, depending on the lifeguard agency. These approaches have included employing police, sheriff, fire department and US Coast Guard helicopters, using static lines and winches to retrieve victims. No US lifeguard organization has its own helicopter, although as lifeguard organizations have merged into fire departments with helicopters, the helicopter services are more directly integrated with lifeguard operations.

Lifeguard towers

Lifesavers primarily respond based upon their own observations of people in distress. This procedure differentiates them from other public safety providers, who more typically respond to reports of emergencies conveyed by others. It has long been recognized that water observation is enhanced by a raised point of observation, which has brought about the creation of various types of elevated viewing platforms.

The simplest solution to providing an elevated viewpoint was a raised lifeguard chair. These are quite common in some areas of the world. They have the benefit of low cost and portability, and they can easily be moved to remain close to the water's edge at beaches with large tidal fluctuations. In some areas, raised platforms or 'perches' made of cement or other materials were created.

Larger towers, some with enclosed areas, have been constructed of wood in various parts of the world. They provide varying degrees of shade and protection from the elements to lifesavers, as well as storage for lifesaving equipment.

In the 1980s, a fibreglass design was introduced by several manufacturers and trialled in Southern California. This design proved popular, especially since it was fully enclosed with windows for viewing, along with shutters to secure the towers after hours. The towers were all initially moveable via skids, when towed by a vehicle. The designs evolved over time to include space for multiple lifeguards. They have become the primary tower solution in many areas of the world, sometimes moveable and sometimes permanently installed. Their design, which protects lifeguards from the elements, may help maintain the alertness of lifesavers.

The most sophisticated towers, commonly found in California, involve permanently constructed, multi-storey buildings with an upper glass-enclosed viewing deck and, in some cases, additional facilities such as offices, changing rooms, training areas and garages. Budgets for construction of some of these buildings can exceed $8 million. Some lifeguard agencies have also built observation towers on piers, allowing for unique visibility within the surf zone.

MEDICAL RESPONSE

Medical care (first aid) was a responsibility of lifesavers from the start. It was perhaps inevitable that resuscitation was a primary expectation of lifesavers. Over the years, many techniques and devices have been employed by lifesavers. Resuscitation methods reflected the concepts of the time, such as the Shafer method and the Sylvester method, which involved various manipulations of the human body in an effort to restart breathing.

One of the early resuscitation devices was the pulmotor. In a 1918 article on an incident resulting in the death of 13 people at Ocean Beach in San Diego, the local newspaper reported, 'The pulmotor at the beach was put in use and a telephone call rushed out a lung motor from police headquarters at San Diego' [40]. (The lifeguards were part of the police department at the time.) Similarly in 1921, SLSA was recommending use of a pulmotor [25]. Various improvements to what came to be called *resuscitators* occurred over the years, including demand valves.

In 1956, Peter Safar and James Elam invented mouth-to-mouth resuscitation [41]. Shortly thereafter, cardiopulmonary resuscitation (CPR) was invented. The uptake by lifesaving organizations occurred at different times in different places. CPR was first introduced to the Los Angeles County lifeguard programme in 1957 [35]. In Australia, volunteers were anesthetized and revived to demonstrate the efficacy of mouth-to-mouth, but it was not until 1969 that the older methods were completely discontinued by SLSA in favour of CPR [25].

Medical care procedures for other injuries also evolved in accordance with public understanding and local acceptance. As well, lifesaving organizations were faced with decisions regarding the level of care to provide, ranging from the most basic to the most advanced. In most countries medical aid and CPR training are basic requirements. The Bronze Medallion, for example, requires first aid training to a level tailored to common injuries and ailments likely to be found at the beach.

In Rio de Janeiro, specialized medical teams staff three separate medical care centres (drowning resuscitation centres). These centres are pre-hospital emergency facilities at the beach, developed in the 1960s to deal with aquatic emergencies. They help reduce the dispatch time and the need to refer the patient to a hospital. They provide a key link between pre-hospital services and hospitals and also provide support for lifeguards' work. David Szpilman, MD, of Brazil, devised a drowning classification system based on the severity of cardiopulmonary involvement in 1972, which offers lifeguards confidence in recognizing signs to let them know the drowning severity, treatment and outcome (David Szpilman, MD, Sobrasa, personal communication via e-mail, 9 March 2015).

Paramedic lifeguard services were initiated by Los Angeles County in the mid-1970s due to the relative isolation of some lifeguarded areas, and they continue today [35]. About that time some California lifeguard agencies began training their lifeguards as emergency medical technicians (EMTs). The USLA presently certifies lifeguard agencies at two levels. To qualify for the advanced level, agencies must train all seasonal (part-time) lifeguards to a standard of care similar to a basic ambulance attendant. Year-round (full-time) lifeguards must be trained and certified EMTs, which is standard for ambulance attendants in most major population areas. As of April 2015, 46 US lifeguard agencies were certified to this standard [42].

STANDARDS

SLSA pioneered the concept of a national standard for beach lifesaving. The Bronze Medallion has been in existence since 1910. Most other countries follow a similar model, involving nationally credentialed instructors who in turn train and credential lifesavers. The United States is a notable departure. Since its lifesaving developed locally, without oversight of a national organization, standards have always been up to the employer. It was not until 1980 that the USLA published minimum recommended standards and not until 1993 that it developed a system of certifying (accrediting) employers, leaving them to continue to train their own employees to the minimum standards. The ARC had managed a national lifeguard certification system since 1914, used to varying extents by some beach lifeguard agencies.

However, in 1997, after discussions with the USLA, the ARC declared that they would not be developing a surf-specific lifeguard course, leaving the USLA programme the only one for surf beaches (ARC Vice President Susan Morrisey Livingstone to USLA President Bill Richardson, personal communication via letter, 4 September 1996). The International Life Saving Federation (ILS), which is introduced later in this chapter, has developed international standards in an effort to encourage standardization and to offer a model to countries lacking them. While it is notable that no two countries appear to have identical standards, it is clear that the international exchange of information has encouraged many countries to recognize various minimums.

EXPANDED SERVICES

The breadth of services provided by lifesavers around the world varies. Every lifesaving service with rescue boats provides some level of assistance to boaters in distress, whether simple towing or evacuation. In some areas of California, this includes marine firefighting using appropriately equipped boats, firefighting training and equipment that allows for attacking fires aboard affected boats.

Enforcement of beach rules is a standard role of lifesavers, although the level of involvement and authority varies dramatically. In some areas of the world, lifesavers may limit their involvement to advice and encouragement. In others, some lawful authority is granted. Full-time lifeguards working for the State of California; Volusia County, Florida; and Galveston, Texas, are also police officers who carry firearms, with a responsibility for the full gamut of law enforcement responsibilities.

It is not surprising that lifesavers are sometimes asked to assist in flood and underwater rescue, given their aquatic skills. The German DLRG has primary responsibility for flood rescue response in the country. A number of lifesaving organizations in the United States provide primary flood, swift water and dive rescue teams for their communities, and, as previously noted, in San Diego the lifeguards are responsible for coastal cliff rescue. In Australia, various lifesaving resources, including helicopters, have been used in flooding.

Lifesaving in areas with changing seasons has traditionally centred around summer months, as this is when the climate is most favourable and the beach most highly utilized. In areas with consistently warm climates, year-round lifeguard protection is typically provided for most or all of the year. It is not unusual for lifesaving organizations to offer call-back systems whereby lifesavers are available to respond at night; but in 1945 Los Angeles County began assigning two lifeguards to work through the night year-round, responding to emergency calls. The county expanded this crew to four in 1950. The City of San Diego Lifeguard Service followed with 24-hour staffing in the mid-1980s. Both services continue to this day. San Diego also maintains a 24-hour dispatch centre staffed by one or more lifeguards at all times.

WOMEN IN LIFESAVING

The involvement of women as lifesavers was certainly not something that occurred from the early days in many places. SLSNZ was an outlier in welcoming women from the beginning, but it was not without barriers [26]. They acknowledge,

> Though they were originally welcomed into clubs as full clubbies, the 1930s saw the heroic bronzed and tanned man become the idealised image of the beach. When those young men went overseas to fight and die in World War II, women again found their rightful place. They took up the reel and patrolled the beach on summer weekends. Surf history shows a string of mass rescues performed by women lifesavers in New Zealand in the 1940s. However when the men returned, those women were often relegated to fundraising, tea making and cake baking. Many broke off and started 'ladies' lifesaving clubs, often near the clubhouses of their former colleagues. These days women stand alongside men on surf patrols throughout New Zealand and compete in all the same events. [21]

In the United States, the USLA was not the controlling body for decisions of this nature. They were solely in the hands of employers. Women were first hired in New Jersey in the 1960s [10]. San Diego began hiring women in the 1970s [43].

Los Angeles County hired its first two women in 1973. These transitions were not always smooth. In 1992, after years of work in a male-dominated environment, a female California lifeguard was quoted as saying, 'The lifeguard service is a men's club – it is, was and always will be' [44]. There has been progress, but statistics are hard to come by and at most US beach lifeguard agencies it appears that women represent a distinct minority of the overall staff.

SLSA started a bit later than most. It was not until 1980 that women were allowed to receive the Bronze Medallion. Even then, clubs were permitted but not required to admit them as full members [45]. Once that happened, they were not all welcoming. In fact, hostility was evident at some clubs [46]. It was not until the early 1990s that women were allowed to compete in the full range of disciplines in competitions [45]. Interestingly, part of SLSA's decision involved membership, which had been on the decline in the all-male patrol scheme. By 2007, membership by women qualified for patrol approached 40% and that continued in 2014 [45,47]. Moreover, at the national level, 50% of executive managers, senior managers and managers were reported to be women as of 2014 [47].

NIPPERS AND JUNIOR LIFEGUARDS

The Chicago Park District faced a staffing problem thanks to World War I and the great influenza epidemic. They solved the problem in 1919 by establishing a junior lifeguard corps to help patrol the beaches. They would alert duty lifeguards of problems; they received shirts or swim trunks in return for their service [48]. By 1926, a senior lifeguard named Sam Leone had 40 junior lifeguards at his beach alone and decided to formalize the programme. He did so, and it grew from there. The Los Angeles City lifeguards established the first West Coast junior lifeguard programme in 1927 [48]. That programme grew as well, and other agencies there adopted the concept.

In Australia, beginning in the 1930s, a few clubs took on what they called 'nippers'. The concept grew in the 1960s as recruitment vehicles, with a hope that the nippers would stay on as adult club members. In fact, many did. Free from restrictions on gender, these programmes brought in girls and their parents, who would later contribute strongly to the push to accept women as surf lifesavers [46].

Many other countries also created these programmes. It was reported in 2014 that Australia had over 60,000 participants, the United States 35,000, South Africa 25,000, New Zealand 15,000, Great Britain 10,000, Canada 3,000, Sri Lanka 900 and Mexico 300 [48].

INTERNATIONAL LIFESAVING

The Fédération Internationale de Sauvetage Aquatique (FIS) began in 1910 in France. Founding nations included Belgium, Denmark, France, Great Britain, Luxembourg and Switzerland. It was to provide continuous leadership, primarily in Europe and primarily for pool and still-water lifesavers, for over 80 years, adding many nations as the time passed. Surf lifesavers, though, did not unite for decades.

As early as 1919, the forerunner of SLSA asserted, 'It is the intention of your Executive to further negotiate for the formation of similar bodies in other states of the Commonwealth and New Zealand' [26]. The goal was not just altruistic. The organization was battling with the RLSS for dominance in surf lifesaving. Indeed, SLSA's official history relates, 'Between the 1920s and 1970s, there appear to have been four principles guiding surf lifesaving's expansion overseas. The first was a determination to advocate its methods at the expense of the RLSS', while the others were to promote lifesaving generally, introduce lifesaving methods and promote lifesaving overseas [26].

In those early years, SLSA members toured many places with a missionary zeal for spreading the word of lifesaving, most notably Great Britain, South Africa, New Zealand and Hawaii. They also worked with Egypt and Palestine. After 20 years, however, according to SLSA's official history, 'There was some knowledge of Australian methods in possibly ten countries, but little beyond that. RLSS methods were still widely used within the British Empire, the United States had an efficient lifeguard system and elsewhere there was only occasional interest' [26].

SLSA's Allan Kennedy has been mentioned previously here as the organizer of surf lifesaving in Great Britain. He travelled elsewhere as well and became familiar with lifesaving in many nations. In 1954, he proposed to the SLSA National Council the formation of a world surf lifesaving body [26]. His vision was to promote Australian

surf lifesaving methods globally [26]. On the occasion of the Australian Olympic International Surf Championships in 1956, delegates were invited to attend a meeting in Melbourne, which resulted in agreement to form the International Council of Surf Lifesaving [26].

The International Council of Surf Lifesaving appears to have existed mostly in name. There was an International Convention on Life Saving Techniques in Sydney in 1960 and a meeting of the original signatories in 1969, but no meaningful initiatives [26]. Eventually, in 1971 in Sydney, Australian businessman Kevin Weldon was elected president and Alan Whelpton was elected secretary of what would be called the WLS Council. The founding members were Australia, Great Britain, New Zealand, South Africa and the United States [49].

Weldon was not one to sit on his hands. He and SLSA chief superintendent Jack Dearlove, who headed the WLS education committee, embarked on a tour of South Africa, Ireland, England, Wales, Portugal, France, Germany, Greece and Hong Kong; and also attended an FIS meeting in the Canary Islands of Spain [26]. It is notable that according to SLSA's history Dearlove considered this an opportunity to sell the concept of Australian surf lifesaving [26]. (This was an issue WLS was to grapple with for much of its existence. In 1978, the then-president of WLS, Vince Moorehouse of the United States, remarked that 'Australia needs to start promoting World Life Saving instead of Australian Lifesaving' [26].)

The presidency of the Council rotated from 1974 forward, with presidents from South Africa, the United States and New Zealand [26]. The constitution was approved on 14 June 1977 with a formal agreement among the founding nations [49]. One of the successes of WLS was to cause each of the signatories to review their own practices in light of the other nations. This led, among other things, to SLSA re-evaluating the use of the reel, line and belt, which it had so tenaciously retained for so many years [26].

The Australian passion for lifesaving competition, which has always been something of a glue binding SLSA, was not shared in the United States. On the one hand, there were Australian volunteers organized into clubs who greatly enjoyed surf carnivals. On the other hand, there were US paid professionals mostly interested in improving the quality of the services they provided to the public who paid them. Vince Moorehouse and others wanted an emphasis on education programmes, while Australians wanted more competition [26]. In the end, a compromise was reached to address both.

The first WLS competition was conducted in Bali in 1981. It did not involve national teams, but rather club teams. In events in later years, some teams cancelled their participation due to issues related to participation of the South African team during South Africa's period of apartheid. In fact, this led to the cancellation of the event in 1986 [26]. The end of apartheid led to a resolution of the problem and resumption of robust international lifesaving competition. WLS also held several world conferences aimed at current rescue and medical techniques, equipment and lifesaving standards. This was a critical contribution at a time without instant Internet exchange of ideas and methods. This balance of education and competition continues to this day, with biennial international competitions and drowning prevention conferences conducted by the organization into which WLS later merged.

It was well understood that there could be no truly international lifesaving body until WLS and the FIS merged. This merger was a long and complicated process of diplomacy requiring a variety of trade-offs, but on 24 February 1993 the FIS and WLS were merged into a single, worldwide lifesaving organization known as the International Life Saving Federation under the presidency of Kevin Weldon. The constitution was subsequently approved on 3 September 1994 in Cardiff, UK [49].

As he had done with WLS at the start, Weldon chaired the ILS with a firm hand. He was not one to mince words or tolerate extensive debate. Indeed, his implementation of the democratic process envisioned under the constitution involved certain expediencies. (He was initially reluctant to allow board members to exercise their vote.) Such are the realities of international organizations; they bring with them a myriad of approaches and views. The measure of his success, and that of many who have contributed over the years, is that the ILS has continued ever since that time, growing and thriving.

There are now more than 120 member federations of the ILS. In many countries, new lifesaving federations (associations) have been created under the encouragement and support of the ILS. In others, existing federations have been strengthened.

While competition continues to be a hallmark of international lifesaving exchange, so does education and the promotion of appropriate standards in lifesaving. The Lifesaving World Championships (Rescue Series) are held biennially, as is the World Conference on Drowning Prevention, in opposite years.

VOLUNTEERISM AND PROFESSIONALISM

The volunteer ethos that originated in the earliest days of lifesaving remains in some areas, but the complexion has changed. In nations that retain a volunteer model, it is often supplemented by some degree of professionalism. In less developed nations, where few people have free time to donate, it has been difficult or impossible to utilize a volunteer system. In developed countries with consistent workweeks, it is challenging to find volunteers on traditional workdays, especially in areas with high tourism that need continual daily protection.

In the United States, volunteer lifesaving was all but ended by the mid-1900s. Even Australia, the champion of the volunteer system, accepted the limits of relying entirely on volunteers decades ago. According to its annual report for 2014, 'Surf Life Saving, through the State and Territory Centres, operates the Australian Lifeguard Service, the country's largest lifeguard service, providing cost recovery lifesaving services to local government and other coastal land managers' [47]. SLSA is not the only provider of paid beach lifeguards in Australia, but more than 23% of patrol hours by SLSA volunteers and paid lifeguards are provided by the paid staff [47].

Whether the trend towards more paid lifeguards versus volunteers will continue is unknown. It is difficult to imagine the culture of lifesaving volunteerism that SLSA created ending anytime in the foreseeable future.

CURRENT DATA

There are many ways to appraise the advancement of beach lifesaving around the world. The following is a small effort focused on two of the pioneers of beach lifesaving.

Australia has little more than half the population of California, but through SLSA it maintains the best known and probably the most influential national lifesaving organization in the world. For 2014, SLSA reported a consolidated operating budget of A$69.5 million [47]. (This figure does not include the budgets of the individually run state centres.)

Here are some SLSA metrics for 2013–2014 from its annual report, which includes all of its members and its professional lifeguard service:

11,711 rescues from drowning
1,016,037 preventive actions
31,797 medical aids (first aids)

In the United States, where the first beach lifesavers came to protect beachgoers, but where there was no national organization until US lifeguards learned of the concept from SLSA, the USLA turned 50 in 2014, just a few years after SLSA turned 100. The USLA's operating budget for 2015 was a little over $350,000, an amount dwarfed by many of the individually managed, mostly municipal lifeguard operations affiliated with the USLA. Los Angeles County Lifeguards, for example, reported a 2015 operating budget of $42 million, and the City of San Diego's lifeguards reported a 2015 budget of $19.7 million [50,51].

Here are some USLA metrics for 2013 (with 127 lifeguard agencies reporting) from its published statistics:

68,320 rescues from drowning
6,725,264 preventive actions
329,385 medical aids (first aids)

CONCLUSION

At the time of publication of this book, beach lifesaving is less than 130 years old. In the history of humankind, that's a very short time. A public safety discipline that didn't exist has evolved quickly and admirably to its present state. The police and firefighting professions have existed for many hundreds, perhaps thousands, of years. We are a new discipline, no less important in the protection and preservation of human life. We have achieved levels of professionalism, be we paid or volunteer, that leave people willing to place their safety and that of family and friends in our hands. And indeed we deliver.

The USLA has consistently found that the chance of drowning death in an area protected by affiliated beach lifeguards is 1 in 18 million beach visits. There is little reason to think that similarly trained lifesavers in other countries fail to achieve similar safety records. We contribute, primarily, by preventing accidents and responding to those that occur before they can have dire consequences. The nobility of our service is undeniable.

Innumerable dedicated people have contributed over the years to ensuring that lifesaving is the best it can be. Some have died in the effort to rescue others. Many have been injured. The face of lifesaving is not the same everywhere, but the heart of lifesaving beats at the same rhythm. We are one.

REFERENCES

1. U.S. Census. Population 1790 to 1990. Available at https://www.census.gov/population/censusdata/table-4.pdf.
2. Hembry PM. *The English Spa, 1560–1815: A Social History*. London: Athlone; 1990.
3. The Margate Charter Trustees. The Bathing Machine. Available at http://www.mayormargate.plus.com/bathing-machine.html (accessed 28 March 2015).
4. Goddard I. Sea Bathing. Available at http://www.isabellegoddard.com/sea-bathing-regency-period.html (accessed 28 March 2015).
5. Brawley S. Surf bathing and surf lifesaving: Origins and beginnings. In Jaggard E (ed.). *Between the Flags: One Hundred Summers of Australian Surf Lifesaving*. Sydney: University of New South Wales Press; 2007.
6. Shanks R, York W. *The U.S. Life-Saving Service: Heroes, Rescues and Architecture of the Early Coast Guard*. 3rd ed. Petaluma, CA: Costano; 1998.
7. Royal National Lifeboat Institution. Available at http://rnli.org/aboutus/historyandheritage/Pages/timeline-flash.aspx (accessed 12 April 2015).
8. Methot J. *Up & Down the Beach*. Navesink, NJ: Whip; 1988.
9. Talese G. And now, another spin of the wheel for Atlantic City. *The New York Times*, 8 September 1996.
10. Fowler M, Olsen BA, Olsen E. *Lifeguards of the Jersey Shore*. Atglen: Shiffer; 2010.
11. Talese G. Century by the sea. *The New York Times*, 25 August 1956.
12. *Single Handed Rescues Seven from Drowning*. Los Angeles Herald, 17 December 1908.

13. United States Treasury, Life-Saving Service. *Record of Medals Issued 1910, Form #86.* Washington, DC: United States of America, National Records and Archives Administration; 1910.
14. United States Lifesaving Association. *Lifesaving and Marine Safety.* D'Arnall DG (ed.). Piscataway, NJ: New Century; 1981.
15. Kucher K. A century of lifesaving for city lifeguards. *UT San Diego*, 2 January 2015. Available at http://www.sandiegouniontribune.com/news/2015/jan/02/lifeguards-city-100-years-rescues/
16. American Red Cross. *Swimming and Water Safety*, 3rd ed. 2009. Available at http://editiondigital.net/publication/?i=55928 (accessed 9 June 2015).
17. Mitchell B. Australian Dictionary of Biography. Available at http://adb.anu.edu.au/biography/gocher-william-henry-6408 (accessed 28 March 2015).
18. Booth D. *Australian Beach Cultures: The History of Sun, Sand and Surf.* London: Frank Cass; 2001.
19. 'Life-Saver' is held for endangering life. *The New York Times*, 13 August 1938.
20. Phillips M. Dissension and challenges in surf lifesaving: Amateurism and professionalism. In Jaggard E (ed.). *Between the Flags: One Hundred Summers of Australian Surf Lifesaving.* Sydney: University of New South Wales Press; 2007.
21. Surf Life Saving New Zealand. Available at http://www.surflifesaving.org.nz (accessed 29 March 2015).
22. Lifesaving South Africa. Available at http://www.ilsf.org/about/members/lsa (accessed 29 March 2015).
23. Wake-Walker E. *Break Through: How the Inflatable Rescue Boat Conquered the Surf.* Cambridge, UK: Granta Editions; 2007.
24. Jaggard E. From Bondi to Bude: Allan Kennedy and the Exportation of Australian Surf Lifesaving to Britain in the 1950s. *Sport in History* 2011; 31: 62–83.
25. Best A. Saving lives, changing methods: Surf lifesaving technology. In Jaggard E (ed.). *Between the Flags: One Hundred Summers of Australian Surf Lifesaving.* Sydney: University of New South Wales Press; 2007.
26. Ford C, Jaggard E. *Between the Flags: One Hundred Summers of Australian Surf Lifesaving.* Sydney: University of New South Wales Press; 2007.
27. United States Lifesaving Association. *The United States Lifesaving Association Manual of Open Water Lifesaving.* Brewster BC (ed.). Upper Saddle River, NJ: Prentice-Hall; 2003.
28. Long Beach Lifeguard Association. History of the Long Beach Lifeguards. Available at https://www.youtube.com/watch?v=Zy7cXJ5dOvE (accessed 31 March 2015).
29. Kahanamoku helps save 13 in launch. *The New York Times*, June, 1925.
30. National Film and Sound Archive. Australian Screen. 1957. Available at http://aso.gov.au/titles/sponsored-films/service-in-the-sun/notes/ (accessed 30 March 2015).
31. Ampol Petroleum. *Service in the Sun* (film). T3Media; 1957. Available at http://bit.ly/1BYW0z6
32. Jaggard E. From beach to boardroom: Governing surf lifesaving. In Jaggard E (ed.). *Between the Flags: One Hundred Years of Surf Lifesaving.* Sydney: University of New South Wales Press; 2007.
33. United States Coast Guard. Lifeboat History. Available at http://www.uscg.mil/d1/stachatham/Lifeboat%20History.asp (accessed 1 April 2015).
34. Surf Life Saving Australia. *Between the Flags: One Hundred Summers of Australian Surf Lifesaving.* Jaggard E (ed.). Sydney: University of New South Wales Press; 2007.
35. County of Los Angeles Fire Department. Lifeguard History. Available at http://www.fire.lacounty.gov/lifeguard/lifeguard-history/ (accessed 31 March 2015).
36. Los Angeles County Fire Department. Catalina Paramedic Operations. Available at http://www.fire.lacounty.gov/portfolio/catalina-paramedic-operations/ (accessed 12 April 2015).
37. Martino MT. *Lifeguards of San Diego County.* Charleston, SC: Arcadia; 2007.
38. Auckland Rescue Helicopter Trust. Available at http://rescuehelicopter.org.nz/who-we-are (accessed 12 April 2015).

39. Goulart CPRM. Helicopter sea rescue in Rio de Janeiro. In Brewster BC (ed.). *International Medical-Rescue Conference*. San Diego, CA: International Life Saving Federation; 1997.

40. 2 Drown, 11 missing, 60 are saved at Ocean Beach. *The San Diego Union*, 6 May 1918.

41. American Heart Association. History of CPR. Available at http://bit.ly/1xJQCEH (accessed 3 April 2015).

42. United States Lifesaving Association. Available at http://www.usla.org (accessed 3 April 2015).

43. San Diego Lifeguard Service. History. Available at http://www.sandiego.gov/lifeguards/about/history.shtml (accessed 1 April 2015).

44. Kowsky K. Turning the tide: Female lifeguards have gained a foothold in the male-dominated profession. But they still battle sexism—sometimes even from swimmers they are trying to help. *The Los Angeles Times*, 30 August 1992.

45. Galton B, Jaggard E. The luck of the surf? In Jaggard E (ed.). *Between the Flags: One Hundred Summers of Australian Surf Lifesaving*. Sydney: University of New South Wales Press; 2007.

46. Booth D. Managing pleasure and discipline. In Jaggard E (ed.). *Between the Flags: One Hundred Years of Surf Lifesaving*. Sydney: University of New South Wales Press; 2007.

47. *Surf Life Saving Australia*. Annual Report 2013–14.

48. Burnside R. To Australia With Tears, *American Lifeguard Magazine* 2014 Winter, 31(2). 8–9.

49. International Life Saving Federation. World Life Saving. Available at http://www.ilsf.org/about/history/wls (accessed 3 April 2015).

50. Los Angeles County. 2014–2015 Recommended Budget. 2014.

51. City of San Diego. FY 2015 Adopted Budget; 2015.

2

Lifeguard effectiveness*

JULIE GILCHRIST AND CHRISTINE BRANCHE

INTRODUCTION

Lifeguards play an important role in protecting patrons as they swim in and spend time around recreational bodies of water. They provide vital information to patrons on how to prevent drowning and other injuries and also assist those in distress and provide emergency medical care when needed. Few studies have examined the effectiveness of lifeguards; however, a consistent water safety message from public health and safety organizations is to choose swimming locations with lifeguard supervision. This chapter explores drowning burden, prevention strategies, lifeguard effectiveness, efforts towards improved lifeguard standards and training and other interventions to improve patron safety.

DROWNING BURDEN

While time in and around water should be fun and contribute to fitness, it also puts patrons at risk of fatal or nonfatal drowning and other injuries. Drowning is a serious and neglected public health threat worldwide [1]. More than 90% of drownings occur in low- and middle-income countries [1]. In the United States, almost 4,000 people die from drowning each year [2]. Of these, about 18% of drownings occur in swimming pools and 51% in natural water settings [3].

Nonfatal drowning is also a public health concern because drowning survivors often sustain permanent disabling conditions, ranging from learning disabilities and memory impairment to loss of basic cognitive functioning (i.e., a persistent vegetative state). In the United States, hospital emergency departments annually treat about 6,500 victims [4] and more than 50% require hospitalization or additional medical care [3]. In contrast, the hospitalization rate for all unintentional injuries treated in the emergency department is approximately 6% [4].

Medical treatment of drowning victims is expensive. For all cases of drowning in the United States in 2000, researchers estimated the lifetime medical costs, including emergency department, hospital, and outpatient treatment, to be more than US$95 million [5]. These estimates do not include on-site costs incurred by lifeguarding staff

---

* The findings and conclusions in this chapter are those of the authors and do not represent the official views of the US Department of Health and Human Services (DHHS) and the Centers for Disease Control and Prevention (CDC). The inclusion of individuals, programmes or organizations in this article does not constitute endorsement by the US federal government, DHHS or CDC.

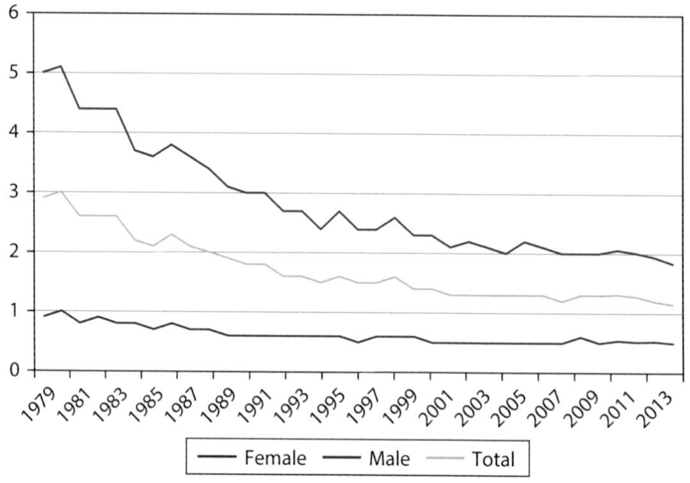

Figure 2.1 Fatal unintentional drowning rates (per 100,000 population) by sex – United States, 1979–2013. Includes drowning events while boating. (From National Vital Statistics System ICD codes: E830, E832, E910 & V90, V92, W65-W74.)

or emergency medical services. Indirect costs to society from fatal and nonfatal drowning, including lost productivity, totalled more than US$5.2 billion [5].

Research suggests that in-hospital treatment typically does not alter the outcomes of fatal or nonfatal drowning [6,7], whereas immediate removal from the water and prompt initiation of cardiopulmonary resuscitation (CPR) does reduce mortality and improve outcomes [8]. This information on the burden, costs and general ineffectiveness of in-hospital medical care for drowning highlights the importance of active water safety promotion and drowning prevention including an effective on-site response.

Although drowning remains a significant threat to children, the population-based rates of drowning have declined substantially in high-income countries. In 1979, the United States' age-adjusted unintentional drowning rates were 2.9 per 100,000 population (almost 6,900 people); in 2010, this was reduced to 1.3 per 100,000 (or just over 4,000 people) (Figure 2.1) [2]. This represents a 55% reduction in drowning rates over three decades.

PREVENTION STRATEGIES

Swimming is a popular sport and recreational activity, with more than 21.5 million Americans participating [9]. Attendance at swimming pools, water parks, beaches and lakefronts continues to grow.

Public health officials, local officials, owners and operators are all interested in patron safety, and the lifeguard serves as the face of that effort.

Drowning prevention strategies can be classified into three types: (1) improving knowledge or skills of patrons or lifeguards, (2) improving engineering or technology, and (3) altering the physical or sociocultural environment [10]. Examples of improving patron knowledge or skills might include gaining swim skills, understanding aquatic risks like rip currents and the dangers of alcohol use, and understanding and heeding beach safety flags and signs. Lifeguard skills include improving early identification of distressed swimmers and improving recovery and response. Advances in engineering and technology might increase water safety by developing or improving the comfort and usability of life jackets, the means to predict or identify rip currents or the ability to monitor swimmers. Altering the physical environment might include the use of signs and flags, designated swimming areas, lakefront slope gradients to prevent sudden underwater drop-offs or barriers to prevent access to dangerous areas [11]. Finally, improving the sociocultural environment might include enacting or enhancing rules, policies and laws such as those promoting effective measures regarding the following: (1) life jacket wear, (2) swim skill attainment, (3) avoidance of alcohol use and (4) lifeguarding services. Lifeguards are public safety professionals; they play a prominent role in both improving the knowledge of patrons about immediate physical risks (e.g., rip currents, marine life) and ensuring that the physical environment in which patrons swim is as safe as possible (e.g., appropriate flags, signage, swim area markers). Because they are respected in the community, lifeguards also have the opportunity to educate and influence the public beyond the confines of their sight lines.

LIFEGUARD EFFECTIVENESS

In the United States, beach lifeguarding has a long history in public safety. In the late 1800s, recognizing that police officers or other public safety professionals could not perform water safety duties in addition to their regular duties, specifically equipped and trained 'lifeguards' were hired to take on water safety responsibilities. In 1914, the American Red Cross introduced the American Red Cross Lifesaving course, developed by Commodore Wilbert E. Longfellow to train swimmers in lifesaving and resuscitation and to organize them into volunteer corps to protect their communities [12]. The American Red Cross and the YMCA collaborated to promote first aid training, including lifesaving, through community programmes [13].

Through the years, lifeguards became respected public safety professionals. In 1964, lifeguards from several surf lifeguard agencies in California came together to improve lifeguard training and professionalism with the goal of enhancing drowning prevention and other lifesaving efforts. This group standardized beach lifeguard practices and training, and encouraged and improved public water safety education. This organization is now the United States Lifesaving Association (USLA), a non-profit professional association of lifeguards with membership available to any employee of a US ocean, bay, lake, river or other open water rescue service [14]. Today USLA standards are followed by most surf beach lifeguard providers and some larger inland beach lifeguard providers. In addition, the YMCA and the American Red Cross continue to provide nationally standardized training programmes for beach lifeguards, predominantly at inland beaches.

Since the establishment of lifeguarding services, population-based drowning rates have declined as participation in aquatics continues to rise. Research has not been able to measure the specific contribution of lifeguards. However, water safety education, on-site supervision and intervention by lifeguards have undoubtedly contributed to this reduction in drowning rates.

A previous examination of lifeguard effectiveness included data from the USLA and open water rescuers [11]. The USLA compiles statistics for drownings at most ocean beaches and other open water beaches patrolled by USLA lifeguards. In 2001, using 10 years of attendance estimates and drowning counts, the USLA estimated that 'the chance of drowning at a beach protected by lifeguards trained under USLA standards was less than 1 in 18 million per year' [11,14]. This ratio has not changed in the years since ([14], Rick Gould, personal communication, 22 July 2014). Three-quarters of drowning events at protected sites occurred when the lifeguards were not on patrol [11].

USLA data from 2013 suggest that 111 visitors to USLA beaches fatally drowned; 92 (83%) occurred when the beach was unguarded and 19 (17%) when guarded. These 19 fatalities occurred among more than 66,000 rescues. In addition, lifeguards reported 100 times more preventive actions (compared with rescues) to keep patrons safe. Finally, USLA lifeguards report participating in more than 10,000 lectures or presentations to improve public safety [14].

The data from the USLA appear to be comparable to published data from waterparks. A 2011 review of waterpark lifeguard reports included four deaths during 63,800,000 visits or a ratio of one death to 15,950,000 visits [15]. Among 56,000 rescues recorded, 32 involved 'loss of spontaneous respiration,' defined by the authors as 'lifeguard noting loss of consciousness and/or lack of breathing'.

A study from Brazil examined reports from more than 41,000 beach lifeguard rescues over 20 years. The authors found that 5.5% required additional medical care and 0.5% required on-site CPR [16].

Several brief case studies have provided ecological evidence suggesting the effectiveness of lifeguards. These reports are from local jurisdictions and describe the drowning risks on beaches before and after a change in lifeguard policies. Each report demonstrates either a benefit to the public from the presence of lifeguards or negative effects following termination of lifeguard services [11].

Finally, the cost effectiveness of lifeguarding services on coastal beaches was examined in Australia and the United Kingdom [17,18]. In Australia, beach lifeguards are largely unpaid volunteers organized through surf lifesaving clubs and their governing bodies. A study estimated the cost–benefit ratios of lifesaving activities, both with imputed salaries (if salaries were paid: 10.4:1) and without (if they remain unpaid volunteers: 16.5:1). In both scenarios, the cost–benefit ratios are positive, thus substantiating the value to the community of surf lifesaving services. In addition, while not quantified, the authors discussed the added 'social capital' that these volunteer lifesaving units contribute to the community through decreased mortality, decreased crime, a safer natural environment, increased tourism and increased economic performance [17].

Similarly, in the United Kingdom, researchers compared the identified costs of running the Royal National Lifeboat Institution (RNLI) lifeguarding operations with the economic and comprehensive costs of drowning resulting in death, disability or recovery [18]. They estimated the tangible economic costs of drowning, including treatment costs, lost earnings, lost productivity, employer costs and disability allowances. The broader comprehensive costs included all of the tangible costs as well as pain and suffering. The reported costs of the RNLI lifeguarding operations in 2006 was £6.4 million (US$9.9 million), whereas the average annual economic cost of coastal drowning was reported as £211 million (US$327 million) and the average annual comprehensive costs as £308 million (US$477 million). Furthermore, the economic and comprehensive values of a beach lifeguard unit per life saved were reported as £1.8 million (US$2.8 million) and £2.7 million (US$4.2 million), respectively, while requiring £66,000 (US$102,000) annually to function [18]. In addition, the RNLI commissioned a survey to explore further costs and benefits [19]. The researchers identified that the presence of lifeguards was a positive consideration in the selection of locations for recreation and tourism bringing in additional patrons; lifeguards are perceived to keep beaches safer from injuries and drowning as well as from antisocial behaviour and crime. Finally, immediate lifeguard triage and care reduced health care costs by reducing unnecessary emergency transports and emergency department visits [19].

Taken together, these epidemiologic studies from beachfronts, swimming pools and waterparks suggest that lifeguards are effective in reducing situations likely to end in injury, identifying swimmers in trouble and intervening during the drowning process, in most cases in time to avert lasting harmful consequences. Additional data on preventive actions and public education demonstrate the commitment lifeguards show to the primary prevention of drowning. Finally, the economic evaluations suggest that surf lifeguarding is good value for the communities they serve.

IMPROVING LIFEGUARD EFFECTIVENESS

To maximize lifeguard effectiveness, decision-makers must attend to the staffing, training and practice of lifeguards. Drowning is a process that often happens quickly and quietly. Contrary to the versions depicted in popular media, many drowning victims are unable to call out, splash or wave a hand [20,21]. Untrained bystanders would have difficulty recognizing drowning victims. Because drowning happens quickly and with little opportunity for others to know to intervene, patron surveillance is at the core of lifeguard duties. Consequently, policies and practices must include minimizing distractions and competing tasks as well as enhancing a lifeguard's ability to remain vigilant. Such attentiveness allows a lifeguard to identify circumstances that might lead to injury and take action to prevent or minimize the injury [22,23].

In an effort to examine the available science that might inform lifeguard certification, training and practice standards, in 2005 the USLA, the American Red Cross and the YMCA established the US Lifeguard Standards Coalition. Experts from relevant health and safety organizations and agencies worked together to identify key issues in lifeguard training or practice for review to identify best practices and to define the level of the supporting science. Practices were classified as *standards*, *guidelines* or *options* [24]. The 2011 report covered available science regarding topics such as lifeguard scanning and vigilance to identify troubled swimmers; age, hearing, vision and physical requirements of lifeguards; and aspects of resuscitation, first aid and education [24].

The coalition recommended guidelines for training; for example, providing information on scanning methods to maximize attentiveness and minimize distractions, and options for lifeguard support, positioning and staffing. To improve vigilance, recommended standards include regular contact and encouragement while on task. Guidelines include education on the need for sleep and screening for sleep apnea as well as provision of shade and cooling while on task. Options included promoting physical activity and prohibiting the use of recreational drugs. However, it was not possible to recommend an optimal length for a lifeguard shift due to the need to balance risks inherent in frequent lifeguard rotation with optimal vigilance for short periods. Guidelines for minimum lifeguard age were related to the level of stress and risk in the aquatic environment. The coalition identified the need for hearing and vision standards to be developed. The coalition stated, furthermore, that agencies should ensure that lifeguards meet minimum standards for physical fitness, which would be tested using venue-specific water rescue competency exams. Guidelines include testing lifeguards every 10–12 weeks and providing in-service training or exercise programming to ensure continued fitness. Continued periodic efforts to examine the scientific literature and provide guidance to update lifeguard certification, training and practice are necessary and useful [24].

Lifeguard vigilance is critical to their success in protecting the public. Scientific evidence suggests, however, that this is a difficult cognitive and perceptual task [22]. Vigilance requires that the eyes must see and the brain must attend to the information.

Researchers have identified three specific strategies to improve patron surveillance at swimming pools supported by evidence from related health and safety fields [22].

1. *Provide in-service training.* Regular in-service training can remind lifeguards of the importance of their efforts in patron surveillance and assist in problem-solving and overcoming barriers to success. For instance, a brief intervention conducted in midsummer was designed to improve surveillance by (a) increasing lifeguards' perception that a drowning is possible by reporting observed patron risk-taking and the frequency of distracted lifeguards, (b) reviewing a recent drowning fatality in a similar facility to reinforce the

severity of drowning and (c) reviewing scanning techniques and American Red Cross surveillance strategies. This programme resulted in improved observed attention and scanning as well as reduced risk-taking behaviour by patrons throughout the remainder of the season [23].
2. *Practice lifeguarding scenarios.* Similar to other health and safety professionals, lifeguards must routinely practise the skills needed to respond efficiently and effectively during an emergency response [25,26]. Role-playing can improve a lifeguard's ability to respond quickly and appropriately during a stressful situation [22].
3. *Ensure appropriate staffing practices.* The organizational structure must support effective lifeguarding practice by ensuring that a lifeguard's attention is not split between surveillance and other tasks. Establishing adequate staffing, regular rotations and breaks can support lifeguards in maintaining their vigilance [11,22,24].

ENVIRONMENTAL AND OTHER CONSIDERATIONS

The physical aquatic environment can influence the risk of drowning regardless of the presence or absence of lifeguards. Attention to physical details does not remove the need for lifeguards but can enhance their effectiveness. The US Army Corps of Engineers does not use lifeguards at their lakefront facilities but manages drowning risk by establishing specific design criteria to improve safety [27]. Examples of these criteria include using buoys and markers to designate swimming areas, ensuring gradual slope gradients to deeper water, prohibiting diving platforms and other floats and providing safety devices such as rings, buoy lines and poles.

Other possible environmental considerations include appropriate signage and flags to highlight environmental risks, and barriers and fencing to prevent access to particularly hazardous areas. Some of these will not be appropriate for every aquatic setting. For instance, slope gradients cannot be maintained on surf beaches. Careful consideration, however, should be given to modifying the environment when possible to reduce risks [11].

Improving the sociocultural environment around aquatics encompasses improving the relevant rules, policies and laws as well as the public attitudes and beliefs regarding risks and safety around the water. Life jackets are effective [28], yet few people wear them [29]. Basic swim skill is protective [30,31], yet large segments of the US population report limited swim ability [32,33]. Furthermore, few people may understand the identification and avoidance of rip currents, which are the leading reason for rescues at surf beaches [14]. Education and enactment with enforcement of relevant policies and laws can influence risks in each of these areas.

CONCLUSION

Fatal drowning is a preventable public health problem affecting thousands in the United States and hundreds of thousands globally each year. In addition, nonfatal drowning is potentially severe, with an extraordinary hospitalization rate and little hope to improve outcomes through in-hospital care. Preventing drowning incidents and improving on-site response is therefore critical to reducing the burden, costs and consequences of drowning injuries.

Lifeguards are public health and safety professionals. They are positioned well, literally and figuratively, to improve the general public's water safety knowledge, to help patrons avoid drowning risks and to intervene when necessary to improve the outcome of a drowning event.

Lifeguard effectiveness can be improved through enhanced training and organizational support to ensure that they (1) are able to remain appropriately vigilant and undistracted, (2) are empowered to intervene to avert an incident, (3) have the knowledge, skills and confidence to respond appropriately when necessary and (4) can educate and advocate for public safety policies to reduce drowning. At the same time, agencies and organizations should examine the physical and sociocultural environment to address drowning risks. Finally, to provide the evidence base for future recommendations, critical scientific evaluation of the effectiveness of lifeguard training, standards and practices should be ongoing.

REFERENCES

1. World Health Organization. *Global Report on Drowning: Preventing a Leading Killer.* Geneva: WHO; 2014.
2. Centers for Disease Control and Prevention, National Center for Health Statistics. Wide-Ranging Online Data for Epidemiologic Research (WONDER). [cited 3 August 2014]. Available at http://wonder.cdc.gov/mortSQL.html
3. Laosee OC, Gilchrist J, Rudd R. Drowning 2005–2009. *MMWR.* 2012; 61(19): 344–7.
4. Centers for Disease Control and Prevention, National Center for Injury Prevention and Control. Web-based Injury Statistics Query and Reporting System (WISQARS). [cited 3 August 2014]. Available at http://www.cdc.gov/injury/wisqars
5. Finkelstein EA, Corso PS, Miller TR. *The Incidence and Economic Burden of Injuries in the United States.* New York: Oxford University Press; 2006.
6. Cummings P, Quan L. Trends in unintentional drowning: The role of alcohol and medical care. *JAMA.* 1999; 281(23): 2198–202.
7. Spack L, Gedeit R, Splaingard M, Havens PL. Failure of aggressive therapy to alter outcomes in pediatric near-drowning. *Pediatr Emerg Care.* 1997; 13(2): 98–102.
8. Kyriacou DN, Arcinue EL, Peek C, Kraus JF. Effect of immediate resuscitation on children with submersion injury. *Pediatrics.* 1994; 94(2): 137–42.
9. Sporting Goods Manufacturers Association. 2012 Sports, Fitness and Leisure Activities Topline Participation Report. [cited 3 August 2014]. Available at http://assets.usta.com/assets/1/15/SGMA_Research_2012_Participation_Topline_Report.pdf
10. Sleet DA. Injury prevention. In Cortese P, Middleton K (eds.). *The Comprehensive School Health Challenge: Promoting Health through Education.* Santa Cruz, CA: ETR; 1994, p. 459.
11. Branche CM, Stewart S (eds.). *Lifeguard Effectiveness: A Report of the Working Group.* Atlanta, GA: Centers for Disease Control and Prevention, National Center for Injury Prevention and Control; 2001.
12. American Red Cross. *Swimming and Water Safety Manual.* 3rd ed. [cited 3 August 2014]. Available at http://editiondigital.net/publication/?i=55928

13. Freas SJ. A history of drowning and resuscitation. In Fletemeyer JR, Freas SJ (eds). *Drowning: New Perspectives on Intervention and Prevention*. Boca Raton, FL: CRC Press; 1999, p. 10.

14. United States Lifesaving Association. [cited 3 August 2014]. Available at www.usla.org

15. Hunsucker JL, Davison SJ. Analysis of rescue and drowning history from a life-guarded waterpark environment. *Int J Inj Contr Saf Promot*. 2011; 18(4): 277–84.

16. Szpilman D. Near-drowning and drowning classification: A proposal to stratify mortality based on the analysis of 1,831 cases. *Chest*. 1997; 112(3): 660–5.

17. *Valuing an Australian Icon: The Economic and Social Contribution of Surf Life Saving in Australia*. Report to Surf Life Saving Limited. The Allen Consulting Group; 2005.

18. *The Economic Value of Lifeguarding: A Research Study Exploring the Value of Providing Lifeguarding Service in the UK*. Report to the Royal National Lifeboat Institution. Mintel Custom Solutions; 2007.

19. Logan A. The Economic and Social Benefits of Lifeguard Provision. RNLI Research Project ID: 13-1. Available at http://rnli.org/aboutus/aboutthernli/Documents/benefits-lifeguard-provision.pdf

20. Pia F. Observations on the drowning of non-swimmers. *J Phys Edu*. 1974; 71(6), 164–67 and 181.

21. Webber J. Surf lifeguard response to drowning: The SENTINEL system revisited. Oral abstract at *The Lifesaving Foundation Drowning Prevention and Rescue Conference*, Thursday, 27 September 2012, to Saturday, 29 September 2012, Carlow, Ireland. doi: 10.13140/RG.2.1.3844.3041.

22. Schwebel DC, Jones HN, Holder E, Marciani F. Lifeguards: A forgotten aspect of drowning prevention. *J Inj Violence Res*. 2010; 2(1): 1–3.

23. Schwebel DC, Lindsay S, Simpson J. Brief report: A brief intervention to improve lifeguard surveillance at a public swimming pool. *J Pediatr Psychol*. 2007; 32: 862–8.

24. United States Lifeguard Standards Coalition. United States Lifeguard Standards: An Evidence-Based Review and Report by the United States Lifeguard Standards Coalition. 2011. Available at http://www.lifeguardstandards.org/index.php?pg=final_report

25. Anderson M, Leflore J. Playing it safe: Simulated team training in the OR. *AORN J*. 2008; 87: 772–9.

26. Van Hasselt VB, Romaon SJ, Vecchi GM. Role playing: Applications in hostage and crisis negotiation skills training. *Behav Modif*. 2008; 32: 248–63.

27. US Army Corps of Engineers. Engineer Manual [EM-1110-1-400], Recreation Planning and Design Criteria, July 31, 1987.

28. Cummings P, Mueller BA, Quan L. Association between wearing a personal floatation device and death by drowning among recreational boaters: A matched cohort analysis of United States Coast Guard data. *Injury Prev*. 2011; 17: 156–9.

29. Chung C, Quan L, Bennett E, Kernic MA, Ebel BE. Informing policy on open water drowning prevention: An observational survey of life jacket use in Washington state. *Inj Prev*. 2014; 20(4): 238–43.

30. Brenner RA, Taneja GS, Haynie DL, Trumble AC, Qian C, Klinger RM, Klevanoff MA. Association between swimming lessons and drowning in childhood: A case-control study. *Arch Pediatr Adolesc Med*. 2009; 163(3): 203–10.

31. Rahman F, Bose S, Linnan M, Rahman A, Mashreky S, Haaland B, Finkelstein E. Cost-effectiveness of an injury and drowning prevention programme in Bangladesh. *Pediatrics*. 2012; 130: e1621–8.

32. Gilchrist J, Sacks JJ, Branche CM. Self-reported swimming ability in U.S. adults, 1994. *Public Health Rep*. 2000; 115(2–3): 110–11.

33. Irwin CC, Irwin RL, Ryan TD. Urban minority youth swimming (in)ability in the United States and associated demographic characteristics: Toward a drowning prevention plan. *Inj Prev*. 2009; 15: 234–9.

3

Data, risk analysis and evaluation: Their role in advancing the science of beach lifeguarding

MICHAEL WRIGHT

INTRODUCTION

Risk analysis and risk assessment mean many things to different people. This is because risk analysis and assessment serve a wide range of purposes and use a wide range of methods. They take many forms, even within the limited scope of the risk of drowning covered by this book. In their different forms, risk analysis and assessment can help answer national and strategic level questions:

1. Inform national level debates on whether or not to try to reduce the risk associated with an activity
    Is the risk high enough to justify investing society's resources in reducing it? Are there other higher risk areas that deserve priority?
2. Targeting safety work to people most at risk
    Who is at greatest risk? Who are the 'at-risk groups' that require our attention?

These national and strategic questions often entail numerical forms of analysis, drawing on data covering fatalities and participants. It tends to be an occasional form of assessment used to inform strategic decisions.

Risk analysis and risk assessment are also used to help devise safety measures for specific and often local cases, such as safety measures for a specific beach. Moving from national risk assessment to more local assessments, the form of risk analysis tends to become more qualitative, perhaps involving rating schemes and guidance, to support forms of assessment based on expert judgement. Some key examples include the beach risk assessment methods of the Royal National Lifeboat Institution (RNLI) [1,2]. The methods help to identify the hazards on a specific beach, such as rip currents, and identify suitable safety measures. These qualitative and rating forms of risk assessment have been covered elsewhere in this book.

This chapter describes the more 'strategic' forms of numerical risk analysis and how they can support decisions on drowning prevention. It uses two drowning risk assessments, drowning at sea and drowning inland in the United Kingdom, as examples to exemplify the rationale, method and potential use of results. Noting that the two examples are not specific to beach-related water safety, the chapter aims to exemplify methods and rationale that can be drawn upon by the lifeguarding community to advance the science of lifeguarding.

STRATEGIC LEVEL RISK ANALYSIS AND ASSESSMENT

We are exposed to innumerable hazards in our daily lives, at work, at home, when travelling and when at leisure. Sunlight poses a risk of skin cancer. Walking poses a risk of tripping. Water sports pose a risk of drowning. Using gas at home poses a risk of carbon monoxide poisoning. Some risks are far greater than others, with driving being one of the most common forms of accidental death, and being struck by lightning far less so. Many of these activities are an essential part of daily lives, offer many benefits and are often entered into voluntarily. As a society we must decide how to divide our finite time and resources to manage these risks. How can we decide which risks are too high and need to be reduced?

Tolerability of risk criteria

One approach to informing decisions on whether a risk is too high has been developed by the UK Health and Safety Executive (HSE) over the past 40 years [3,4]. The HSE has devised a set of quantitative criteria to help assess whether a risk from a specific activity is high and should be reduced, or whether it is low.

The approach is based on a set of quantitative criteria applied to rates of accidental fatality. The rationale of this approach is that society has, and continues, to 'tolerate' the risk associated with some activities, while demanding action for other risks. By reviewing society's response to risks, it is possible to determine what level of risk has and has not been tolerated.

Thus, the criteria are presented here as representing how society would commonly view various rates of death.

This is of course an inexact science. People often lack awareness of hazards and the actual rate of incidents. Accordingly, the HSE initially based their risk criteria on very familiar activities, driving and (familiar to fishermen) commercial fishing. At the time of review, there was strong public demand to prevent incidents in these activities, indicating intolerance of the risk. The rates of fatality were 1 in 1000 fishermen per year and 1 in 10,000 road users per year, which were used as upper limits for occupational and public safety, respectively. These figures were used as the upper points of tolerated risk. As time went by, the HSE took the view that new activities should be able to achieve higher standards of safety and so set an upper limit of 1 in 100,000 persons per year.

On the other hand, there was no great demand to reduce other forms of risk, such as being struck by lightning. At the same time, risks that are far lower are assumed to be of diminishing concern, being relatively small. This type of risk was defined as 1 in 1,000,000 people per year, with any risk below this being classed as *negligible*.

Risks between the upper limit and negligible level are defined as *tolerated*, but they should be reduced wherever it is reasonably practicable in respect of time, money and resources. This is often termed the *ALARP region*, where risks should be reduced 'as low as reasonably practicable'.

The HSE approach uses a number of measures of risk. As already noted, a common approach is the annual rate of death per person. The HSE categorizes rates of death as shown in Figure 3.1.

Care must be taken in applying these criteria. Negligible risks are not to be forgotten, but monitored and controlled. Indeed, risks might be negligible because of the effect of current safety measures that need to be maintained. A low risk may be testament to the success of safety measures rather than evidence that they are no longer required. Moreover, society often demands action to be taken for risks, despite them being numerically low, especially where it is judged that the casualty was vulnerable or

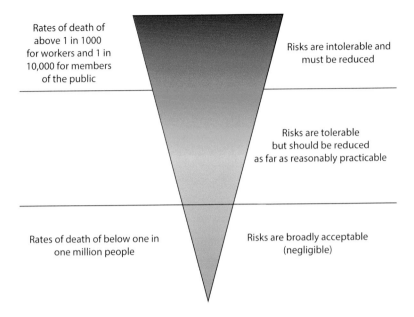

Rates of death of above 1 in 1000 for workers and 1 in 10,000 for members of the public

Risks are intolerable and must be reduced

Risks are tolerable but should be reduced as far as reasonably practicable

Rates of death of below one in one million people

Risks are broadly acceptable (negligible)

Figure 3.1 Health and Safety Executive risk criteria.

where inappropriate actions of a third party caused the incident.

The latter point highlights how numerical risk criteria are but one consideration in the assessment of risk. Society's view of fairness, vulnerability, the benefit of the activity associated with the risk and the practicality of reducing a risk are also equally relevant considerations.

Risks that fall in the ALARP region *should* be reduced. It is only in the assessment of potential risk reduction measures that we consider the balance of possible risk reduction against costs and impacts.

Risks classed as intolerable do not necessarily require activities to be prohibited. Rather the first step is to identify ways of reducing the risk. However, where a risk is classed as intolerable, less weight tends to be given to the cost of options and more weight to the scope for risk reduction.

Finally, it should be noted that in the case of leisure activities these are guidelines and have no legal force.

Benchmarking risks

It is also possible to put risks in perspective by comparing them with other causes of accidental death. Some benchmarks for other activities are as follows:

- One death per 2703 motorbike users[*]
- One in 11,333 UK gliders[†]
- One death per 18,077 cyclists[‡]
- One death per 56,657 car users (assuming 60 million UK car users)
- One death per 120,000 pedestrians (assuming 60 million UK pedestrians)
- One death in 231,343 residents by accidental fire deaths in the home (Great Britain 2010)[§]
- One per every 300,000 to 400,000 horse riders[¶]

Motorbike and cycling safety are particular targets for safety work in the United Kingdom,

[*] http://www.dft.gov.uk/statistics/releases/road-accidents-and-safety-annual-report-2010/
[†] Three deaths in ONS 2010 mortality data and 34,000 UK gliders estimated by British Gliding Association.
[‡] http://www.dft.gov.uk/statistics/releases/road-accidents-and-safety-annual-report-2010/
[§] http://www.communities.gov.uk/publications/corporate/statistics/firestatsgb201011 (accessed 5 December 2014).
[¶] http://news.bbc.co.uk/1/hi/magazine/8339097.stm (accessed 5 December 2014).

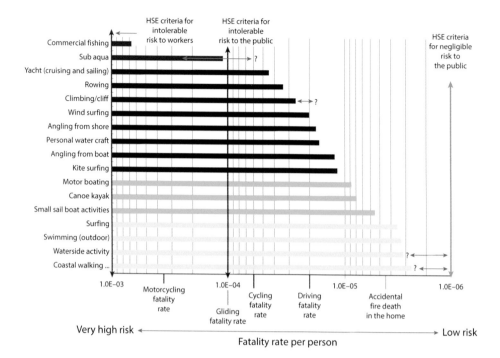

Figure 3.2 Risk of fatal drowning at sea (UK). (From Wright M, et al. *Analysing Causes of Water Related Deaths and Serious Incidents around the Coast: The RNLI's New Causal Analysis Process.* World Congress on Drowning Prevention; 2013. Available at http://www.wcdp2013.org/uploads/media/Sea_Rescue1_1_073_Causes_of_drowning_at_Sea_MichaelWright.pdf [accessed 5 December 2014].)

with ongoing road safety campaigns. Fire safety has been a target for safety for many years. Therefore, these areas can be used to reinforce the judgement of what risk levels are considered to be high or intolerable by society. It is pertinent to note that, despite the risk of drowning in many activities, as shown in Figure 3.2, being greater than the risk of fire deaths in the home, there is not a national drowning prevention campaign in the United Kingdom at the time of writing. This situation may reflect a low level of awareness of the risk of drowning in the United Kingdom.

Clearly, these benchmarks will change over time and need to be refreshed.

Variations on the HSE criteria

The HSE criteria use very broad categories. The risk associated with many water sports falls within the ALARP region, limiting the scope for prioritization. Therefore, an option is to use more bands. In work with the RNLI [5], a six-band categorization has been used to allow for a finer

gradation of risks, for the sake of prioritizing prevention and education work, namely

- Any fatality rate that is within a factor of two of the intolerable criterion is *very high*.
- Any rate between 1 in 20,000 and 1 in 100,000 is *high*.
- Rates between 1 in 100,000 and 1 in 250,000 are *moderate*.
- Rates between 1 in 250,000 and 1 in 500,000 are *low*.
- Rates between 1 in 500,000 and one in one million are *very low*.
- Anything below one in one million is *negligible*.

APPLICATION TO WATER SPORTS AND WATER-RELATED RISKS

How does this somewhat high level framework apply to water safety? A number of organizations have quantified the risk associated with water sports and activities and assessed the results using the tolerability of risk framework, including the

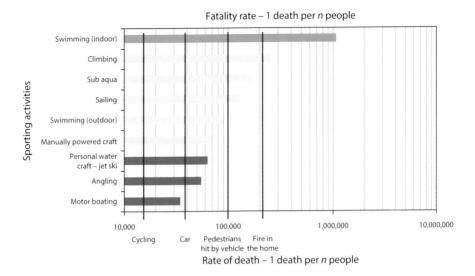

Figure 3.3 **Rates of death for inland water activities.**

RNLI [6] and the Royal Society for the Prevention of Accidents [7]. In both cases the rate of death per person per year was estimated for a range of activities for incidents at sea and inland, respectively.

The rates have been estimated for men and women together (i.e. adults) and then for men alone, as most fatal drownings involve men. These rates have been compared with HSE risk tolerability criteria and our five-band risk categories, grading the activities from *very high* to *very low* risk. In addition, uncertainties in the data have been explored and the implications for the calculated rates have been identified.

Drowning at sea

Some example results for adults drowning at sea around the United Kingdom are shown in Figure 3.2 [4]. The figure presents results as a rate per *n* people, with the highest rate presented by the shortest bar.

The assessment indicated a very wide range of risk estimates for the different activities. This would immediately suggest that the case for additional safety intervention varies, with activities such as scuba diving being a greater priority than, for example, walking by the sea.

In interpreting these results, it is important to note that activities with a relatively small number of deaths may have higher rates of death due to the smaller number of participants. As a result, activities may be prioritized based on the rate (risk) of death rather than the absolute number of deaths.

This logic follows the rationale of a risk-based approach to safety.

An approximation of child deaths at sea was also made. As these are relatively few in number, they were not presented per activity. The fortunately relatively small number of child deaths at sea was assessed as very low (about one per five million each year), less than one per million children participating in water activities at sea. Care must be taken in interpreting this. First, the low rate may reflect high levels of parental supervision, the preventive work of lifeguards and a presumption that children are more limited to activities such as swimming rather than sailing and scuba diving. In addition, as previously noted, society tends to aim for higher standards of safety for vulnerable children; hence a very low rate of death does not necessarily imply no further intervention. Indeed, the UK Water Accident Incident Database* reported 46 deaths of people aged 19 and under in 2013. None of these deaths took place at sea (most in inland outdoor water), but the figures indicate that there remains a need to consider child water safety.

Inland drowning risk assessment

Some sample results for adults drowning inland in the United Kingdom are shown in Figure 3.3 (taken from [7]). These are presented here as an

---

* http://www.nationalwatersafety.org.uk/waid/reports.
  asp (accessed May, 2015).

example of how to complete risk assessment and how the results may inform decision making. As for Figure 3.2, Figure 3.3 presents results as a rate per *n* people, with the highest rate presented by the shortest bar. For example, there was one death per 30,000 motor boating participants, a high rate of death and a short bar in the chart. Indoor swimming had one death per 3,420,000 swimmers, a very low rate of death and so a very large bar.

The rates of death are colour-coded for presentational purposes, with red being very high, orange high, yellow moderate and green very low, following on from the HSE risk criteria. The figure also shows the rates of death in some other activities, such as cycling, as benchmarks. Using this example:

- Motor boating and scuba diving have the highest risk and would be the highest priority for improved safety.
- There are four activities (angling, sailing, jet skis and manually powered crafts) where the rate of accidental death is defined as *high*. These activities would be the second highest priority for improved safety.
- Three activities have a moderate rate of death, namely, outdoor swimming and scuba diving and sailing, with outdoor swimming being in the cusp of moderate to high risk. These activities would be the third priority for improved safety and improvements should be reasonably practicable.
- Swimming indoors has a very low rate of death and the risk would be defined as *negligible* at about one in three million participants.

If the rates of death are compared with the benchmarks, the occasional participation in motor boating, scuba diving, angling, jet skiing, outdoor swimming and manually powered sports have rates of death in the same region as driving a car, which is typically a daily activity. Clearly cycling is a higher risk than all listed activities, but it should be noted that there are demands for improved cycling safety.

The very low (indeed negligible) fatality rate for indoor swimming would be interpreted as indicating that *additional* safety precautions are not a priority for indoor swimming pools. However, as previously noted, the very low risk may reflect the value of lifeguards and other precautions, vindicating their implementation and the need to maintain them. Indeed, the results raise the question of whether extending lifeguarding to selected, inland open waterways and other drowning prevention interventions would help reduce the risk of inland outdoor swimming.

THE ADVANTAGES AND LIMITS OF TOLERABILITY OF RISK FRAMEWORK

This approach has a number of advantages, including the following:

- The criteria are objective and, if agreed prior to an analysis, can be used to inform decisions in an impartial manner.
- The criteria are absolute rather than relative. All risks may be assessed as high or low. This avoids the potential error of prioritizing risks because they are relatively high despite them all being, in absolute terms, very low.
- The criteria are well established and have been used to inform many decisions about public as well as occupational safety.

However, the approach has some weaknesses and limits.

First, it is a data hungry approach, requiring data on fatalities and number of participants. In the absence of robust data, it may not be possible to develop risk estimates of any value.

Second, there has been no significant research into how the voluntary nature of some activities, such as leisure activities, influences the tolerability of risks. The HSE criteria were developed in the context of road safety, which could be said to be a voluntary activity. However, driving may also be defined as an essential activity for daily living, travelling to work and so forth. Participating in open water swimming, sailing and other sports is not necessarily a necessity. Therefore, it is uncertain whether the same criteria would apply to leisure activities that are entirely voluntary.

Similarly, anecdotal evidence and some research suggest that society's tolerance of risk varies according to the vulnerability of the casualty. The tolerance of risk tends to be lower where children are involved, for example. However, it is unknown how the quantitative criteria would be modified, numerically, to reflect these differences in societal values.

Finally, many activities offer benefits as well as risk. Sports offer enjoyment, physical exercise and health benefits, as well as opportunities for social and family engagement. Sports can be educational and help develop a person's sense of self-worth and self-esteem and develop abilities such as teamwork and communication. The tolerability of risk framework does recognize these benefits. Specifically, when a risk is classed as falling in the ALARP region (not intolerable but high enough to require reduction), potential risk reduction options are assessed by comparing the estimated quantity of risk reduction to the costs and impacts, including any impact on benefits such as exercise.

However, the balancing of risk reduction against less tangible benefits such as enjoyment remains a matter of judgement, currently lacking any realistic form of objective comparison. There are, though, some emerging examples of risk–benefit comparison that exemplify how to qualitatively compare options for risk reduction against the benefits of the activity [8,9].

Noting these limits and uncertainties, any quantification of risk can only be an input to what remains a subjective and value-laden decision process. To reduce the possibility of bias and inconsistent decisions, some analysts attempt to articulate all potential impacts, making the costs and benefits explicit, thereby enabling transparent, consistent and balanced decisions.

OTHER MEASURES OF RISK

Societal risk

Anecdotal evidence and research also show that society tends to be particularly averse to incidents that result in many casualties. These types of multi-casualty incidents have been termed *societal risk*, which is defined as the frequency of incidents with a given number of deaths (or other outcomes). Societal risk is measured as a frequency per year rather than as a rate per person. For example, there may be five incidents per year with 10 or more deaths.

There have been some notable coastal societal water-related incidents in the United Kingdom, including the following:

- In February 2004, 21 cockle pickers died from drowning in Morecambe Bay.
- On 20 August 1989, 51 drowned after the sinking of the *Marchioness* on the River Thames in London.
- Five commercial fishermen died in 2007 off Dublin after adverse weather.
- In 1987 the *Herald of Free Enterprise* capsized in the English Channel, killing 193 people.
- In 2000 the *Solway Harvester* fishing vessel sank with the loss of seven lives off the Isle of Man.
- In 2000 the UK-registered fishing vessel *Arosa* grounded on Doonguddle Rock, off the west coast of Ireland, with the loss of 12 crew members.

Thus, there is a real potential for major loss of life at sea.

This topic leads onto the question of how to assess the tolerability of risk of larger scale incidents. The HSE [10] suggested within its document 'Reducing risks, protecting people' that intolerable societal risk for fatal incidents for any single industrial installation can be defined thus:

> ...the risk of an accident causing the death of 50 or more people in a single event should be regarded as intolerable if the frequency is estimated to be more than one in five thousand per annum.

The HSE regulates over 1000 industrial installations [10, p. 3]. Therefore, an option is to multiply the HSE criterion by 1000 to provide an indicative UK-wide societal risk criterion, that is, one event causing 50 or more deaths per five years. Clearly, an intuitive judgement would suggest that any society would view 50 people dying every five years (or five people twice per year) in any one activity, such as sailing, as the very upper limit. If the approach of banding risk into five or more categories were to be applied, then the national societal risk categories would be as follows:

- Upper limit: five deaths twice per year
- High: five deaths between twice per year and every 25 years

- Moderate: five deaths between every 25 years and 62.5 years
- Low: five deaths between every 62.5 years and 125 years
- Very low: five deaths less than once per 125 years

As before, the use of quantitative criteria offers objectivity. However, the calculation of societal risk measures is even harder than for rates of death, due to the infrequency of such events. Typically, societal risk is calculated using data from a very long time period, such as 20 years, in order to build a robust dataset. However, this method leads to any risk estimate, if based on historic data, being dominated by history and hence possibly not indicative of modern day standards. These data problems tend to limit the production and use of societal risk estimates.

The aforementioned RNLI risk assessment looked at societal risk at sea, for all types of water sports, finding it to be high but not intolerable when assessed using the HSE's criteria.

Rates of death per million hours of participation

Some analysts prefer to use another measure of risk, specifically the rate of fatalities per million hours of participation. The rationale is that participation time varies greatly between sports and so any annualized risk measure fails to reflect the duration of participation. The concern is that this method may lead to a false comparison of risk per hour of participation. This line of thinking reflects a focus on trying to assess the relative risk of participating in different activities.

The previous approach of assessing the rate of death per year reflects the idea that it is important to assess activities based on the 'typical' frequency and duration of participation. Scuba diving is likely to have a higher rate of death per hour, as each dive will be less than one hour. Sailing is likely to have a lower rate of death per hour, as each trip may last many hours or days. The previous annualized risk assessments indicate the risk associated with a typical participation profile.

Of course it is entirely possible to produce both risk measures and use them both to inform decisions, while recognizing their respective rationales.

Number of deaths per activity

A relatively simple but still powerful form of assessment is to compare the number of deaths between activities. It is powerful in at least two respects:

- It enables a simple comparison of activities based on the number of deaths.
- The number of deaths for water sports as a whole can be compared with other risks in society to inform judgements of the relative importance of water safety versus (for example) fire safety.

Figure 3.4 shows the number of accidental deaths at sea per activity in the United Kingdom, averaging data for a period of four years (taken from [6]). It is clear that the more common activities such as walking and swimming have the larger number of deaths.

A similar example can be found in the Australian Royal Life Saving Society annual report for 2014 [11]. Within their analysis, they identify that 13% (34 deaths) of fatal drownings occurred on beaches and that 59% of these involved swimming and recreating.

Such data support a simple rationale of targeting those activities in which more deaths occur, thereby maximizing the value of additional safety work.

Figure 3.5 provides a simple comparison of drownings with other causes of accidental death in the United Kingdom. Whereas falls, transport and medical-related incidents are more common, drowning deaths occur more often than deaths from either work-related or fire-related causes. This information would suggest that drowning prevention is as important as work safety and fire safety.

Comparing numbers of deaths with rates of death

The assessment of frequency of deaths can be compared with the results of calculating the rates of death. The comparison reveals a different ordering of activities. Walking has the largest number of deaths but the lowest rate of death. This situation obviously reflects the large number of people

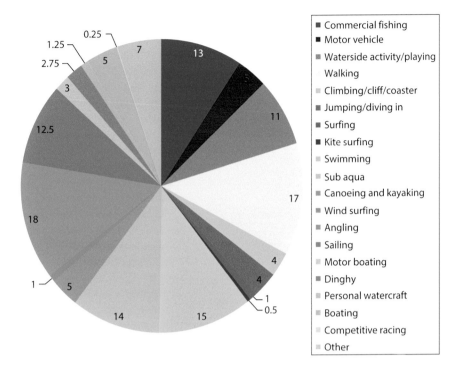

Figure 3.4 Number of deaths at sea by activity. (From Ramm H, Stephens W. *RNLI's Coastal Safety Strategy*. World Congress on Drowning Prevention; 2013. Available at http://www.wcdp2013.org/uploads/media/Sea_Rescue1_3_74_Prevention_Drowning_at_Sea_MichaelWright.pdf [accessed 5 December 2014].)

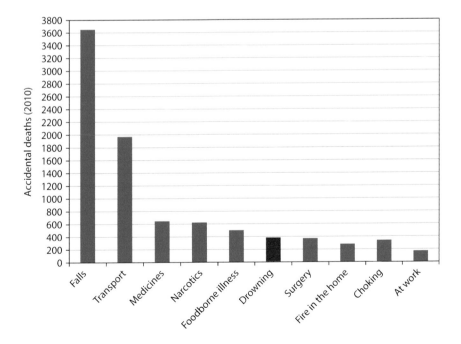

Figure 3.5 Number of accidental water-related deaths (at sea and inland) compared with number of accidental deaths from other causes.

participating in walking. This begs the question of which measure is more important. Unfortunately, there is no simple answer. If the objective is to reduce an individual's risk to a very low level, then activities with higher rates of death such as sailing would be prioritized. If the aim is to reduce the burden on society of accidental deaths, then walking would be the top priority. The answer perhaps lies in the objectives and rationale pursued by decision makers.

DATA

All of the latter strategic forms of risk assessment are reliant on robust data, particularly the following:

- Data on the number of participants per activity
- Data on the number of deaths per year

In the United Kingdom, we are privileged to have the Water Accident Incident Database,[*] which provides data on water-related deaths, injuries and incidents. The database is supplied from a wider range of organizations including the Maritime and Coastguard Agency, RNLI, Royal Society for the Prevention of Accidents, Royal Life Saving Society (UK) and police and fire service. It is the only known source of shared, reconciled and validated data on water-related deaths in the United Kingdom, with data split by activities. The development of such data is a prerequisite for strategic risk assessments as described here.

Other excellent sources of data are as follows:

- The Maritime Accident Investigation Board[†] – for UK deaths within commercial marine activities
- British Sub Aqua Club – for UK scuba diving deaths (National Diving Committee Diving Incidents Report[‡]).

All of the latter sources also note casualties' gender and, usually, their age and whether the death was accidental.

As the number of deaths in any one activity is thankfully small in statistical terms, in most developed countries, it is necessary to have data for a period of years. The number of fatalities needs to be at a level where a valid calculation can be completed. In the United Kingdom, with about 400 accidental deaths per year in the 2010s, a period of four to five years of data has been used to produce risk estimates per activity.

The United Kingdom is also privileged by a consortium of organizations funding annual surveys of water sports participation, namely the Water Sports and Leisure Participation[§] (WSLP) survey. The WSLP survey provides estimates of the number of participants per activity and their age (in bands), gender and frequency of participation. Again the development of such data is a prerequisite for strategic level risk assessments.

The WSLP sample size of 12,000 provides a high level of confidence in the survey as a whole. However, the participation estimates for specific water sports are, in some cases, very small. For example:

- A reported participation level of 2.57% for canoeing equates to 326 respondents.
- A reported participation level of 0.96% for motor boating equates to 122 respondents.

Therefore, some care must be taken in the interpretation of subsequent risk estimates per activity. Small differences in risk estimates might not indicate a true difference in risk when based on uncertain estimates of the number of participants in any one water sport.

The Sports England Active Surveys[¶] provide some data on indoor swimming while the UK census provides local resident data that is of value when assessing the risk from 'everyday' waterside activities such as walking from home to shops.

---

[*] National Water Safety Forum. Water Incident Database. Available at http://www.nationalwatersafety.org.uk/waid/ (accessed 5 December 2014).

[†] Maritime Accident Investigation Board. Available at http://www.maib.gov.uk/publications/annual_reports.cfm (accessed 5 December 2014).

[‡] BSAC annual incident report web page. Available at www.bsac.com (accessed 5 December 2014).

[§] http://www.bcu.org.uk/files/Watersports%20 Participation%20Survey%202012%20-%20 Executive%20Summary.pdf (accessed 5 December 2014).

[¶] http://www.sportengland.org/research/about-our-research/what-is-the-active-people-survey/ (accessed 5 December 2014).

At a practical level, the two datasets need to be aligned to develop activity-based risk assessments.

ASSESSING WHO IS AT GREATEST RISK

The previous example of risk assessment split casualties into adults and children. This practice reflects the notion of segmenting participants in such a way that those people most at risk can be identified. By segmenting people and quantifying the rates of death, it is possible to simultaneously target safety work and assess the risk levels for each subgroup of people.

Common approaches segment people by age and gender. However, at an early stage of research, there might be any basis on which to purposefully segment participants. Therefore, an option is to segment people using an array of criteria and then assess if or how the risk varies. This option is a more exploratory or discovery approach to risk assessment. Its value is that it can provide powerful indicators of who is most at risk, helping to target finite resources to greatest effect.

In the aforementioned inland risk assessments, risk was assessed by local area deprivation, country, age, gender and extent of waterways per area. It was found that risk was associated with age, gender, country and extent of waterway but not deprivation. The following points were apparent:

- The rate of death was about four times higher in areas with more waterways and canals.
- Scotland and Wales had higher rates of death than England, about 50% higher.
- The male rate of death was about three times greater than that for females.
- The rate of drownings increased as children went from infancy to being teenagers, especially for boys, peaking among 20- to 24-year-olds, and then declining as people got older.
- The rate of drowning was not associated with the level of deprivation in an area.

Such results help target safety work, in this case, at boys and men, in areas with more rivers/canals in the countries of Scotland and Wales.

Figure 3.6 shows the results by gender and country for UK inland drownings.

The aforementioned Royal Life Saving Society report for Australia noted that 82% of fatal drowning casualties at beaches were men, aged 18–64, with only two victims aged under 18.

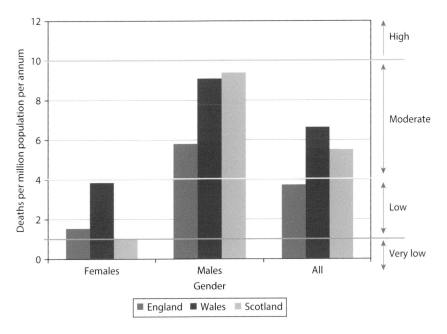

Figure 3.6 Inland rates of drowning in Great Britain, by gender.

The RNLI assessment of drowning risk at sea also found a major gender difference, with adult men accounting for the vast majority of deaths. Indeed, the male rate of drowning while swimming at sea was four times greater than for females. In both cases, the assessments help target interventions at those most at risk and provide some indication of risk factors, such as being exposed to hazards (i.e. being near waterways).

The assessment of who is at greatest risk can be taken further, data permitting. Recent work by the RNLI [12] has started to profile casualties in far greater detail, such as household type, frequency of participation, ethnicity and level of experience, enabling a finer level of identification of people most at risk. The finer the level of identification of people most at risk, the more it will be possible to devote finite resources to saving people, such as through new preventive interventions.

CONCLUSIONS

This chapter has provided an introduction to a form of quantitative risk analysis and assessment that aims to support national level decisions on safety. It has indicated how to provide an empirical and evidence-based comparison of drowning risk against other public safety risks. It has also indicated how to prioritize, using risk assessment, types of water sports and leisure activities for further reduction and has touched upon how to identify those most at risk.

Being a quantitative method, it relies on the availability of robust data on fatalities and participants. Collection of this data is itself no small task, requiring collaboration between stakeholders to share, reconcile and check data for many years. However, being able to provide a robust empirical evidence base on which to make decisions rewards the investment of effort. Where decision makers, such as local and national governments, charities and others have to choose how to invest finite resources across a wide range of safety issues, such analyses can help ensure that water safety is given due consideration.

This chapter has used two examples of risk assessment from the United Kingdom, covering drowning at sea and inland. The benefits of beach lifeguarding have previously been assessed,

with evidence of substantial lifesaving being reported (for example [13]). This evidence could be built upon by quantifying the risk of drowning on beaches and other coastal features, such as piers. This would require data to be collated on the number of people who use beaches and other coastal features, as well as the number of deaths per feature. Ideally data would be split into lifeguarded and not lifeguarded locations as well as by age, activity and gender, to enable comparisons of risk of drowning to be made. Such an assessment would help demonstrate the benefit of lifeguarding and the risk of drowning at unguarded areas. Moreover, it would identify those types of coastal features that could benefit from additional preventative interventions, such as an extension of lifeguarding beyond beaches and extending lifeguarded periods.

The approach draws heavily upon the tolerability of risk framework. The framework has been applied extensively in the United Kingdom and some other countries, such as Holland and Australia, and across many sectors such as road safety, fire safety and occupational safety. However, there is very little research into how to take account of the voluntary nature of water sports and leisure activities. It also needs to be remembered that familiarity with a risk is associated with inaccurate, underestimated, subjective risk assessments [14]. The issue of setting risk criteria for voluntary activities is ripe for further research and would help to inform debates with stakeholders, such as water sports associations, about the case for new drowning prevention interventions.

This chapter has focused on assessing the tolerability of risk and establishing the case for additional safety measures. Such assessment can be built upon by assessing and quantifying the causes of incidents, such as being overcome by waves versus being swept out by rip currents, thereby providing an empirical basis for identifying which causes to prioritize in order to achieve the greatest reduction in casualties. Although beyond the scope of this chapter, examples of such causal analysis can be found in the RNLI's latest work [12]. In addition, it should be noted that while risk assessment may help identify who is at greatest risk, it does not, by itself, identify preventative measures. For example, while the rate of child drowning in the United Kingdom may be relatively low, with most deaths being adult men, school-based water safety education and swimming lessons may nonetheless comprise a preventative measure for adult men (and others), equipping children with the awareness and skills they need as adults.

REFERENCES

1. Fisher L, Lewis D. *RNLI Risk Assessment Report.* Ventor Beach; 2011. Available at http://www.ventnortowncouncil.org.uk/userfiles/risk%20assessment%20rnli%20110831.pdf (accessed 5 December 2014).
2. Wilkens K. *Risk Assessment and Evaluation of Beaches.* World Congress on Drowning Prevention; 2013. Available at http://www.wcdp2013.org/uploads/media/Risk_Assessment1_1_428_Risk_Assessment_Safety_europe_KlausWilkens.pdf (accessed 5 December 2014).
3. Health and Safety Executive. *Proposals for Revised Policies to Address Societal Risk Around Onshore Non-Nuclear Major Hazard Installations.* CD212. HSE; 2007. Available at http://consultations.hse.gov.uk/inovem/gf2.ti/f/4610/130181.1/PDF/-/cd212.pdf
4. Health and Safety Executive. *Reducing Risk Protecting People. HSE's Decision Making Process.* HSE Books; 2001. Available at http://www.hse.gov.uk/risk/theory/r2p2.pdf (accessed 5 December 2014).
5. Wright M, Ramm H, Walters T, Stephens T, Reynolds R. *Assessing the Risk of Water Related (Accidental) Deaths Around the Coast: UK Case Study.* World Congress on Drowning Prevention; 2013. Available at http://www.wcdp2013.org/uploads/media/Prevention7_1_072_Risk_of_drowning_at_sea_MichaelWright.pdf (accessed 5 December 2014).
6. Ramm H, Stephens W. *RNLI's Coastal Safety Strategy.* World Congress on Drowning Prevention; 2013. Available at http://www.wcdp2013.org/uploads/media/Sea_Rescue1_3_74_Prevention_Drowning_at_Sea_MichaelWright.pdf (accessed 5 December 2014).
7. RoSPA. Assessing inland accidental drowning risk. 2013. Available at http://www.rospa.com/leisuresafety/Info/Watersafety/inland-waters-risk-assessment.pdf (accessed 5 December 2014). (Work completed by Michael Wright, Eshani Ghosh and Fowzia Ibrahim of Greenstreet Berman Ltd under the management of David Walker of RoSPA and was funded by the BNFL/RoSPA scholarship fund for safety-related research.)
8. Gill T. Nothing ventured. Balancing risks and benefits in the outdoors. 2010. Available at http://www.englishoutdoorcouncil.org/wp-content/uploads/Nothing-Ventured.pdf (accessed 5 December 2014).
9. Treasury HM. Managing risks to the public: Appraisal guidance. 2005. Available at https://www.gov.uk/government/uploads/system/uploads/attachment_data/file/191518/Managing_risks_to_the_public_appraisal_guidance.pdf (accessed 5 December 2014).
10. Health and Safety Executive. *Societal Risk: Initial Briefing to Societal Risk Technical Advisory Group.* HSE report 703. 2009. Available at http://www.hse.gov.uk/research/rrpdf/rr703.pdf
11. Royal Life Saving Society. National drowning report. 2014. Available at http://www.royallifesaving.com.au/__data/assets/pdf_file/0007/11995/RLS_NDR2014_LR.pdf (accessed May, 2015).
12. Wright M, Ramm H, Walters T, Reynolds R. *Analysing Causes of Water Related Deaths and Serious Incidents Around the Coast: The RNLI's New Causal Analysis Process.* World Congress on Drowning Prevention; 2013. Available at http://www.wcdp2013.org/uploads/media/Sea_Rescue1_1_073_Causes_of_drowning_at_Sea_MichaelWright.pdf (accessed 5 December 2014).
13. Branche CM, Stewart S. (eds.). *Lifeguard Effectiveness: A Report of the Working Group.* Atlanta, GA: Centers for Disease Control and Prevention, National Center for Injury Prevention and Control; 2001.
14. Schmidt M. Investigating risk perception: A short introduction. 2004. Available at http://www.markusschmidt.eu/pdf/Intro_risk_perception_Schmidt.pdf (accessed 5 December 2014).

PART 2

Physical Environment

4

Beach types, hazards and risk assessment

ANDREW SHORT AND ADAM WEIR

INTRODUCTION

Beaches and their associated surf zones are hazardous locations. The physical, biological and, in places, chemical hazards associated with beaches have been well documented by Short [1,2]. However, these hazards only become a concern to people when they venture onto the beach and in particular into the water. At that point the combination of a hazardous environment and human interaction produces a level of risk. The greater the hazard and number of people, the greater the risk.

While humans have been at risk in the beach environment since they first ventured to the water's edge, it is only in the last century that society has formally reacted to this risk with attempts to mitigate the hazard and/or level of risk. The most obvious reaction has been the development of beach lifeguarding services, as recorded by Walker [3]. Developed initially in North America and Australia, lifeguarding is now a highly visible global response to beach hazards and public risk.

Beach hazards are aspects of the beach and surf zone that expose the public to injury. Some, such as

rip currents, can be accurately identified, mapped and measured, at least by experienced observers, whereas others (such as variable water depth, trough and bars) can be difficult to see, let alone predict. Biological hazards are even harder to accurately assess, except to say they may be present. All beaches will have some level of hazard from the simple fact that they provide access to deep water. As risk is a function of both the level of hazard and the level of beach usage, a mechanism is required to quantify or rate the level of hazard and the level of usage and combine the two to rate the level of risk (R), where

$$R = f(\text{beach hazard} \times \text{beach usage})$$

Beach risk therefore involves an assessment of beach hazards together with the type and level of public beach usage. Just as all hazards can be difficult to quantify, so too is any assessment of the number and type of beach users. Users can range from very experienced and competent surfers to the naive tourist who cannot swim and may have never seen a beach. Risk assessment is all about bringing these two factors together in a meaningful way so as to quantify or at least rate the level of hazard and risk.

The formal response to beach risk and endeavours to mitigate it date back to the establishment of the first professional lifeguards in the United States in the late nineteenth century and volunteer lifesaving clubs in Australia from about 1903. However, attempts to measure and quantify both the hazards and risk of beaches are a more recent phenomenon.

Rip currents as beach hazard were first mentioned in the scientific literature during a debate about the 'undertow myth' by Hite [4], Davis [5] and Jones [6], with Shepard [7–9,11] suggesting the use of the term *rip current*. Shepard [8–10] went on to conduct the first rip current studies at La Jolla; he emphasized the hazardousness of rips in a paper titled 'Dangerous currents in the surf' [11]. In Australia, the first detailed publication on rips was by McKenzie [12], who described what we now call *beach rips, topographic* or *boundary rips* and *mega-rips* in the Sydney region. While rips continued to be studied in the United States as part of general beach science (e.g. Arthur [13], Bowen and Inman [14], Cook [15], Sonu [16]), it was their study in Australia during the 1970s and 1980s that ultimately led to them being incorporated into the quantification of beach hazards and risk.

Detailed studies of rip current occurrence commenced in Australia with Eliot [17], followed by Short [18] and Wright et al. [19] and cumulating in the first classification of beaches and surf zones by Wright and Short [20] and rip current types by Short [21]. Rip currents however are only one of a number of physical hazards in the surf zone. In order to address the full range of hazards and to bring the growing scientific awareness of rip currents and beach hazards to lifesavers and the beach-going public, in 1986 Short and Hogan [22] in collaboration with Surf Life Saving New South Wales (NSW) initiated the NSW Beach Safety Program. Following its successful application in NSW, in 1990 the programme was transferred to Surf Life Saving Australia (SLSA) as the Australian Beach Safety and Management Programme (ABSAMP) [23]. ABSAMP and its application in Australia is discussed in Part 3 of this book.

This chapter is to briefly outline the range of beach systems present globally, then to review the ABSAMP programme and its application to Australia beach systems and elsewhere to beach hazard and risk assessment. We then examine risk management and the International Life Saving Federation (ILS) Drowning Prevention Framework and how they apply to beach risk assessment. Finally, we will use case studies from Australia to apply the ABSAMP and ILS framework to practical risk assessment and response.

BEACH SYSTEMS

Beaches are wave-deposited accumulations of sediment at the shoreline. They are a product of breaker wave height and period acting on the sediment (sand through boulders). Most beaches are also affected by tides. Using these parameters, they can be classified using the relative tide range (RTR):

$$RTR = TR/H_b$$

where TR is the spring tide range (m) and H_b is the breaker wave height (m) (Table 4.1). In the table, the influence of waves decreases from the wave-dominated to tide-dominated types (as the tide range increases), as well as within each beach type from the dissipative to the reflective states.

Table 4.1 Simplified classification of beach types and states

RTR[a]	Beach type	Beach state	Comments
<3	Wave-dominated (six beach states)	Dissipative	Wide, multi-bar surf zone
		Intermediate	Rip-dominated, bars and channels
		Reflective	Steep barless
3–10	Tide-modified (three beach states)	Ultradissipative	Wide, low gradient intertidal
		R + low-tide rips	Wide, rips and bars at low tide
		R + low-tide terrace	Wide low-tide bar/terrace
10–50+	Tide-dominated (four beach states)	Beach + sand flats	Beach plus wide intertidal sand/tidal flats

[a] RTR, relative tide range.

For a full description and classification of beach states in Australia see Short [24] and in the United Kingdom see Scott et al. [25]. In nature, beaches will also be affected by wave direction and a range of factors including the presence of headlands, reefs, inlets and human structures such as groynes, seawalls and breakwaters. Each will have a predictable impact on the beach and its behaviour, as discussed by Short and Masselink [26] and Masselink et al. [27].

BEACH TYPES, STATES AND HAZARDS

All beaches are hazardous as they provide an environment where deep water lies close to shore. Water depth is however just one of a range of hazards that can be permanent or variable. Variable hazards include passive variables such as the increasing water depth away from the shore and the variable water depth where bars, troughs, channels and inlets are present. Active variables include breaking waves, wave set-up and set-down, surf zone currents and especially rip currents, together with tide stage and tidal currents; water temperature and water pollution; and biological hazards. Permanent hazards relate to the boundary geology where present and include headlands, rocks, reefs, inlets and human structures including groynes, breakwaters, jetties, seawalls and storm water pipes.

All of these hazards produce an environment where there is deep water, turbulence and currents, all of which can transport bathers out of their comfort zone, as well as being a solid physical hazard in themselves.

The beach types and states listed in Table 4.1 can be used to review the range of hazards that occur on these beaches. Wave-dominated beaches are produced by larger waves (0.5–3 m) and are the most hazardous of the beach types. Such wave types maintain energetic surf zones potentially containing bars, troughs and channels; breaking waves; and surf zone currents that move onshore (broken waves), longshore (rip feeder currents) and offshore (rip currents). They range from the most hazardous dissipative (H_b > 2.5 m) through the rip-dominated intermediate beaches, to the least hazardous, the barless reflective state. The morphology and surf zone dynamics of each of the six beach states is described in detail by Short [1,2].

Tide-modified beaches have higher tide ranges and may also have large waves. These beaches undergo substantial tidal modulation of the beach, its processes and its hazards. At high tide, water is deeper and waves may not break until they reach a reflective high tide beach, while at low tide the near stationary surf zone can produce the full range of bars and troughs and strong rip currents present in the wave-dominated surf zones. Scott et al. [25] mapped and classified the full range of tide-modified beaches in the UK, and Brander and Scott [28] discussed the tide-modulated rip currents associated with these beaches, as well as rip currents in general. In Australia, tide-modified beaches generally have lower waves (<0.5 m) and less hazardous conditions, as discussed by Short [24].

Australian tide-dominated beaches are characterized by low waves (<0.5 m) and high tides and are the least hazardous beach type. They vary considerably between high tide when water covers the tidal flats and low tide when the flats are exposed. One of their major hazards relates to people walking out across the wide flats and possible ridges at low tide and being trapped by the rising tide.

Each of these beach types will be affected by geological, biological and human structures located in the beach environment. Structures crossing the surf zone will lead to the formation of strong topographic (boundary) rip currents; structures in the surf zone will produce greater wave breaking, turbulence and currents; and structures backing the beach can generate strong wave reflection and turbulence. All will increase the type and level of hazard and risk.

THE AUSTRALIAN BEACH SAFETY AND MANAGEMENT PROGRAM

The ABSAMP is a joint project between SLSA and the Coastal Studies Unit of the University of Sydney. The main aims of the programme are as follows:

- Develop a comprehensive, standardized and scientific information base on all Australian beaches with regard to their location, physical characteristics, access, facilities, usage, rescues, physical and biological hazards and level of public risk under various wave, tide and weather conditions [23].
- Expand and improve the management and safety services of all Australian beaches and assist other countries to develop similar programs.

The beach investigations were undertaken between 1990 and 2004; they included all 10,796 mainland and 1583 beaches on 30 major islands. These results made up the core of the ABSAMP database. The beach descriptions were also published in a series of eight books, one on each state and territory, the last of which was by Short [29], while photos and descriptions of every beach are also available on the free iPhone app Beachsafe.

Beach hazard rating

One of ABSAMP's major aims was to assess the nature and level of hazards on every Australian beach. To do this in a quantifiable way, the beach hazard rating of Short and Hogan [22] was developed into the beach hazard matrix (for wave-dominated beaches) by Short [30], with beach hazards rated from low (1) to extreme (10). Two types of rating were defined – modal and prevailing. The *modal beach hazard rating* refers to 'the beach hazards associated with that beach state during the typical (or modal) wave conditions' together with permanent local factors. The *prevailing beach hazard rating* is based on the prevailing beach state and wave conditions, together with local factors such as presence of headlands, wave direction and state of tide, some of which will vary throughout the day, causing associated changes in the hazard rating.

Short [26] defined the ratings as follows:

modal hazard rating
= f(modal beach state × modal wave height + fixed local hazards)

prevailing hazard rating
= f(prevailing beach state × prevailing wave height + fixed and variable local and regional hazards)

Next Short [31] developed a matrix to allow the impact of wind on beach hazards to be included. This study was followed by an expansion of the wave-dominated beach hazard matrix to include tide-modified and tide-dominated Australian beaches (Figure 4.1) [32]. In this extension into Australia's higher tide range and generally more northern and tropical waters, a range of deadly biological hazards (e.g. crocodiles, sea snakes, marine stingers) were also discussed but were not incorporated in the hazard rating. The modal hazard ratings for wave-dominated, tide-modified and tide-dominated beaches were then used in ABSAMP to hazard rate all Australian beaches under their average conditions.

Beach risk

Short and Hogan [22] acknowledged the impact of beach usage on public risk when they attempted to calibrate the level of beach hazard using the number of rescues per thousand beach goers. They found that some of the more hazardous Sydney beaches had 10 times more rescues per thousand beach goers than the less hazardous beaches. However, the first formal definition of beach risk was provided by Short and Hogan [33], who defined public risk as a function of beach hazards and the number and type of beach users. This definition implies that, in order to accurately gauge beach risk, an assessment of both the range and type of hazards present, as well as the number and nature of beach users, is required. While hazards can be readily assessed using Figure 4.1, assessing the level and nature of beach usage is far more difficult. Numbers can be counted, although this task becomes very difficult on crowded beaches and as beach population varies through the day. Determining the age, sex, level of beach experience and so on is far more difficult and apart from occasional surveys can only be estimated. For this reason, risk level is far more difficult to accurately assess than hazards.

Short and Hogan [33] went on to provide a framework for risk mitigation (Figure 4.2) that involves undertaking a beach safety impact assessment and using the result to allocate beach safety resources starting at the coastal planning stage and including education, signage, equipment, lifeguards and so on. This framework fits well within the MOVE framework proposed by Birkmann et al. [34] for assessing societal vulnerability to a wide range of environmental hazards (Figure 4.3). The MOVE framework can be readily adapted to the beach environment using Figure 4.2. The beach environment presents a range of *hazards*, while *society* is represented by the beach users who will have a range of *vulnerability* based on age, sex, beach experience and so on. These factors combine as in Figure 4.2 to present a level of public *risk*, with *risk governance* presented in the right-hand column in the form of coastal planning and safety assessment, which is then mitigated through *vulnerability intervention* through the allocation of beach safety resources.

BEACH HAZARD RATING GUIDE

Impact of changing breaker wave height on hazard rating for each beach type

WAVE-DOMINATED BEACHES

Beach type	<0.5 (m)	0.5 (m)	1.0 (m)	1.5 (m)	2.0 (m)	2.5 (m)	3.0 (m)	>3.0 (m)
				Wave height				
Dissipative	4	5	6	7	8	**9**	**10**	10
Long shore bar trough	4	5	6	**7**	**7**	**8**	9	10
Rhythmic bar beach	4	5	6	**6**	**7**	8	9	10
Transverse bar tip	4	4	**5**	**6**	7	8	9	10
Low-tide terrace	3	**3**	**4**	5	6	7	8	10
Reflective	**2**	**3**	4	5	6	7	8	10

TIDE-MODIFIED BEACHES
(at high tide – at low tide add 1)

Beach type	<0.5 (m)	0.5 (m)	1.0 (m)	1.5 (m)	2.0 (m)	2.5 (m)	>3.0 (m)
			Wave height				
Ultradissipative	1	2	4	6	8	10	10
Bar and rips	1	2	3	5	7	9	10
Beach and low-tide terrace	1	1	2	4	6	8	10

TIDE-DOMINATED BEACHES
(at high tide – at low tide add 1)

Beach type	<0.5 (m)	0.5 (m)	1.0 (m)	Waves unlikely to exceed 0.5–1 m
			Wave height	
Beach + sand ridges	1	1	2	
Beach + sand flats	1	1		*Note: If adjacent to tidal channel, beware of deep water and string tidal currents.*
Tidal sand flats	1			

Beach hazard rating	Key to hazards
Least hazardous: 1–3	☐ Water depth and/or weak currents
Moderately hazardous: 4–6	☐ Shorebreak (high tide only)
Highly hazardous: 7–8	☐ Rips and surf zone currents
Extremely hazardous: 9–10	☐ Rips, currents and large breakers

Note: All hazard level ratings are based on a bather being in the surf zone and will increase with increasing wave height or with the presence of features such as inlet, headland or reef-induced rips and currents. Rips also become stronger with falling tide.

Bold grading indicate the average wave height usually required to produce the beach type and its average hazard rating.

Figure 4.1 Table for calculating the beach hazard rating for Australian wave-dominated, tide-modified and tide-dominated beaches based on beach state, wave height and tide range. Note that modification may need to be made for beach systems outside Australia. (From Short AD, *Beaches of the Queensland Coast: Cooktown to Coolangatta*, Sydney University Press, Sydney, 2000, p. 360.)

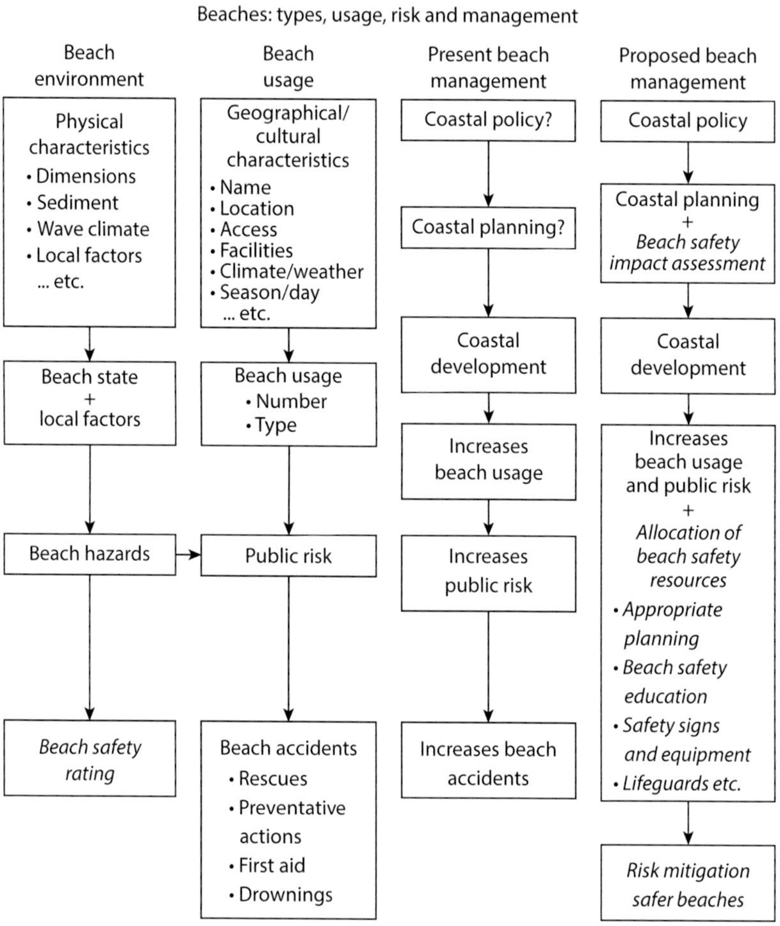

Beaches: types, usage, risk and management

Figure 4.2 A flow chart for assessing beach risk based on beach hazards and usage, and how this can be incorporated in a range of risk mitigation programs. (From Short AD, Hogan CL, J Coast Res, 12, 197–209, 1994.)

Application

At the 2002 World Congress on Drowning, it was agreed that the Australian approach to beach hazard rating and risk assessment be 'implemented as the world-wide standard to enable the development of appropriate drowning prevention strategies at beaches' [35].

The ABSAMP approach to assessing beach hazards has been applied to all Australian beaches [29,31,32]. It has also in a modified fashion been applied in New Zealand (NZ), as part of the 1997 NZ Coastal Survey; in Hawaii as part of the 2003 Hawaii Beach Safety*; in Brazil [36]; and has been adapted in the United Kingdom by the Royal

National Lifeboat Institution as part of their beach management program.[†] Its ongoing application in Australia is discussed in Section 5.5

The most ambitious attempt to model risk however was undertaken by CoastalCOMS in 2009 who in collaboration with SLSA developed an automated real-time beach risk index. The flow chart presented in Figure 4.4 shows how the risk is assessed. Beach type is central to the calculations, together with, on the left-hand side, input from lifeguards with regard to their assessment of beach usage, wave height, beach state and any recent incidents. On the right-hand side is

* http://oceansafety.soest.hawaii.edu

[†] http://rnli.org/safetyandeducation/stayingsafe/beach-safety/Pages/Beach-management.aspx

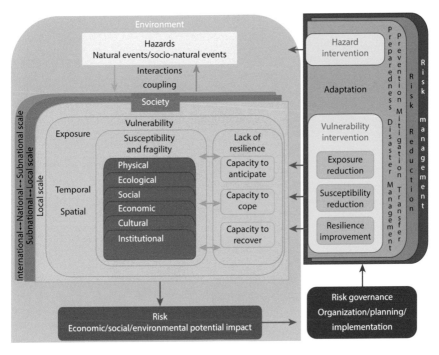

Figure 4.3 The MOVE (Methods for the Improvement of Vulnerability Assessment in Europe) framework for assessing society's vulnerability and response to environmental hazards. (Reprinted from Birkmann J, et al., *Nat Hazards*, 67, 193–211, 2013. With permission.)

input from beach video cameras with regard to measurements of people counted, breaker wave height and period, infragravity waves and beach state. These are integrated in the central column and enter the data process together with real-time wave, weather and tide data (lower right) to produce the final risk index, which ranges from 1 to 20. This model is presently being evaluated as part of SLSA's 'Surf Hazard Rating Framework', which aims to produce a real-time risk assessment module by 2017.

RISK MANAGEMENT AND THE INTERNATIONAL LIFE SAVING DROWNING PREVENTION FRAMEWORK

Risk management, as defined in ISO 31000:2009, *Risk Management: Principles and Guidelines*, is 'coordinated activities to direct and control an organization with regard to risk' [37]. Further, the risk management process is a 'systematic application of management policies, procedures and practices to the activities of communicating, consulting, establishing the context, and identifying, analysing, evaluating, treating, monitoring and reviewing risk' [37].

On beaches, lifeguards are commonly required to assess risk and determine an appropriate response to mitigate the assessed risk. A risk assessment is a systematic process of identifying hazards, assessing the risks posed to the public by those hazards and then controlling or mitigating those risks. Assessments can be documented and formal or more informal as part of the proactive, day-to-day process of a lifeguard to identify potential issues and reduce the likelihood of injuries from happening before they can cause harm [38].

ISO 31000:2009 is the recommended standard to which the ILS coastal public safety risk assessment process is benchmarked. In summary, the standard provides a generic framework for the application of a risk management process (Figure 4.5) and also contains definitions of terminology, flow charts of the risk management process and sample documentation. This flow chart in principle is similar to the MOVE framework in Figure 4.3.

The implementation of an effective risk management programme may reduce the incidence of injury and death on the coast. The importance of

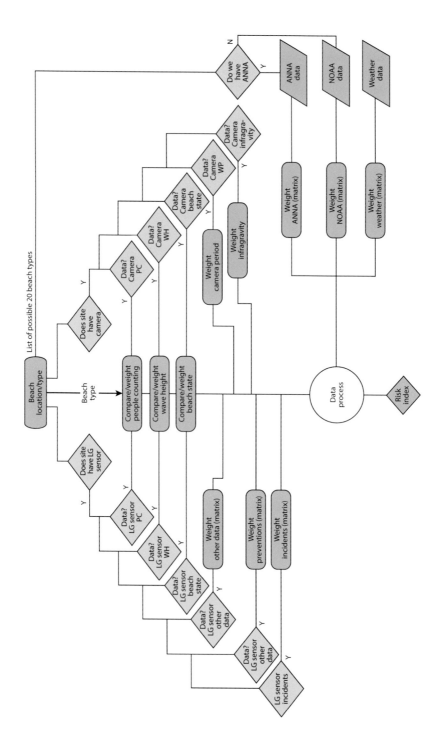

Figure 4.4 Flow chart for beach risk assessment based on real-time hazards and environmental parameters, together with input from lifeguards. (Reprinted with permission from C.L. Lane, CoastalCOMS Gold Coast, QLD, Australia.)

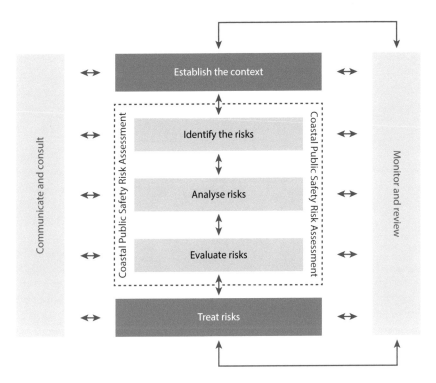

Figure 4.5 The Coastal Public Safety Risk Assessment process. (Adapted from ISO 31000:2009. Standards Australia, *AS/NZS ISO31000:2009 Risk Management Principles and Guidelines*, Standards Australia, 2009.)

drowning as a public health issue is emphasized in the WHO *Global Report on Drowning*, which states that 'drowning is preventable' [39]. Effective and specific drowning prevention strategies are vital in preventing drowning [39,40].

There are many different techniques that may be used to assess risk. ISO 31010:2009, *Risk Management – Risk Assessment Techniques*, provides details on 31 different risk assessment techniques. Risk is often expressed in terms of a combination of the consequences of an event (including changes in circumstances) and the associated likelihood of occurrence. In the context of beach lifeguarding, risk can be viewed as a combination of the physical hazardousness of a beach (consequence) and the exposure to that level of hazard, derived from the number of people at the beach and their susceptibility to the hazard [41]. More simply, this may be expressed as follows:

$$\text{Risk} = f(\text{hazard} \times \text{exposure} \times \text{vulnerability})$$

In the context of drowning, risk management can and should be applied at all levels. This includes operationally in the provision of lifesaving services

and also in the frontline delivery of drowning prevention strategies. The ILS drowning chain (Figure 4.6) provides the framework for identifying the fundamental causes of accidental drowning deaths in the coastal aquatic environment and the strategies to mitigate each causal factor [42].

A gap in any of the factors shown in Figure 4.6, or any combination of the factors, may contribute to accidental drowning deaths. To prevent drowning, it is helpful to gain an understanding of which factors are the key contributors to drowning incidents and focus on prevention strategies targeted at these factors. In some nations/regions, a multiple factor approach would be needed. In other nations/regions, a focus on one factor may be the best use of available resources. The ILS has identified key strategies for each of these factors in order to help reduce drowning deaths in the aquatic environment [42].

It is important to note that the critical link between the causal factors and implementing effective drowning prevention strategies is a comprehensive risk assessment process (Table 4.2). The risk assessment process helps us identify the gaps and also enables us to set priorities.

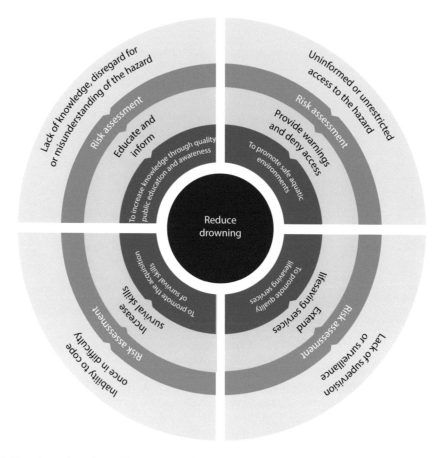

Figure 4.6 The drowning chain. (From Kennedy DM, et al., *Ocean Coast Manag*, 82, 85–94, 2013.)

Table 4.2 Factors causing, and strategies to prevent, accidental drowning

Causal factor		Prevention strategy
Lack of knowledge, disregard or misunderstanding of the hazard	Comprehensive risk assessment	Education and information
Uninformed or unrestricted access to the hazard		Denial of access, improvement of infrastructure and/or provision of warnings
Lack of supervision or surveillance		Provision of supervision
An inability to cope once in difficulty		Acquisition of survival skills

Source: Data from International Life Saving Federation, *A Framework to Reduce Drowning Deaths in the Aquatic Environment for Nations/Regions Engaged in Lifesaving*, International Life Saving Federation, Belgium, 2011.

COASTAL PUBLIC SAFETY RISK ASSESSMENT – CASE STUDIES

SLSA's Coastal Public Safety Risk Assessment programme evolved from the ABSAMP programme discussed above. The resulting database, beach models and classification system [29] form the foundation of SLSA's Coastal Public Safety Risk Management Program. Used in conjunction with the international standard for risk management [37] and other relevant industry compliance and guidelines, the programme provides SLSA with an internationally recognized

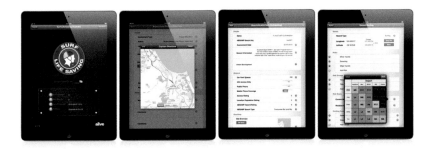

Figure 4.7 Screenshots of the iRisk Assessor platform. (Image courtesy of Surf Life Saving Australia, Sydney, NSW, Australia. With permission.)

scientific core system for the management and understanding of risks to public safety and the management of these risks around the Australian coast.

As described in the previous section, the coastal public safety risk assessment process is designed to provide a comprehensive risk-based analysis of the causal factors of preventable drowning in a region, identify gaps in the drowning prevention strategies being implemented and provide the evidence and prioritization for recommended strategies to minimize the risk of preventable drowning in the future.

Central to our ability to quantify and compare levels of risk on beaches is the beach hazard rating [2,41] discussed above. However, it is important to understand that hazardousness is only the first part of the overall risk equation. Once we have determined the level of hazard, we are then able to combine it with elements of other factors describing exposure and vulnerability in order to quantify the level of risk. One method for accomplishing this goal is the Action Planning Priority Index (APPI) [43]. The index seeks to identify the risks associated with the broader coastal environment under assessment, rather than the specific risks of an individual hazard

APPI = (2 × beach hazard rating) + (2 × population rating) + (human activity and interaction rating) + (access rating)

The total score for the APPI is intended to be used for the purpose of prioritizing risk mitigation strategies.

In recent times, SLSA has invested in cost-efficient technological solutions to improve the delivery of coastal public safety risk assessments. The system, known as *iRisk Assessor*, has been rolled out across the country and allows assessors to collect highly detailed spatially located

assessment data and produce reports through a semi-automated system (Figure 4.7).

Currently, this process is being implemented across the Australian state of New South Wales through a NSW government-funded project known as 'Project Blueprint'. This project is applying the coastal public safety risk assessment framework across every accessible beach and rock platform along the NSW coastline. The project has already assessed more than 70% of the coast including 1230 locations covering 1239 km of the 1990 km [44] NSW coastline. A vast amount of spatial data has been collected on aspects of the coast which have traditionally been seen as contributing to the risk of drowning along the coast, including data on 21,341 identified coastal hazards, 4651 coastal access points, 12,258 coastal signs, 316 items of publicly accessible rescue equipment, and 12,154 coastal amenities and facilities. This evidence is being used to provide support for the next generation of drowning intervention strategies.

DISCUSSION

Beach systems are inherently hazardous and when people enter the beach environment they are exposed to a level of risk. In order to mitigate this risk, we need to know about the physical beach systems and their hazards; the number and type of people using the beach; and then, after determining the level of risk, what mechanisms can be put in place to minimize the risk. The three components therefore – the beach, the beach users and risk reduction – all need to be addressed to achieve the optimal outcome.

Beach systems are now reasonably well understood. We can classify the world's beaches based on their wave, tide and sediment characteristics (e.g. Table 4.1); we can quantify their modal and prevailing hazards associated with permanent and variable hazards (Figures 4.1 and 4.4); and we can quantify the size and nature of the beach population (Figure 4.4). While it is simple to qualify the links between hazards, users and risk, quantifying and then applying this knowledge is far more involved and difficult.

In Australia, the APPI is used to prioritize risk mitigation strategies. These strategies are primarily designed to address the modal hazards and risk, not the prevailing level of risk.

In terms of preventing drowning, ILS has developed the drowning chain (Figure 4.6 and Table 4.2), which identifies four major causes of drowning and proposes prevention strategies for drowning reduction. These strategies are undertaken within a generic framework for the application of a risk management process (Figure 4.5), which is in agreement with the MOVE framework for identifying environmental hazards and risk and developing risk governance and adaption strategies (Figure 4.3). The above contain elements that address both modal and prevailing hazards, with prevailing hazards and risk levels being the most difficult to address owing to their high degree of variability in time and space. To overcome this difficulty, beach risk managers are increasingly turning to new technologies to assist in this process. SLSA uses the semi-automated iRisk Assessor to plot both beach hazards and risk levels. In collaboration with a range of stakeholders, SLSA is developing a 'Surf Hazard Rating Framework', which will incorporate information from cameras, lifeguards and external environmental sources to provide real-time hazards and risk levels that can be delivered globally via iCloud. We now have the capability to closely and accurately monitor the beach environment and rate its hazards in real time using largely remote technology. We also have the ability to assess public vulnerability with additional input from lifeguards. When these are combined, we have the elements of real-time risk assessment. The next stage is in assisting beach managers to utilize this information, both in a planning and real-time framework.

REFERENCES

1. Short AD. Wave-dominated beaches. In Short AD (ed.). *Beach and Shoreface Morphodynamics*. Chichester: Wiley; 1999, pp. 173–203.
2. Short AD. Beach hazards and safety. In Short AD (ed.). *Beach and Shoreface Morphodynamics*. Chichester: Wiley; 1999, pp. 293–304.
3. Walker EW. History of beach lifeguarding. In Tipton M, Wooler A, Reilly T (eds.). *The Science of Beach Lifeguarding*. Boca Raton, FL: CRC Press; 2016.
4. Hite M. The "undertow." *Science*. 1925; 62: 31–3.
5. Davis WM. The "undertow." *Science*. 1925; 62: 33.
6. Jones WC. The undertow myth. *Science*. 1935; 61: 444.
7. Shepard FP. Undertow, rip tide or "rip current." *Science*. 1936; 84: 181–2.
8. Shepard FP, Emery KO, La Fond EC. Rip currents: A process of geological importance. *J Geol*. 1941; 49: 337–69.
9. Shepard FP, Inman DL. Nearshore water circulation related to bottom topography and wave refraction. *Trans Am Geophys Union*. 1950; 31: 196–212.
10. Inman DL, Quinn WH. Currents in the surf zone. *Proceedings of the 2nd Conference on Coastal Engineering Council on Wave Research*, 1952, American Society of Civil Engineers, Washington, pp. 24–36.
11. Shepard FP. Dangerous currents in the surf. *Phys Today*. 1949; 2: 20–9.
12. McKenzie P. Rip-current systems. *J Geol*. 1958; 66: 103–13.
13. Arthur RS. A note on the dynamics of rip currents. *J Geophys Res*. 1962; 67: 2777–9.
14. Bowen AJ, Inman DL. Rip currents, 2. Laboratory and field observations. *J Geophys Res*. 1969; 74: 5479–90.
15. Cook DO. The occurrence and geologic work of rip currents off southern California. *Mar Geol*. 1970; 9: 173–86.
16. Sonu CJ. Field observation of nearshore circulation and meandering currents. *J Geophys Res*. 1972; 77: 3232–47.
17. Eliot I. The persistence of rip current patterns on sandy beaches. *Proceedings of the 1st Australian Conference on Coastal Engineering*, The Institute of Engineers, Australia, 1973, pp. 29–34.
18. Short AD. Three dimensional beach stage model. *J Geol*. 1979; 87: 553–71.

19. Wright LD, Chappell J, Thom BG, Bradshaw MP, Cowell P. Morphodynamics of reflective and dissipative beach and inshore systems: Southeastern Australia. *Mar Geol.* 1979; 32: 105–40.

20. Wright LD, Short AD. Morphodynamic variability of surf zones and beaches: A synthesis. *Mar Geol.* 1984; 56: 93–118.

21. Short AD. Rip current type, spacing and persistence, Narrabeen Beach, Australia. *Mar Geol.* 1985; 65: 47–71.

22. Short AD, Hogan CL. Sydney's southern beaches—Characteristics and hazards. In Fabbri P (ed.). *Recreational Uses of Coastal Areas*. Kluwer Academic; Dordtrecht, 1990, pp. 199–209.

23. Short AD, Williamson B, Hogan CL. The Australian Beach Safety and Management Program—Surf Life Saving Australia' approach to beach safety and coastal planning. *11th Australasian Conference on Coastal and Ocean Engineering*, National Conference Publication 93/4, Townsville, The Institution of Engineers, Australia, 1993, pp. 113–18.

24. Short AD. Australian beach systems—Nature and distribution. *J Coast Res.* 2006; 22: 11–27.

25. Scott T, Masselink G, Russell P. Morphodynamic characteristics and classification of beaches in England and wales. *Mar Geol.* 2011; 286: 1–20.

26. Short AD, Masselink G. Embayed and structurally controlled beaches. In Short AD (ed.). *Beach and Shoreface Morphodynamics*. Chichester: Wiley; 1999, pp. 230–50.

27. Masselink G, Hughes MG, Knight J. *Coastal Processes and Geomorphology* (2nd ed.). London: Hodder Education; 2011, 416 p.

28. Brander R, Scott T. Rip currents. In Tipton M and Wooler A (eds.). *The Science of Beach Lifeguarding*. Boca Raton, FL: CRC Press; 2016.

29. Short AD. *Beaches of the New South Wales Coast* (2nd ed.). Sydney: Sydney University Press; 2007, 398 p.

30. Short AD. *Beaches of the New South Wales Coast*. Sydney: Sydney University Press; 1993, 356 p.

31. Short AD. *Beaches of the Victorian Coast and Port Phillip Bay*. Sydney: Sydney University Press; 1996, 298 p.

32. Short AD. *Beaches of the Queensland Coast: Cooktown to Coolangatta*. Sydney: Sydney University Press; 2000, 360 p.

33. Short AD, Hogan CL. Rips and beach hazards, their impact on public safety and implications for coastal management. *J Coast Res.* 1994; 12: 197–209.

34. Birkmann J, Cardona OD, Carreño ML, Barbat AH, Peling M, Schneiderbauer S, Kienberger S, et al. Framing vulnerability, risk and societal responses: The MOVE framework. *Nat Hazards.* 2013; 67: 193–211.

35. Bierens JJLM. (ed.). *Handbook on Drowning: Prevention, Rescue, Treatment*. Berlin: Springer; 2006, pp. 713.

36. Klein AHF, Santana GG, Diehl FL, De Menezes JT. Analysis of hazards associated with sea bathing: Results of five years work in oceanic beaches of Santa Catarina state, Southern Brazil. *J Coast Res.* 2003; 35: 107–16.

37. Standards Australia. *AS/NZS ISO31000:2009 Risk Management Principles and Guidelines*. Standards Australia; 2009.

38. Surf Life Saving New South Wales. *Guidelines for Safer Surf Clubs*. Sydney: Surf Life Saving NSW; 2013.

39. World Health Organization. *Global Report on Drowning: Preventing a Leading Killer*. World Health Organization; 2014, pp. vii–ix.

40. World Health Organization. *Guidelines for Safe Recreational Water Environments. Volume 1: Coastal and Fresh Waters*. World Health Organization; 2003, pp. 20–35.

41. Kennedy DM, Sherker S, Brighton B, Weir A, Woodroffe CD. Rocky coast hazards and public safety: Moving beyond the beach in coastal risk management. *Ocean Coast Manag.* 2013; 82: 85–94.

42. International Life Saving Federation. *A Framework to Reduce Drowning Deaths in the Aquatic Environment for Nations/Regions Engaged in Lifesaving*. Belgium: International Life Saving Federation; 2011.

43. Surf Life Saving Australia. *Coastal Public Safety Risk Assessor Learner Guide*. Sydney: Surf Life Saving Australia; 2011.

44. Commonwealth of Australia. *Geodata Coast 100K 2004*. Canberra: Geoscience Australia; 2004.

5

Science of the rip current hazard

ROBERT BRANDER AND TIM SCOTT

INTRODUCTION

Many ocean, inland sea and lake beaches are characterized by waves breaking across a wide surf zone. On these beaches, the greatest hazard to bathers and most significant management challenge for lifeguards is arguably the presence of rip currents. These strong, narrow and concentrated offshore flows of water can quickly carry unsuspecting bathers of all swimming abilities offshore into deeper water, where they may become exhausted and begin to panic. On lifeguarded beaches, this scenario is typically pre-empted through preventative measures or by lifeguard-assisted rescue. Tragically, however, this is not always the case, particularly on beaches lacking lifeguard presence. Too often, rip currents are a factor in drowning deaths, near-miss drowning, injuries and trauma and therefore represent a serious global public hazard and health issue with significant personal, societal and economic costs [1].

Unfortunately, there are many common misconceptions and a degree of complacency about rip currents that have contributed to an overall lack of understanding and awareness by the general beach-going public. While it is likely that experienced lifeguards have a good understanding of rip current behaviour and identification, this may not be the case for inexperienced trainee or junior beach lifeguards. Rip current flow behaviour is extremely complex and can vary within a given rip over time, between adjacent rip current systems and between different types of rip currents on the same beach. Improved understanding of rip current behaviour is therefore critical for any lifeguard who works on surf beaches.

Recently, there has been renewed interest in the rip current hazard from both physical and social scientists and new findings have important implications for lifeguards and bathers alike. The aim of this chapter is therefore to describe our present understanding of the rip current hazard for the benefit and interest of lifeguards. The chapter provides an overview of physical aspects of rip current behaviour including formation, types and spatial and temporal morphologic and flow characteristics. It also describes recent social science efforts that have been undertaken to understand what beachgoers and the general public know about rip currents and identifies some of the limitations and challenges associated with rip current educational outreach efforts, which many lifeguards are involved in. By providing more information on the science of rip currents, beach lifeguards and their managers will have a better appreciation of how to manage this important beach hazard.

THE RIP CURRENT HAZARD

On beaches where they occur, rip currents are the main cause of rescue and drowning. The United States Lifesaving Association (USLA) estimates that rip currents account for 81% of the approximately 43,000 surf rescues in the United States each year from reporting beaches [2]. In Australia, 89% of rescues are related to rip currents [3] and, in the United Kingdom between 2006 and 2011, 67% of incidents reported by Royal National Lifeboat Institution (RNLI) lifeguards on 163 patrolled beaches were related to rip currents [4]. Confirmed numbers of rip current–related drowning fatalities are often underestimated or unknown, particularly in developing countries, due to the inherent difficulty in accurate incident reporting, but it is likely that hundreds of people drown annually in rip currents globally. In the United States, the USLA estimates that around 100 rip current fatalities occur each year [5], exceeding the number of fatalities caused by more publicized hazards such as floods, hurricanes and tornados [6]. In Australia, an average of 21 confirmed fatal rip current drownings occur each year [7]. This figure is greater than the annual average number of fatalities in Australia caused by bushfires, floods, cyclones and sharks combined [8]. In the United Kingdom, incidents of accidental coastal drowning where rip currents may be implicated are estimated to be 20 per year [9]. In this context, the severity of the rip current hazard should not be underestimated.

Rip currents are hazardous because of their ability to physically move bathers from a position of relative safety to a region of greater hazard (e.g. deeper water, further offshore, a region of heavy breaking waves or a collision hazard). While rip currents clearly present a hazard to water users, it is not uniform across the beach-going demographic. The ability of a water user to safely respond to the movement of a rip current will be significantly controlled by many factors including their swimming ability, surf experience, knowledge and risk perception [10,11]. This complex variability in rip current risk between demographic groups is alluded to by analysis of lifeguard incident records in the United Kingdom, which found 66% of rip victims to be male and 67% teenagers, with the greatest probability of incident occurring outside the lifeguard flags [4].

Male-dominated beach-related drownings are also dominant in Australia [12].

A robust evaluation of rip risk must also consider bather exposure to the rip current hazard. An example of the importance of considering exposure as well as hazard is highlighted by Scott et al. [13], who found that the highest risk rip current conditions in the United Kingdom often occurred under small and medium swell waves, when rip currents were still relatively strong and large numbers of bathers could interact with the surf, increasing their exposure to rip current hazards. To gain a complete picture of rip current threat to bathers, it is important to consider the implications of the human behavioural aspects of rip current risk in conjunction with the identification and assessment of the physical rip current hazard.

RIP CURRENT DEFINITION, FORMATION AND CIRCULATION

Despite being common features, rip currents have traditionally been poorly understood and misinterpreted. The term 'rip current' was first coined by Shepard [14] to distinguish these concentrated offshore surface flows from the potentially misleading terms 'rip tide' and 'undertow', which were gaining popularity at the time [15]. Unfortunately, both terms are still sometimes used incorrectly to describe rip currents today. 'Rip tide' is a misnomer as rip currents are not tides and tidal rips are associated with tidal inlets during the ebbing and flooding tide [6]. The use of the term 'undertow' is also not appropriate. Coastal scientists refer to undertow as a steady offshore drift of water near the seabed that occurs along relatively flat beaches – or flat sections of beaches, such as the seaward slope of sand bars – at velocities much lower than rip currents. Undertow is not considered a hazard to bathers [16]. Taken out of context, the term may also imply that bathers can be pulled underwater and taken offshore, which is not true.

Rip currents are generated by breaking waves across surf zones and occur regularly on exposed swell-dominated beaches and episodically on beaches in more sheltered environments, such as inland seas or large lakes, during strong winds or storms. Breaking waves transport water towards the shoreline and rip currents help return that water offshore in order to maintain a mass balance (Figure 5.1). The actual process is more complex as the degree of wave breaking can vary in both the alongshore and cross-shore directions.

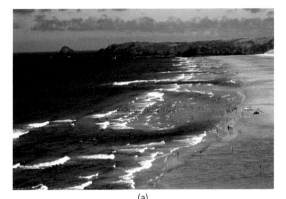

(a)

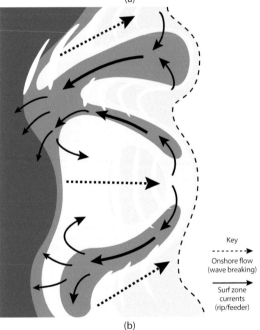

Key

------► Onshore flow (wave breaking)

——► Surf zone currents (rip/feeder)

(b)

Figure 5.1 **(a)** A low-tide photograph of Perranporth Beach in Cornwall, UK, a complex low-tide bar/rip channel system. Breaking waves occur over shallow sandbars, with rip currents in the darker, deeper channels. There is a busy bathing zone over the shallow sandbars between the red/yellow flags. (Photo courtesy of T. Scott. With permission.) **(b)** A diagram based on the Perranporth image, illustrating the characteristic flow patterns on a beach with bar/rip channel morphology.

Breaking waves result in localized increases in water level termed 'wave set-up'. Higher breaking waves generate higher set-up and lower waves generate lower set-up. Rip currents are therefore most common on beaches with varying patterns of sand bars, channels and troughs. As illustrated in Figure 5.1, wave breaking is intensified in the shallow regions and minimized, or restricted to larger waves, in deeper regions. Currents are then formed as water flows from regions of intense wave breaking (e.g. bars) to regions with fewer waves breaking (e.g. channels) that are often relatively deeper [17]. Changes in water level during a tidal cycle will also affect the intensity of wave breaking over sandbars and deeper channels, resulting in temporal variability of rip current flow, particularly in environments with large tidal ranges [18].

Rip currents also occur on beaches that are relatively flat without pronounced bar and channel morphology [19]. The spatial variability in wave breaking that drives rip current formation on these beaches is related to factors other than sandbar morphology, such as (1) the interactions between different waves and wave groups (sets), often when approaching from different directions, and (2) waves approaching beaches at large angles generating strong longshore currents in the surf zone that can shed rip currents as they become unstable and meander. These mechanisms can create unpredictable offshore-directed, but short-lived, whirlpool-like rip current flows. The location of some rip currents can also be determined by offshore geologic controls such as submarine canyons, offshore shoals, ridges and reefs, which influence wave refraction and focusing and hence the location and height of breaking waves.

RIP CURRENT OCCURRENCE, TYPES AND IDENTIFICATION

Given the variability of rip current formation described previously, it is not surprising that different types of rip currents exist (Figure 5.2). Unfortunately, the terminology used to describe rip current types varies, posing a potential problem for public education efforts (Table 5.1). In general, rip currents fall into two broad categories: (1) those that are relatively fixed in location for varying periods of

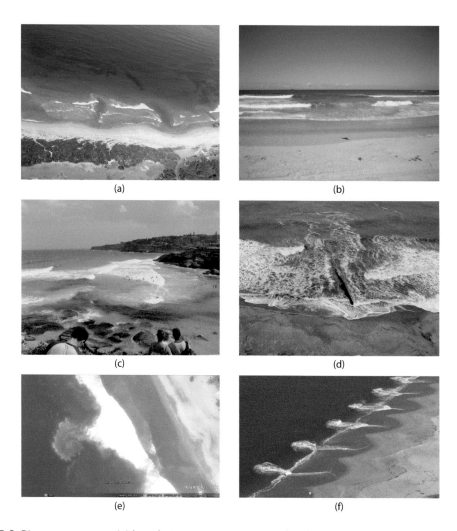

Figure 5.2 Rip current types: **(a)** beach rip currents associated with transverse bar and rip morphology at Shelly Beach, NSW, Australia; **(b)** beach rip current at Soldiers Beach, NSW, Australia, illustrating dark gap visual identifier; **(c)** boundary rip current adjacent to a headland at Tamarama Beach, NSW, Australia – the purple dye is part of a community rip current demonstration; **(d)** boundary rip current adjacent to a groyne at Cape Hatteras, NC, USA; **(e)** flash rip current at Puerto Escondido, Mexico, evident by sediment plume and turbulent water extending seaward from the surf zone; **(f)** swash rips formed by backwash from beach cusp embayments at Pearl Beach, NSW, Australia. ([a] photo courtesy of Wyong Shire Council, with permission; [b, c] photos courtesy of R. Brander, with permission; [d] photo courtesy of S.P. Leatherman, with permission; [e, f] photos courtesy of A. Short, with permission.)

time and (2) those that tend to be more transient and variable in occurrence, both spatially and temporally. The former are strongly controlled by the morphology of the beach, surf zone and the geological configuration of the coastline and can be described as *beach rip currents* and *boundary rip currents*. Both types flow offshore through deeper channels. In contrast, transient rips tend to be controlled more by hydrodynamic factors related to waves and are

often referred to as *flash rips*. All types are potentially dangerous to swimmers, but have distinct visual characteristics to assist in identification.

Beach rips

Beach rip currents occupying deep channels between adjacent shallow sand bars (Figure 5.2a and b) are the most commonly occurring type of

Table 5.1 Rip current types, key characteristics and terminology

RIP current type	Characteristics	Terminology
Beach	• Occupy deeper channels between adjacent sand bars • Relatively stationary in position for various periods of time • Associated with decreasing or lower wave energy conditions • Most common type	Accretion, low energy, linear bar-trough, semi-enclosed, fixed, bar-gap, cusped-shore, scalloped
Boundary	• Fixed in location adjacent to natural (headland, rock reef, platform) or anthropogenic (groyne, jetty, pier) structures; usually channelized	Topographic, structural, headland, permanent
Megarip	• Large-scale boundary rip current associated with large wave conditions • Most common on embayed beaches adjacent to headlands or mid-beach • Erosional with high flow velocities and offshore extent	Megarip Undertow
Swash	• Strong backwash in embayments of shoreline beach cusps • Limited seaward extent	
Flash	• Associated with rising or higher wave energy conditions, confused sea states, wave groups • Episodic/quasi-periodic and can migrate along beach; channels mostly absent • Generally limited offshore flow extent and velocity	Erosional, transient, travelling

Note: See Figure 5.2 for photographic examples.

rip current [20]. Their shapes and sizes are determined by the type of beach and associated sand bars, and they are an important part of the beach evolution following erosion events caused by large storm waves [21]. Storms transport sand from the beach offshore, typically forming a longshore, or shore-parallel, outer sand bar separated from the beach by a deep trough. Under lower wave conditions, the sandbar migrates landward, becoming rhythmic in shape, eventually merging with the beach face as transverse bars before reaching a low-tide terrace, or merged bar state (Figure 5.3). Rip current channels are present during all of these evolving beach states, with the transverse bar and rip state (Figure 5.3) being more prevalent in terms of both occurrence and number of rip channels [22].

While individual beach rip currents may persist for several months, their location and orientation can vary as channels may migrate along the beach at rates ranging from 2 to 50 m/day, particularly when storm waves approach at a high angle to shore [23]. Rip current channels are not necessarily oriented transverse, or perpendicular, to the shoreline, but are commonly oblique or sinuous in the offshore direction. Beach rip current channels tend to be irregularly spaced along the beach, ranging from 50 m to more than 500 m apart.

Example sandbar change

High (storm)

Longshore outer bar

Wave energy

Rhythmic outer bar

Rhythmic attached bar

Transverse bar

Low (swell)

Merged bar

Figure 5.3 An example of the different types of sandbar formations often associated with beach rip currents. Arrows illustrate typical rip current flow patterns. Note that rip current activity, and thus rip current hazard, is controlled to a large extent by the type of bar morphology, which in turn is related to the wave energy conditions.

Beaches with consistently higher waves tend to have bigger rip currents which are spaced greater distances apart [24]. Their offshore extent also increases as the prevailing wave height increases. Beach rip channels can vary in width from several metres to tens of metres and their depth can vary from 1 to 10 m. Rip current channels are also present on low-tide bar/rip and low-tide terrace and rip beach states in multi-barred meso- and macro-tidal environments (Figure 5.4) [25].

As wave breaking is reduced over deeper rip channels, beach rip currents usually appear as darker green gaps between areas of white water over adjacent shallow sandbars (Figure 5.2b).

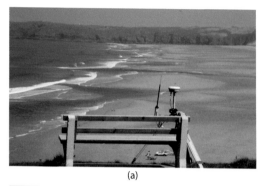

(a)

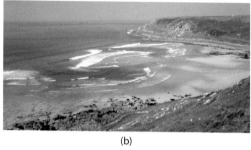

(b)

Figure 5.4 Examples of popular, macro-tidal, low-tide bar/rip and low-tide terrace and rip beaches in Cornwall, UK, at (a) Perranporth Beach and (b) Gwenver Beach. (Courtesy of T. Scott. With permission.)

Other visual indicators include agitated surface water due to the interaction between outgoing rip flow and incoming waves and pronounced shoreline rip embayments (Figure 5.2a). Anecdotally, beach rip currents are considered by lifeguards to be the most dangerous in terms of drowning and rescues as they typically exist during ideal beach-going weather conditions, which promote large beach crowds, and low to moderate wave energy conditions, which are more attractive for swimming. Their appearance can also be deceptive to inexperienced beachgoers, who may choose to swim in the 'calmer' water away from breaking waves. Beach rips have also been referred to in literature as accretionary, low energy, linear bar-trough and fixed rip currents (Table 5.1).

Boundary rips

Many rip currents also occupy deep channels adjacent to natural boundaries such as headlands, rock platforms, outcrops and reefs (Figure 5.2c) or rigid artificial structures (Figure 5.2d) such as groynes, jetties and piers [19]. Various combinations of wave shadowing and refraction processes and the deflection of longshore currents can act to create permanent rip current channels against the boundaries that become active during periods of wave breaking. Some studies have suggested that flow against headlands and rock platforms may be relatively stronger and more confined and extend further offshore than beach rip currents, representing further potential risk to bathers [26,27]. As they occupy deeper channels, they also appear as areas of darker water between the structure and adjacent sandbar and have an additional risk to bathers posed by collision with solid features (Figure 5.2c). Boundary rips are also described synonymously in the literature as permanent, topographic, structurally controlled and headland rip currents (Table 5.1).

Flash rips

Rip currents can also be episodic in nature, both temporally and spatially, lasting in the order of one to tens of minutes at a particular location or migrating slowly alongshore. These flash rips (Figure 5.2e) have been referred to as *transient*, *erosional* and *travelling rips* (Table 5.1) and are generally not channelized, occurring on beaches or sections of beaches (e.g. sand bars) that are fairly flat. Their formation is associated with variable wave set-up gradients caused by incident waves of different frequencies and direction, combined interactions of breaking wave vortices in the surf, wave groups, rising wave conditions and shear instabilities in alongshore currents [19,28–31]. Flash rips can initiate at any location within a surf zone, typically appearing as narrow bands of choppy churning water with streaky, turbulent and sediment-laden rip head plumes extending seaward (Figure 5.2e). They generally have smaller flow velocities than beach rip currents, but still represent a hazard to bathers due to their unpredictability [19].

Other types

During high-wave conditions, where wave heights exceed approximately 3 m, *megarips* can develop that extend hundreds of metres offshore. They are more common on embayed beaches, adjacent to headlands or in the centre of longer embayed beaches [19,31] and are not generally considered a hazard to bathers due to associated inclement weather or obvious dangerous bathing conditions.

In contrast, on steep beaches characterized by pronounced shoreline beach cusps, the backwash associated with wave uprush can form *swash rips* in the middle of the cusp embayments [19]. Although they do not extend far offshore, they represent a hazard to beachgoers, who can lose their footing and be washed into deeper water just seaward of the shoreline. These rip currents are often referred to and perceived by the public as 'undertow' [5]. Swash rips can be identified by the semi-regular spacing of cusp embayments and associated plumes of turbulent water and sediment (Figure 5.2f).

RIP CURRENT FLOW AND IMPLICATIONS FOR BATHERS

A major factor in the level of risk presented by rip currents is the nature of rip current flow, which is extremely variable spatially and temporally within and between different rip current types. This section describes the implications for bather safety due to known rip current flow behaviour. For further information on physical rip current flow behaviour, see reviews by MacMahan et al. [32] and Dalrymple et al. [19].

Spatial circulation patterns

Our conventional generic understanding of rip current flow circulation originated from early observations and experiments made at the Scripps Institution of Oceanography in La Jolla, California [33,34]. These studies described rip currents as part of an idealized nearshore circulation cell (Figure 5.5) consisting of alongshore *feeder currents* close to shore that carry water towards a narrow and fast offshore-flowing *rip neck*, which extends through the surf zone. Rip current flow extends well beyond the surf zone, decelerating as an expanding *rip head*. This water can return shoreward through wave action, completing the cell (Figure 5.5a). This traditional view is found in most coastal textbooks and beach safety material, but it is now being challenged, with important implications for both bathers and lifeguards.

In reality, rip currents do not necessarily simply flow alongshore and then offshore. Studies have shown that lateral flow of water across shallow sand bars may contribute more water entering the rip neck than the idealized alongshore feeder currents shown in Figure 5.5a [35,36]. This situation has

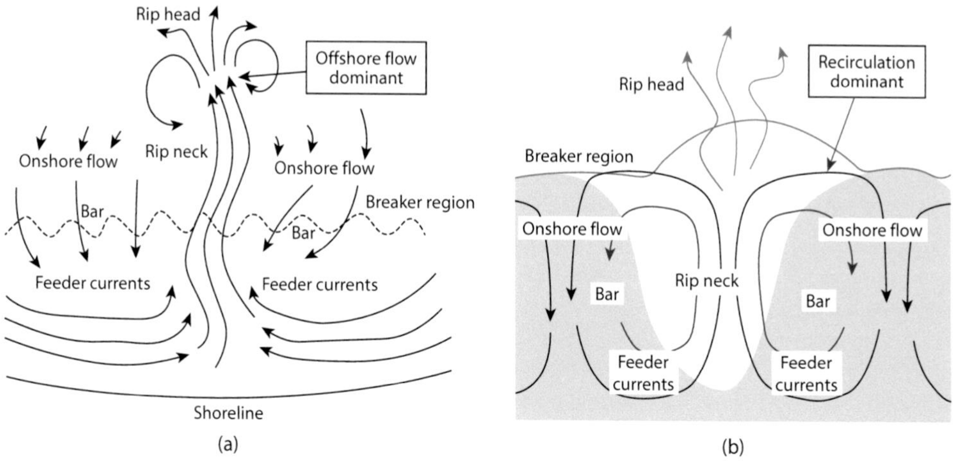

Figure 5.5 The traditional view of rip current flow circulation patterns, based on early observations showing **(a)** dominant offshore flow and a more recent view showing **(b)** dominant flow recirculation within the surf zone with only occasional exits. (Modified from McCarroll RJ, et al., Evaluation of swimmer-based rip current escape strategies. *Nat Hazards*, 71, 1821–46, 2014.)

implications for bathers, who may be swept alongshore into rip currents while standing on shallow sand bars. Recent measurements using low-cost global positioning system (GPS) devices attached to constructed drifters [37] have also shown that rip currents often exhibit a predominantly closed 'eddy' circulation within the surf zone characterized by both clockwise and counterclockwise rotations that vary in shape, orientation and flow magnitude (Figure 5.5b) [13,26,38].

Nevertheless, offshore exits of water and drifters (and hence bathers) beyond the surf zone do occur, often in episodic bursts (Figure 5.5b). Measurements in beach rip currents in California, England and France [36,38] showed that when waves approach parallel to the beach, approximately 15%–20% of drifters per hour exited offshore. However, measurements in Florida have shown that when subject to higher wave angles, exits per hour from beach rip currents can reach 55% [39]. Exit rates between 0% and 73% per hour were reported in active beach rip currents on macro-tidal beaches in the United Kingdom, where circulation was controlled by variable tidal levels and wave conditions [13]. Some of the highest recorded exit rates (up to 90% per hour) were recorded from boundary rip currents adjacent to headlands and rock platforms in Australia [26,27]. In general, the degree of surf zone exits associated with rip current circulation is dependent on a complex series of factors including the type of beach,

surf zone morphology and rip current, as well as the characteristics of wave energy dissipation.

Temporal characteristics of rip current flow

Rip current flow is inherently unsteady, which has significant impacts on bather safety. While typical beach and boundary rip currents can flow at average speeds of 0.3–0.5 m s^{-1}, they can have short-lived bursts in excess of 2 m s^{-1}. To put this in perspective, competent swimmers can easily swim at speeds of 0.5 m s^{-1} and competitive swim times for the 50 m freestyle equate to swimming speeds of 2.3 m s^{-1}. Most measurements of rip flow have been obtained in beach rip currents, but flash rips have been shown to have lower flow speeds, on the order of 0.2–0.3 m s^{-1} [38]. Megarips and beach rips under higher energy wave conditions can flow consistently at speeds of up to 2 m s^{-1} or more [31,40].

Rip flow speeds tend to increase with wave height, and hence wave energy dissipation (breaking), but the characteristics of surf zone sandbar morphology and the geometry of the rip channels are also a controlling factor. The beach morphology dictates (1) the spatial (alongshore and cross-shore) location of wave breaking driving rip circulation, (2) tidal levels which maximize wave breaking and (3) the extent of flow compression through rip channel geometry, which is increased for narrower channels. As such, it is important to consider the temporal variation in rip hazard on timescales of beach morphological change (multi-annual, seasonal and storm scales).

On a shorter timescale, many studies have shown that rip currents generally flow faster around low tide as a result of increased wave breaking due to shallower depths and reduced channel width and cross-sectional area [32]. However, on beaches with large tidal ranges (>4 m), this effect is magnified, meaning rip systems are sometimes only active for limited periods. In the United Kingdom, this is commonly at mean low water on intermediate macro-tidal beaches (Figure 5.6) [13], but examples from

France show nearshore bathymetry can sometimes enhance rip current flow towards mid-high tide [41]. Recent field observations of rip flow from a range of beach environments show that even subtle changes in water levels can have significant impacts on rip current flow characteristics, from the weekly spring–neap cycle to daily diurnal or semi-diurnal tidal oscillations.

Finally, on even shorter timescales, rip current flow has also been observed to pulsate following the arrival and breaking of sets of larger waves called wave groups (Figure 5.6). Breaking wave groups can cause fluctuations in shoreline water levels and, combined with instabilities in the

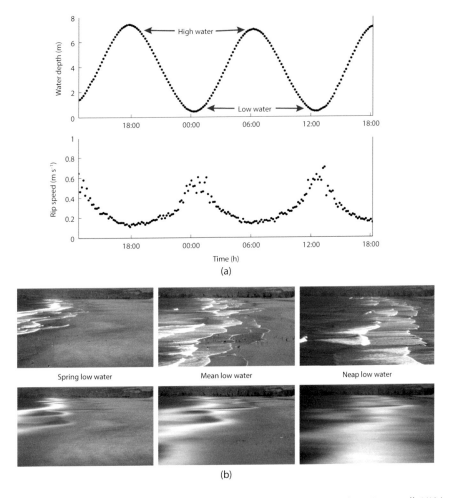

Figure 5.6 (a) Water depth over the low-tide sandbars at Perranporth Beach in Cornwall, UK (greatest water depth is high water), below which is the speed of the rip current in a channel next to the sandbar. Note how the rip flow speed peaks at low water. (b) Examples from Perranporth of low water under neap, mean and spring tidal conditions. This illustrates the significance of the spring–neap tidal cycle for rip current activity and hazard on beaches with large tidal range. Lower images are 10-minute time-lapse videos highlighting wave breaking patterns and the darker rip channels.

current flow, can cause dramatic instantaneous variations in rip current flows and water depths in the surf zone. These pulsations occur over periods of 25–250 seconds and can add or subtract from the average rip flow, often resulting in periods of below average flow followed by a rapid acceleration to instantaneous rip current speeds of over 1 m s^{-1} (Figure 5.6) [32]. Flow velocity within rips tends to increase away from the bottom, reaching a maximum just below the surface, but overall these differences are not significant.

Implications for bather safety

The characteristics of the rip current flow behaviour described above have significant safety implications for bathers and lifeguards. Although it is not well documented how bathers actually find themselves caught in rip currents, it is not surprising that so many do, given the potential for rapid increases in rip current flow speeds from being relatively manageable to very dangerous. Under these circumstances, bathers can lose their footing and become caught in strong rip current flow where their only options are to be rescued by lifeguards or bystanders or to self-escape.

RIP HAZARD ASSESSMENT

Recent studies in the United Kingdom by Plymouth University and the RNLI have combined rip flow measurements, detailed topographic surveys of beaches and surf zones with a five-year record of lifeguard rip current incident, beach population and physical environmental statistics to show that individual and mass rescues of bathers are significantly linked to wave, tide and weather conditions associated with rip activity. Furthermore, they demonstrated through exhaustive rip current measurements that specific rip flow characteristics and their associated wave, tide and beach morphological conditions were correlated with high-risk mass rescue events. In general, high-risk rip current incidents were associated with relatively small swell-wave conditions (<1 m) with a long wave period (>10 seconds) occurring around mean low water tidal level. Under these conditions, rip flow speed, exits and pulsations were maximized. Furthermore, rip current flow speed increased with wave height until there was significant wave breaking across the rip channel. The proportion of rip exit flow patterns also decreased as wave height increased.

On macro-tidal beaches, Scott et al. [13] noted the sensitivity of rip activity to tidal level and the spring–neap cycle with rips being typically active for one to two hours on either side of low water and 'switching off' outside of this period. During large spring tides, the rip system could be inactive at both high tide and for a short period at low tide (dried out), activating only for a limited period as the shoreline swept past the rip morphology on the flood and the ebb tides [42,43]. Conversely, they found that during neap tides the water level might never become low enough to allow sufficient wave breaking around the rip current system to activate significant flows. It is important to note that on many beaches across all tidal ranges, the exposure of sand bars at spring low tide can cause rip current flow to be reduced, or stop, for a short period of time [32,44].

As highlighted by Scott et al. [13,42], mass rescues are also related to many other factors such as attractive weather and wave conditions, where apparently benign surf conditions attract large numbers of bathers while rip currents remain relatively strong. Under these situations, wave groups can increase rip current hazard. Significant mass rescue events also occur on micro-tidal beaches with similar bar/rip channel morphology. In both the United Kingdom and Australia, these incidents are often reported incorrectly as being caused by 'collapsing sand bars'. Sand bars do not collapse. Rather, the arrival of a large wave group can cause sudden increases in water level, which may cause bathers to lose their footing and be carried into a rip current by a combination of subsequent lateral flow off the bars and rip current pulsations that carry them offshore. Rapid rip current flow pulsations, at any time, are clearly hazardous to bathers and can quickly take them significant distances offshore. Under low to moderate wave energy conditions, competent swimmers are hypothetically able to swim out of beach rip currents over short distances to reach safety, but this may not be possible during short-lived rip pulsations of 2 m s^{-1} or more. The implication here is that non-swimmers and poor swimmers are at greatest risk. However, this conclusion does not take into consideration swimmer behaviour and response when presented with an unfamiliar situation. Even strong swimmers can panic when caught in a rip current [45].

BATHER RIP CURRENT ESCAPE STRATEGIES

Traditional advice on how bathers should respond when caught in a rip current generally follows variations of four key points: (1) don't panic; (2) do not swim against the rip; (3) escape the rip by swimming parallel to the beach; or (4) stay afloat and signal for help [20]. While there is common agreement over the importance of the first and second points, there has recently been significant debate over the appropriate order of the third and fourth. The long-adopted advice promoted has been to escape a rip by 'swimming parallel to the beach'. This is largely based on the established view of circulation shown in Figure 5.5a, where rip currents are narrow and flow straight offshore. Theoretically, swimming parallel will get a swimmer out of the rip current without swimming directly against the strong flow and avoiding being carried significant distances offshore. However, this option may be problematic for weak swimmers or non-swimmers and, as many rip currents flow at angles to shore, for competent and experienced swimmers.

Based on recent findings described previously that rip circulation may be dominantly restricted to the surf zone, it has been suggested that *floating* might be a more appropriate escape strategy as bathers would have a high probability of recirculating onto the relative safety of shallow sandbars within minutes while conserving energy. Moreover, as recirculation can occur in different directions (Figure 5.5b), a bather caught in a 'circular' rip current flow pattern would find it difficult to choose the correct direction to swim parallel, particularly as these flow patterns are largely hidden to the naked eye by breaking waves, and may mistakenly swim against an alongshore component of the circulation cell [19,20].

A recent study conducted on beaches in New South Wales, Australia, by the University of New South Wales (UNSW) and Surf Life Saving Australia (SLSA) has rigorously tested different rip current escape strategies using GPS drifters and GPS-equipped swimmers (Figure 5.7) [26]. Floating was found to be a longer duration, but more variable escape strategy than swimming parallel, but both strategies failed in some instances. Swim parallel failures were related to swimming against the alongshore component of cellular rip circulation. Float failures related to surf zone exits and instances where the person recirculated without being able to attain safe footing on the shallower sand bar. McCarroll et al. [26] showed that no single escape strategy action is appropriate for

all instances, making safety recommendations difficult, and suggested that a combined approach involving elements of both floating and swimming and constant assessment of the situation could be adopted by bathers caught in rip currents.

PUBLIC UNDERSTANDING AND AWARENESS OF RIP CURRENTS

While coastal scientists and beach safety organizations are well aware of the hazards that rip currents represent to beachgoers, it is a major concern that many studies have shown that awareness and understanding of rip currents by beachgoers is poor [10,11,46–50]. It is likely that scientific differences between rip current types and their flow characteristics are largely meaningless to most beachgoers. Instead, the risk posed by rip currents primarily depends on beachgoers' ability to identify and avoid them, particularly if they choose to swim away from lifeguarded areas or on unpatrolled beaches [50,51]. However, despite the visual indicators described previously, most beachgoers are unable to spot rips. In a study of domestic and international students' knowledge on beaches in Queensland, Australia, Ballantyne et al. [52] found that two-thirds who claimed to know what a rip current was were unable to recognize one. Only 18% said that rip currents could be identified by the presence of calm water between breaking waves. Furthermore, when shown a photograph of a beach with two beach rip currents, 61% of all students selected the rip currents (dark gaps between white water) as places they would swim. Similarly, Sherker et al. [10] found that 93% of surveyed Australian beachgoers thought they could identify a rip current, but only 33% could when shown a picture of one. Half the survey respondents selected the rip current as the safest place to swim.

Recent studies in the United States have shown beachgoer rip identification is lower than in Australia. Caldwell et al. [49] conducted surveys of beachgoers at Pensacola Beach, Florida, using pictures. While the majority of respondents said they could identify rip currents, less than 20% were able to do so. On three popular beaches in Texas, Brannstrom et al. [50] found that when shown a picture of a groyne with a boundary rip current on one side and breaking waves (with no rip current) on the other, only 13% of beachgoers correctly identified the location of the rip current.

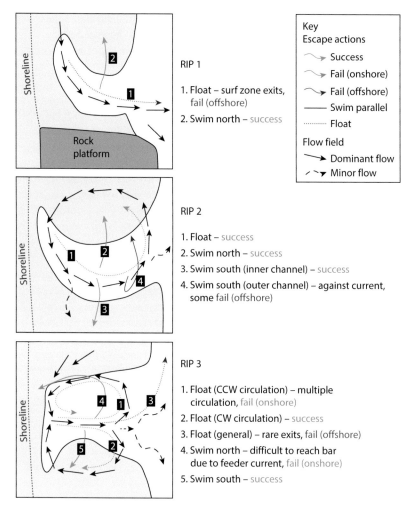

Figure 5.7 Idealized representation of GPS measurements of rip current flow and swimmer escape strategies at Shelly Beach, NSW, Australia: RIP 1 = boundary rip current; RIP 2 = adjacent beach rip current; RIP 3 = beach rip current further up the beach; *success* and *fail* refer to outcomes of swimmer strategy. North is to the top of the figure. CW and CCW refer to clockwise and counterclockwise circulation. (Modified from McCarroll RJ, et al., *Nat Hazards*, 71, 1821–46, 2014.)

In both studies, the majority of respondents identified regions of breaking waves as representing the most hazardous surf conditions and potential for rip current development.

A recent Australian study [11] used online surveys and interviews of rip current survivors to learn more about their experiences being caught in rip currents. In a largely informed and self-rated experienced ocean swimming group, the main recalled escape message when caught in a rip current was to swim parallel (40% of respondents) compared to staying afloat (10%). However, in terms of their actual response, more respondents reacted by swimming against the rip current back to shore rather than swimming parallel, which reflected the dominant reported emotional response of panicking. Of those that self-escaped, 33% did so by swimming parallel compared to 18% who floated. Across the whole study demographic, preliminary results suggest that swimming parallel is the most recalled message by the general public compared to stay afloat. However, regardless of swimming ability and understanding of rip currents, panic tends to override most recalled rip current safety advice, suggesting that more efforts should be made to reinforce the 'don't panic' message to beachgoers.

RIP CURRENT HAZARD MITIGATION AND OUTREACH

Given the range and number of factors involved in the rip current hazard, significant challenges exist for beach safety organizations in terms of mitigation, particularly as existing public awareness of rip currents is poor. Furthermore, despite causing significant long-term loss of life, the severity of rip currents is often overlooked by governments and the general public compared to more catastrophic and episodic natural hazards, such as floods and hurricanes, which have the capacity to cause large loss of life in a single event [8].

Efforts to mitigate the rip current hazard in the developed world are often borne by regional and national beach lifeguarding services, local authorities and various voluntary and community organizations. By contrast in developing countries, where rip hazards can be severe and swimming ability poor, there is often very little mitigation at all outside of more popular tourist destinations (Steve Wills, RNLI, personal communication, 28 May 2014 [53]). Mitigation strategies to break the drowning chain typically fall into pre-arrival and post-arrival measures, the former being through public education and awareness strategies, and the latter through lifeguard provision and signage. Slowly, physical environmental and social behavioural research is beginning to influence approaches to rip current hazard mitigation.

Education and awareness strategies

Most regions with popular recreational beaches characterized by rip currents engage in various forms of public rip current education and awareness strategies targeting a range of demographic groups, including schoolchildren, adults and tourists, with variable surf skills, knowledge and cultural backgrounds [20]. Rip current outreach has traditionally involved distribution of generic material, often with associated slogans, to tourist contact points and other public amenities near beaches with rip currents. The effectiveness of this approach is not generally known. However, recent Australian studies [47,48] have shown improved public understanding, awareness and identification of rip currents through dedicated campaigns involving posters, postcards and brochures, the latter of which achieved the highest message recall.

While beach and surf education is rarely compulsory for schools, numerous beach safety programs deliver rip current education to school students. Based on USLA statistics, between 2008 and 2012, an average of 313,000 students per year received beach safety education across the United States by USLA lifeguards [54]. In Australia, SLSA estimates they provide beach safety education to 240,000 students per year and RNLI statistics from the UK suggest their outreach programs were delivered to an average of 74,000 students per year, between 2009 and 2013. Providing rip current education to the adult population remains more of a challenge. Aside from generic outreach material, other approaches have ranged from public service announcements to highway billboard advertising. Significantly, there is little evidence of dedicated rip current information being provided to tourists on inbound airlines at destinations where rip currents are considered to be a problem.

More recently, online access to information about rip currents has increased globally through popular social communication networks such as YouTube, Facebook and Twitter. Dedicated beach safety sites are proliferating globally and now often provide real-time updates of wave, tide, weather and hazard conditions at popular beaches. The UK (RNLI) and Australia (SLSA) have the Beach Finder and Beachsafe apps, respectively, developed for mobile platforms so beach users can easily find information on lifeguarded beaches and prevailing conditions while on the move. As of May 2015, there were more than 300 YouTube videos related to rip currents with over two million total views. In particular, a 4-minute YouTube video titled 'How to Survive Beach Rip Currents', created in December 2008 by UNSW Australia, has over 1.3 million views as of May 2015. The use of social media will no doubt increase and has the additional advantage of quickly conveying visual information about the rip current hazard to a large global audience [55].

Several countries have developed national rip education programs, which focus outreach efforts around core standardized content. In the United States, a collaboration between the USLA, the National Oceanic and Atmospheric Administration's National Weather Service and the National Sea Grant Programme resulted in the implementation of the 'Break the Grip of the Rip' campaign and Rip Current Awareness

Week in 2005, with a standardized slogan and graphic (Figure 5.8) for all material and signage. Recently, SLSA also launched a three-year campaign in 2009 to educate all Australians about rip currents, based on the slogan 'To Escape a Rip, Swim Parallel to the Beach', also with an accompanying National Rip Current Awareness Day. Unfortunately, it is difficult to assess the effectiveness of these national programs without rigorous evaluations of programme awareness and changes in public understanding; therefore, future campaigns must incorporate formal programme evaluation as a key objective.

Signage provision often represents the final opportunity for the beach safety manager to raise awareness of the rip current hazard. The presence and type of rip current warning signs on beaches can vary greatly regionally between different local governments, states and countries. Often erected for legislative and liability purposes, signs are typically placed permanently near public beach access points on both patrolled and unpatrolled beaches or in front of rip currents by lifeguards during patrols. In general, rip current signs consist of text-based hazard warning messages, which may or may not use the term 'rip current' or include

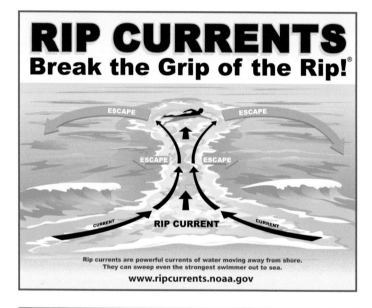

Figure 5.8 The standardized 'Break the Grip of the Rip' slogan and graphic used for rip current educational information and as beach warning signage at many public beach access points in the United States. (Courtesy of National Weather Service, Silver Spring, MD.)

information about how to identify them and react if caught in one (Figure 5.8). However, beach warning signs are rarely evaluated in terms of their use and effectiveness. In a study of Australian beachgoers, Matthews et al. [56] found less than half of those surveyed observed beach warning signs when present and those that did were more likely to notice hazard symbols rather than textual or diagrammatic information. They cautioned that beach signage may have less of an immediate effect on beachgoers than the responsible authorities may assume and that it was unclear whether recognition of hazard symbols translated into specific knowledge of the hazard. There has been an effort in the United Kingdom and Europe, led by the RNLI, to standardize signage format to present a common and clear message and symbology [57].

Over the long term, many rip current mitigation strategies have clearly been successful. For example, in the United States, both beach attendance and surf rescues have risen since 1960, but the total number of drownings has remained relatively stable [58]. In Brazil, a regional safety education campaign led to an 80% reduction in the number of fatal accidents over several years [59]. However, the incidence of global rip current drowning remains high and understanding of long-term drowning trends is restricted by the lack of accurate rip current incident and beach visitation statistics. As such, it is not known whether the incidence of rip current drowning is presently decreasing.

Implications for lifeguarding

The advances in the scientific understanding of the rip current hazard described in this chapter have potentially significant implications for operational lifeguarding practice. In some cases, improved science-informed understanding of the complex rip current hazard can complement years of observational experience of rip current dynamics and hazards, enabling experienced lifeguards to better interpret and predict rip current activity, educate inexperienced trainee lifeguards and protect the public. Once the regionally relevant knowledge is embedded into basic lifeguard training, key concepts can be taught more effectively by experienced lifeguards in support of invaluable practical experience of rip currents.

The complex nature of the rip current hazard means that accurate rip prediction models,

which could indicate when and where rip currents will form and identify particularly dangerous rip current flow behaviour, could potentially help provide rip warnings under high-risk scenarios [60,61]. While developments in numerical rip current modelling, technology and understanding of the rip hazard are improving rapidly, developing effective 'added-value' predictive outputs requires detailed localized meteorological, bathymetric and offshore wave input data [62]. Although these data are not always available, recent developments in remote video monitoring of surf zones are beginning to provide high-resource coastlines with vital information on surf zone bathymetry required to generate accurate rip predications [63]. However, despite these significant efforts, no generic rip current risk forecasting techniques exist that have proven applicable to all beaches with rip currents.

In lieu of expensive monitoring of extensive stretches of coastline, the RNLI in the United Kingdom, in collaboration with the UK Met Office and Plymouth University's DRIBS (Dynamics of Rips and Implications for Beach Safety) project, has begun developing an approach which empowers lifeguards to make use of freely available wave, wind and tidal predictions within a structured, but lifeguard-driven, rip hazard assessment procedure (informed by scientific research). Lifeguards are guided through a simple hazard assessment framework, applying contemporary understanding of rip current dynamics and hazards within an operational 5-day marine weather forecast to predict daily and weekly rip hazard hotspots. The assessed rip hazard indices provide a basis for resource management decisions and public hazard awareness strategies (from information boards to regional media press releases). Importantly, the lifeguards have ownership of this process, which combines their local knowledge of beach morphology with a guided observational methodology and high-quality wave, tide and weather forecasts. In the United States, lifeguard services provide daily updates regarding rip current conditions to local National Weather Service offices to assist in their rip current hazard forecasts.

Traditionally, the primary form of rip current hazard mitigation has been beach lifeguard services, the value of which is significant. The chance of death by drowning on beaches in the United States patrolled by lifeguards is 1 in

18 million [58], and in Australia almost all rip current–related drowning occurs on unpatrolled beaches or outside of supervised areas and lifeguard patrol times [12]. However, the vast majority of global beaches characterized by rip currents are either unpatrolled by lifeguards or only patrolled seasonally during warmer swimming months, and it is logistically and economically impossible to provide lifeguarding services on all beaches all of the time [20]. Therefore, engagement with public rip risk mitigation and outreach strategies beyond patrolled lifeguarded beaches is crucially important in the reduction of global rip current drowning rates.

CONCLUSION

Rip currents are common features on many global beaches and represent a significant hazard to beachgoers, being responsible for a high number of drownings and rescues each year. Global interest in rip current science and improving rip current outreach programs has never been higher, as evidenced by the recent establishment of the biennial International Rip Current Symposium in 2010. Ongoing development and expansion of regional and national rip education campaigns is a major step forward to mitigating the rip current hazard, but a major challenge for beach safety practitioners must be to evaluate the effectiveness of these programs in a meaningful way. The ultimate challenge for rip current outreach is to improve beachgoers' awareness and understanding of the rip current hazard so that they are increasingly motivated to seek out and only swim at beaches supervised and patrolled by lifeguards. Lifeguards now have improved, up-to-date scientific information and weather forecast tools with which to interpret their observations and improve dynamic rip hazard assessment and prediction. However, given that people will continue to swim outside of patrolled areas, it is important to promote rip avoidance by improving rip current identification skills, which comes with its own communication challenges. Reducing the number of global fatalities due to rip currents can only be achieved through continued collaborative efforts between rip current scientists, lifeguard organizations and local communities, particularly in developing countries. This endeavour will take time, but more importantly it will require significantly more global recognition and dedicated funding towards this important coastal hazard.

REFERENCES

1. Sherker S, Brander RW, Finch C, Hatfield J. Why Australia needs an effective national campaign to reduce coastal drowning. *J Sci Med Sport*. 2008; 11: 81–3.
2. Brewster BC, Gould R. Comment on "rip current related drowning deaths and rescues in Australia 2004–2011" by Brighton et al. (2013). *Nat Hazards Earth Syst Sci*. 2014; 14: 2203–4.
3. Short AD, Hogan CL. Rip currents and beach hazards: Their impact on public safety and implications for coastal management. *J Coast Res*. 1994; 12: 197–209.
4. Woodward E, Beaumont E, Russell P, Wooler A, Macleod R. Analysis of rip current incidents and victim demographics in the UK. *J Coast Res*. 2013; 65: 850–5.
5. Brewster BC. Rip current misunderstandings. *Nat Hazards*. 2010; 55(2): 161–2.
6. Leatherman SP. Rip currents. In Finkl CW (ed.). *Coastal Hazards*. Coastal Research Library 6. Springer, New York, 2013; 811–832.
7. Brighton B, Sherker S, Brander RW, Thompson M, Bradstreet A. Rip current related drowning deaths and rescues in Australia 2004–2011. *Nat Hazards Earth Syst Sci*. 2013; 13: 1069–75.
8. Brander RW, Dominey-Howes D, Champion C, Del Vecchio O, Brighton B. A new perspective on the Australian rip current hazard. *Nat Hazards Earth Syst Sci*. 2013; 13: 1687–90.
9. Green Street Burnham. *GSB CL2541 RNLI Programme Review Stage 1 & 2 R5 V1 Draft Final*. ADCR, London, UK; 2012.
10. Sherker S, Williamson A, Hatfield J, Brander RW, Hayen A. Beachgoers' beliefs and behaviours in relation to beach flags and rip currents. *Accid Anal Prev*. 2010; 42: 1785–804.
11. Drozdzewski D, Shaw W, Dominey-Howes D, Brander RW, Walton T, Gero A, Sherker S, Goff J, Edwick B. Surveying rip current survivors: Preliminary insights into the experiences of being caught in rip currents. *Nat Hazards Earth Syst Sci*. 2012; 12: 1201–11.

12. SLSA (Surf Life Saving Australia). *National Coastal Safety Report 2013*. Sydney: SLSA; 2013.

13. Scott TM, Masselink G, Austin MJ, Russell P. Controls on macrotidal rip current circulation and hazard. *Geomorphology*. 2014; 214: 198–215.

14. Shepard FP. Undertow, rip tide or rip current. *Science*. 1936; 84: 181–2.

15. Davis WM. Undertow and rip tides. *Science*. 1931; 73: 526–7.

16. Brander RW. *Dr Rip's Essential Beach Book; Everything You Need to Know about Surf, Sand and Rips*. Sydney: UNSW Press; 2010.

17. MacMahan JH, Reniers A, Brown JA, Brander R, Thornton E, Stanton T, Brown J, Carey W. An introduction to rip currents based on field observations. *J Coast Res*. 2011; 274: iii–vi.

18. Masselink G, Austin M, Scott T, Russell PE. Rip currents: Researching a natural hazard. *Geogr Rev*. 2014; 27(3): 37–41.

19. Dalrymple RA, MacMahan JH, Reniers A, Nelko V. Rip currents. *Ann Rev Fluid Mech*. 2011; 43: 551–81.

20. Brander RW, MacMahan JH. Future challenges for rip current research and outreach. In Leatherman S, Fletemeyer J (eds.). *Rip Currents: Beach Safety, Physical Oceanography and Wave Modeling*. Boca Raton, FL: CRC Press; 2011.

21. Wright LD, Short AD. Morphodynamic variability of surf zones and beaches: A synthesis. *Mar Geol*. 1984; 56: 93–118.

22. Ranasinghe R, Symonds G, Holman RA. Morphodynamics of intermediate beaches: A video imaging and numerical modelling study. *Coast Eng*. 2004; 51: 629–55.

23. Turner IL, Whyte D, Ruessink BG, Ranasinghe R. Observations of rip spacing, persistence and mobility at a long, straight coastline. *Mar Geol*. 2007; 236: 209–21.

24. Short AD, Brander RW. Regional variations in rip density. *J Coast Res*. 1999; 15(3): 813–22.

25. Scott TM, Masselink G, Russell P. Morphodynamic characteristics and classification of beaches in England and Wales. *Mar Geol*. 2011; 286: 1–20.

26. McCarroll RJ, Brander RW, MacMahan JH, Turner IL, Reniers A, Brown JA, Bradstreet A, Sherker S. Evaluation of swimmer-based rip current escape strategies. *Nat Hazards*. 2014; 71: 1821–46.

27. McCarroll RJ, Brander RW, Turner IL, Power HE, Mortlock TR. Lagrangian observations of circulation on an embayed beach with headland rip currents. *Mar Geol*. 2014; 355: 173–88.

28. Slattery MP, Bokuniewicz H, Gayes P. Flash rip currents on ocean shoreline of long Island, New York. In Leatherman S, Fletemeyer J (eds.). *Rip Currents: Beach Safety, Physical Oceanography and Wave Modeling*. Boca Raton, FL: CRC Press; 2011.

29. Johnson D, Pattiaratchi C. Transient rip currents and nearshore circulation on a swell-dominated beach. *J Geophys Res*. 2004; 109: C02026.

30. Feddersen F. The generation of surfzone eddies in a strong alongshore current. *J Phys Oceanogr*. 2014; 44: 600–17.

31. Short AD. Australian rip systems—Friend or foe? *J Coast Res*. 2007; 50: 7–11.

32. MacMahan JH, Thornton EB, Reniers A. Rip current review. *Coast Eng*. 2006; 53: 191–208.

33. Shepard FP, Emery KO, Lafond EC. Rip currents: A process of geological importance. *J Geol*. 1941; 49: 338–69.

34. Shepard FP, Inman DL. Nearshore circulation related to bottom topography and wave refraction. *Trans Am Geophys Union*. 1951; 31(4): 196–213.

35. Brander RW, Short AD. Flow kinematics of low-energy rip current systems. *J Coast Res*. 2001; 17(2): 468–81.

36. Austin M, Scott T, Brown JA, Brown J, MacMahan J, Masselink G, Russell P. Temporal observations of rip current circulation on a macro-tidal beach. *Cont Shelf Res*. 2010; 30: 1149–65.

37. MacMahan J, Brown J, Thornton E. Low-cost handheld global positioning system for measuring surf-zone currents. *J Coast Res*. 2009; 25: 744–54.

38. MacMahan J, Brown JA, Brown J, Thornton E, Reniers A, Stanton T, Henriquez M, et al. Mean lagrangian flow behavior on an open coast rip-channeled beach: A new perspective. *Mar Geol*. 2010; 268: 1–15.

39. Houser C, Arnott R, Ulzhöfer S, Barrett G. Nearshore circulation over transverse bar and rip morphology with oblique wave forcing. *Earth Surf Proc Landforms.* 2013; 38: 1269–79.

40. Brander RW, Short AD. Morphodynamics of a large-scale rip current system, Muriwai Beach, New Zealand. *Mar Geol.* 2000; 165: 27–39.

41. Bruneau N, Castelle B, Bonneton P, Pedreros R, Almar R, Bonneton N, Bretel P, Parisot JP, Senechal N. Field observations of an evolving rip current on a meso-macrotidal well-developed inner bar and rip morphology. *Cont Shelf Res.* 2009; 29: 1650–62.

42. Scott TM, Russell PE, Masselink G, Wooler A. Rip current variability and hazard along a macro-tidal coast. *J Coast Res.* 2009; 50: 1–6.

43. Scott TM, Russell PE, Masselink G, Austin MJ, Wills S, Wooler A. Rip current hazards on large-tidal beaches in the United Kingdom. In Leatherman S, Fletemeyer J (eds.). *Rip Currents: Beach Safety, Physical Oceanography and Wave Modeling.* Boca Raton, FL: CRC Press; 2011.

44. Austin MJ, Masselink G, Scott TM, Russell PE. Water level controls on macro-tidal rip currents. *Cont Shelf Res.* 2014; 75: 28–40.

45. Brander RW, Bradstreet A, Sherker S, MacMahan J. The behavioural responses of swimmers caught in rip currents: New perspectives on mitigating the global rip current hazard. *Int J Aquat Res Educ.* 2011; 5: 476–82.

46. Wilks J, DeNardi M, Wodarski R. Close is not enough: Drowning and rescues outside flagged beach patrol areas in Australia. *Tour Mar Environ.* 2007; 4(1): 57–62.

47. Hatfield J, Williamson A, Sherker S, Brander R, Hayen A. Development and evaluation of an intervention to reduce rip current related beach drowning. *Accid Anal Prev.* 2012; 46: 45–51.

48. Williamson A, Hatfield J, Sherker S, Brander R, Hayen A. A comparison of attitudes and knowledge of beach safety in Australia for beachgoers, rural residents and international tourists. *Aust N Z J Public Health.* 2012; 36: 385–91.

49. Caldwell N, Houser C, Meyer-Arendt K. Ability of beach users to identify rip currents at Pensacola Beach, Florida. *Nat Hazards* 2013; 68: 1041–56.

50. Brannstrom C, Trimble S, Santos A, Brown HL, Houser C. Perception of the rip current hazard on Galveston Island and North Padre Island, Texas. *Nat Hazards* 2014; 12: 1123–38.

51. Brander RW. Thinking space: Can a synthesis of geography save lives in the surf? *Aust Geogr.* 2013; 44(2): 123–7.

52. Ballantyne R, Carr N, Hughes K. Between the flags: An assessment of domestic and international university students' knowledge of beach safety in Australia. *Tour Manage.* 2005; 26(4): 617–22.

53. Hammerton CE, Brander RW, Dawe N, Riddington C, Engel R. Approaches for beach safety and education in Ghana: A case study for developing countries with a surf coast. *Int J Aquat Res Educ.* 2013; 7(3): 254–65.

54. USLA (United States Lifesaving Association). *Statistics.* 2013. Available at http://arc.usla.org/statistics/public.asp

55. Brander R, Drozdzewski D, Dominey-Howes D. "Dye in the water": A visual method of communicating the rip current hazard. *Sci Commun.* 2014; 36: 802–10. doi: 10.1177/1075547014543026.

56. Matthews B, Andronaco R, Adams A. Warning signs at beaches: Do they work? *Saf Sci.* 2014; 62: 312–18.

57. RNLI (Royal National Lifeboat Institution). *A Guide to Beach Safety Signs and Symbols.* UK: RNLI, Poole, UK; 2007.

58. Branche CM, Stewart S (eds.). *Lifeguard Effectiveness: A Report of the Working Group.* Atlanta, GA: Centers for Disease Control and Prevention, National Center for Injury Prevention and Control; 2001.

59. Klein AH, Santana GG, Diehl FL, Menezes JT. Analysis of hazards associated with sea bathing: Results of five years work in oceanic beaches of Santa Catarina State, Southern Brazil. *J Coast Res.* 2003; 35: 107–16.

60. Dusek G, Seim H. Rip current intensity estimates from lifeguard observations. *J Coast Res.* 2013; 29(3): 505–18.

61. Dusek G, Seim H. A probabilistic rip current forecast model. *J Coast Res.* 2013; 29(4): 909–25.

62. Austin MJ, Scott TM, Russell PE, Masselink G. Rip current prediction: Development, validation, and evaluation of an operational tool. *J Coast Res.* 2013; 29(2): 283–300.

63. van Dongeren AL, Sasso SR, Austin MJ, Roelvink JA, van Ormondt M, van Thile de Vires J. Rip current prediction through model-data assimilation on two distinct beaches. In *Coastal Dynamics 2013.* Bordeaux. P. Bonneton, T. Garlan, A. Sottolochio, B.Castelle (eds.), France: ASCE; 2013; 1775–1786.

6

Cold water immersion

MIKE TIPTON

INTRODUCTION

Cold water can, somewhat arbitrarily, be defined as water at a temperature of less than 15°C. Immersion in cold water represents one of the greatest stresses to which the body can be exposed and immersion is the second most common cause of accidental death in many countries of the world. However, it is a relatively hidden killer with many of the over 3000 immersion-related deaths that occur each day worldwide going unnoticed. Despite the fact that drowning kills more children than many high-profile diseases, it receives a fraction of the attention and funding obtained for these conditions.

In this chapter, we examine the physiological responses to cold water immersion, particularly those hazardous responses that can be a precursor to pathophysiological consequences such as drowning and cardiac arrest. The importance of understanding these physiological responses lies in the insight it gives to 'the cause of the cause of death'. This insight is likely to help target and promote interventions such as training, equipment and treatment protocols that reduce immersion deaths.

BACKGROUND

Despite a century-long preoccupation with hypothermia that originated with the sinking of the *Titanic* in 1912 and was perpetuated by the immersion-related deaths that occurred during the Second World War, anecdotal, statistical and experimental evidence point towards other causes of death.

Anecdotal accounts of people succumbing quickly on immersion in cold water to cardiac problems or drowning were common enough for the term *hydrocution* to evolve. The report of the UK Home Office Working Party on Water Safety [1] found that approximately 55% of the annual open-water immersion deaths in the United Kingdom occurred within 3 m of a safe refuge (42% within 2 m) and two-thirds of those who died were regarded as good swimmers. The statistics, in terms of death occurring early on immersion, remain about the same today [2]. As early as 1884, Falk [3] mentioned in a scientific report the respiratory responses to cooling of the skin of the hand. The report of the infamous experiments conducted at the Dachau concentration camp during World War II [4] included reference to the initial increase in ventilation seen on immersion in cold water. It was this range of evidence that led Golden and Hervey [5] to propose the four stages of immersion associated with particular risk:

Stage 1: Initial responses (first 3–5 minutes)
Stage 2: Short-term immersion (5–30+ minutes):
    neuromuscular dysfunction leading to physical

incapacitation caused by cooling of superficial nerves and muscle

Stage 3: Long-term immersion (over 30 minutes): hypothermia

Stage 4: Circum-rescue collapse: just before, during or just after rescue

This remains the most valid categorization of the hazards to be faced by those immersed in cold water and provides the definitive framework for the understanding and interpretation of accidents involving cold water immersion.

THE PHYSIOLOGICAL RESPONSE TO IMMERSION

Stage 1: Initial responses to immersion in cold water

In 1989, Tipton reviewed the initial responses to cold water immersion in humans [6] and used the term *cold shock*, with 'shock' relating to the stimulating, emotive aspect of the response rather than any reference to the medical definition of 'shock'. In that review, it was also concluded that 'the cold shock response can result in the death or serious incapacitation of an individual long before general hypothermia develops'.

The cold shock response comprises a range of cardiorespiratory responses (Figure 6.1) initiated by the stimulation of skin cold receptors on rapid cooling of skin temperature [7–11]. The superficial subepidermal location of these receptors (about 0.18 mm below the surface of the skin) explains the rapidity of the cold shock response and why subcutaneous fat does not protect against it. Within limits, the magnitude of the cold shock response is related to the rate of change of skin temperature (temporal summation) and the surface area of the body exposed (spatial summation) [12]. In naked individuals, the response peaks in water between 10°C and 15°C [13].

In Figure 6.1, the pre-immersion data are typical of someone who is slightly anxious (e.g. resting heart rate of 96 bt min^{-1}). The rapid increase in the response on immersion is indicative of the involvement of the dynamic response of the cutaneous cold receptors. The adaptation of these receptors to lowered skin temperature explains why the cold shock response subsides by five minutes of immersion.

The strength of the respiratory drive, represented in particular by the sudden increase in respiratory frequency [13], is indicated by the fact that it is not diminished by prior hyperventilation – an intervention that normally decreases respiratory dive and extends breath-hold time. There is an inspiratory gasp response followed by uncontrollable hyperventilation, indicated by the reduction in end-tidal carbon dioxide concentration. The gasp response reduces, and in some people prevents, breath holding: in comparison with an average maximum breath-hold time in air of about one minute, maximum breath-hold time on immersion in 10°C water varies greatly between individuals, but averages about 5 seconds when normally clothed, rising to about 20 seconds in those wearing uninsulated immersion drysuits [14]. Goode et al. [11] measured a mean inspiratory gasp of 2 L on initial immersion in 28°C water, rising to 3 L in water at 11°C [6]. To put this into context, the lethal dose for drowning in seawater for a 70-kg individual is approximately 1.5 L [15]. The uncontrollable hyperventilatory response to immersion in cold water can result in tetany. A reduction in cerebral blood flow is also observed, but it is not as great as that seen with a similar reduction in end-tidal carbon dioxide concentration when not immersed [16].

The cardiovascular component of the cold shock response includes an increase in heart rate, cardiac output and blood pressure. These responses increase the likelihood of a cerebrovascular accident during the first minutes of immersion. The hazard associated with the cardiac responses has probably been underestimated because most of the experimental studies on cold shock have been undertaken with young, fit and healthy volunteers. Moreover, although the initial incapacitation may be caused by a cardiac problem, agonal gasps close to death may result in the aspiration of water and apparent drowning. Finally, some of the cardiac problems are electrical disturbances and not therefore detectable at post mortem, so other causes of death are sought. During head-out immersion with young, fit and healthy individuals, the incidence of ECG arrhythmias is about 1%. This figure rises to over 80% if the immersion includes face immersion due, it is hypothesized, to 'autonomic conflict'.

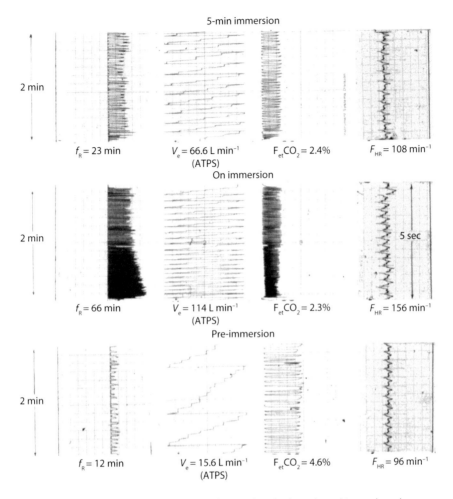

5-min immersion

$f_R = 23$ min $V_e = 66.6$ L min^{-1} (ATPS) $F_{et}CO_2 = 2.4\%$ $F_{HR} = 108$ min^{-1}

On immersion

$f_R = 66$ min $V_e = 114$ L min^{-1} (ATPS) $F_{et}CO_2 = 2.3\%$ $F_{HR} = 156$ min^{-1}

Pre-immersion

$f_R = 12$ min $V_e = 15.6$ L min^{-1} (ATPS) $F_{et}CO_2 = 4.6\%$ $F_{HR} = 96$ min^{-1}

Figure 6.1 The initial responses to immersion of an individual undertaking a head-out, seated, resting immersion in water at 10°C. f_R = respiratory frequency (breaths min^{-1}); V_e = minute ventilation (L min^{-1}); $F_{et}CO_2$ = end-tidal fractional concentration of carbon dioxide (%); F_{HR} = heart rate (bt min^{-1}); ATPS = ambient temperature pressure saturated. The rate of immersion was 8 m min^{-1} (slow).

The recent theory of autonomic conflict [16–19] suggests that the high incidence of arrhythmias seen during submersions, particularly around the time of the release of a breath hold, is caused by concurrent stimulation of both divisions of the autonomic nervous system. Normally the sympathetic and parasympathetic divisions of this system act reciprocally, but during submersion sudden and profound cooling of the skin initiates the cold shock response, including a sympathetically driven tachycardia (increased heart rate). At the same time, cooling of the oronasal region of the face evokes a 'diving response', which includes a vagally induced bradycardia (decreased heart rate) [20]. It is this conflicting input to the heart

from the two divisions of the autonomic nervous system that is thought to produce dysrhythmias and arrhythmias; these are normally asymptomatic and harmless but, in the presence of cofactors such as heart disease, can result in fatal arrhythmias [19]. This is a new, but compelling, theory which we are still in the process of elucidating. There are two major questions: first, what factors provoke, attenuate and potentiate autonomic conflict? Second, what conditions must coexist to cause the arrhythmias caused by autonomic conflict to deteriorate into fatal arrhythmias? Our current understanding is presented in Figure 6.2.

A summary of the cold shock response is presented in Figure 6.3.

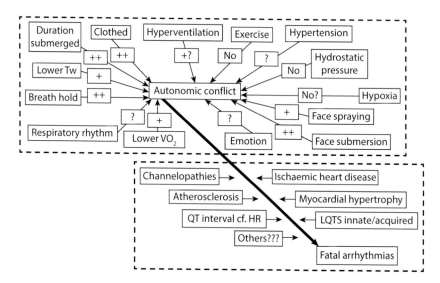

Figure 6.2 Current understanding of the potential conditions influencing autonomic conflict (upper box) and the cofactors necessary to cause the arrhythmias produced by autonomic conflict to descend into fatal arrhythmias (lower box). ++ = strong factor; + = weak factor; No = no influence; ? = unknown influence; LQTS = Long Q-T syndrome; QT = electrocardiogram Q-T wave interval; cf. = compare; HR = heart rate; Tw = water temperature.

Stage 2: Short-term immersion

After the skin, the next body tissues to cool are the superficial nerves and muscles; this cooling can lead to significant incapacitation in the form of decrements in muscular strength, dexterity and coordination in a short period of time. The limbs, especially the arms, are particularly susceptible to cooling because they are thin cylinders with a large surface area to mass ratio and superficially running nerves and muscle.

In nerve tissue below a local temperature of 20°C, the rate of conduction and amplitude of action potentials is slowed. For example, the conduction velocity of the ulnar nerve falls by 15 m/s/10°C fall in local temperature and nerve block can occur at a temperature of 5–15°C for 1–15 minutes. The maximum power output of muscle falls by 3% per degree centigrade fall in muscle temperature, and below a muscle temperature of 27°C fatigue occurs earlier and force production is reduced [21–23]. The reasons for this decreased muscle function include the following [24]:

- Reduced enzyme activity
- Decreased acetylcholine and calcium release
- Slower rates of diffusion
- Decreased muscle perfusion

- Increased viscosity
- Slower rates of conduction and depolarization of action potentials.

Deep muscles in the forearm can cool to 27°C in as little as 5–10 minutes in water at about 5°C, and in 10–20 minutes in water about 12°C [25]. Limb cooling can impair swimming performance and actions essential to survival. The inability to swim or keep the back to oncoming waves can result in drowning. Swim failure is a common feature during the early stages of immersion in cold water; it occurs in strong as well as weak swimmers. Swimming ability in a swimming pool does not equate with swimming ability in open cold water; fatigue and failure occur much sooner in cold water. Swim failure is a significant part of the 'physiological pathways to drowning' (Figure 6.4).

Stage 3: Long-term immersion

In normal circumstances, cooling of the deep tissues of the body and hypothermia will not represent a problem before about 30 minutes following immersion in cold water. Consistent with the vast majority of biological activity, cooling slows down and therefore impairs physiological function. Hypothermia affects cellular metabolism, blood

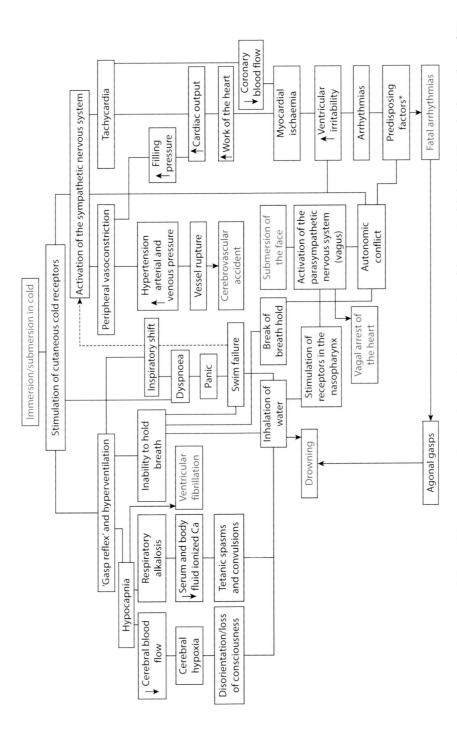

Figure 6.3 A contemporary view of the initial responses to immersion and submersion in cold water (cold shock). *See the lower box of Figure 6.2. [Based on Tipton MJ. *Clin Sci.* 1989; 77: 581–8; Datta A, Tipton MJ. *J Appl Physiol.* 2006; 100(6): 2057–64; Tipton MJ, et al. *Undersea Hyperb Med.* 1994; 21(3): 305–13; Tipton MJ, et al. *Aviat Space Environ Med.* 2010; 81: 399–404; and Shattock M, Tipton MJ. *J Physiol.* 2012; 590(Pt 14): 3219–30.]

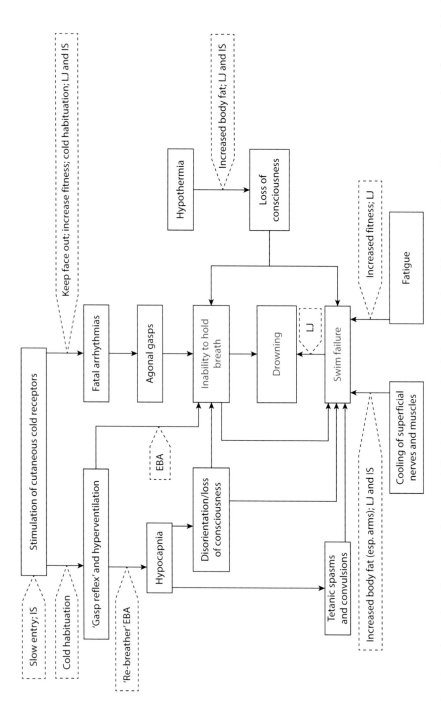

Figure 6.4 The physiological 'pathways' to drowning following immersion/submersion in cold water, with possible interventions for partial mitigation (dashed). IS, immersion suit; LJ, life jacket; EBA, emergency breathing aid.

Table 6.1 Average (50% survive) survival times (hours) for lightly clad males, from various authors

Water temperature (°C)	Molnar	Hayward	Golden	Tikuisis
5	1.0	2.2	1	2.2
10	2.2	2.9	2	3.6
15	5.5	4.8	6	7.7

Source: Data from Golden F, Tipton M, *Essentials of Sea Survival*, Human Kinetics, Champaign, IL, 2002.

flow and neural activation. Progressive hypothermia can cause the following signs and symptoms – deep body temperatures given in parentheses [26]:

- Confusion, disorientation, introversion, aggression (35°C)
- Amnesia (34°C)
- Cardiac arrhythmias (33°C)
- Clouding of consciousness (33°C–30°C)
- Loss of consciousness (30°C)
- Ventricular fibrillation (28°C)
- Cardiac arrest and death (25°C)

It is important to note that drowning occurs with loss of consciousness unless the airway is supported clear of the water. Even then, the legs can act as a sea anchor and turn the body to face the oncoming waves. Therefore, in rough seas the addition of a splash guard to a lifejacket is required to prevent the aspiration of water.

Below a deep body temperature of about 28°C, the following may be observed [27]:

- Decreased spontaneous depolarization of pacemaker cells of the heart.
- Fluid shifts out of the vascular space.
- Renal function is depressed; decreased glomerular filtration, augmented osmotic diuresis.
- Hypovolaemia and increased blood viscosity.
- Hepatic metabolism is impaired.
- Opening and closing of membrane channels is slowed.
- Sodium channel conduction is decreased.
- Potassium ion regulation is impaired.
- Function of the brain stem is impaired.
- Enzyme reaction times are reduced.
- Gastrointestinal smooth muscle motility is decreased.
- Cold-induced collapse of the microvasculature has occurred.
- Role of insulin-dependent glucose transport ceases.

The deep body temperatures associated with the signs and symptoms of hypothermia are only approximations; great variation exists between individuals. This variation is due to well-known factors such as the level of internal (body fat) and external (clothing) insulation, fitness and sex, as well as a wide range of more subtle non-thermal factors, such as blood sugar levels, age and motion illness. Drugs can also influence the way the temperature regulation system functions and consequent cooling rates [28].

The variation in the rate at which different people cool also explains why the average survival times given in Table 6.1 should only be regarded as a guide. It is important to note that these times are for those immersed with their head out of the water (see section on submersion* below).

Stage 4: Circum-rescue collapse

Approximately 17% of immersion deaths occur just before, during or immediately following rescue; the term *circum-rescue collapse* has been given to these deaths [29]. While many of these deaths are likely to be the consequence of the delayed effects of the aspiration of water when immersed, other physiological mechanisms also appear to be involved. These mechanisms are briefly discussed below.

PRE-RESCUE COLLAPSE

The mechanism causing pre-rescue collapse remains unclear, but the sudden deterioration in the condition of some survivors is suggestive of a cardiovascular mechanism, perhaps a variant of autonomic conflict. In addition, catecholamines, particularly noradrenaline, have been

* *Submerged (submersion)* means with the head (airways) underwater. This term should not be confused with *immersed (immersion)*, where the head remains above the water and survival time can be much longer.

shown to have a protective effect in hypothermia via the assistance they give to the maintenance of blood pressure. It is possible that the sense of relief engendered by imminent rescue results in a reduction in catecholamine secretion and the consequent withdrawal of their protective effect [30]. To reduce this problem, those rescuing immersion victims should encourage them to keep fighting for their survival and avoid statements like 'relax, you are safe now'.

DURING-RESCUE COLLAPSE

This sudden deterioration in the condition of previously conscious subjects is too rapid and requires too great a fall in deep body temperature to be caused by thermal changes. An alternative, cardiovascular mechanism was proposed by Golden and Hervey in 1981 [5]. Head-out immersion produces profound changes in cardiovascular, renal and endocrine functions. These effects are a direct result of the high density of the water and the differences in hydrostatic pressure over the immersed body. A negative transthoracic pressure of about 14.7 mmHg is established, which increases central blood volume by up to 700 mL very soon after immersion [31]. This state is associated with enhanced diastolic filling, raised right atrial pressure and a 32%–66% increase in cardiac output, due entirely to an increase in stroke volume [32]. Most of the renal responses following immersion are due to the shift in blood volume, which the body senses as hypervolaemia. These responses include a significant diuresis within the first hour of cold water immersion. A similar set of responses may also occur in those who have endured cold air environments with limited food and water supplies [30].

In these situations, circulatory collapse and cardiac arrest may occur during rescue as a result of a number of factors, including the following:

- Less venous return caused by loss of hydrostatic assistance and the reimposition of the full effects of gravity on removal from the water
- Hypovolaemia caused by diuresis and inter-compartmental fluid shifts
- Increased blood viscosity as a result of cooling of blood
- Diminished work capacity of the hypothermic heart and reduced time for coronary filling

- Dulled baroreceptor reflexes
- Unattainable demands to perfuse skeletal muscle when asked to assist in the rescue
- Psychological stress
- Pre-existing coronary disease
- Possible reduction in catecholamine production

To reduce the problem during rescue, and assuming that the airway is not under threat, hypothermic* casualties who are going to be lifted over a significant distance (i.e. into a helicopter or up a high-sided ship) should, where possible, be removed from the water in a horizontal rather than vertical posture and treated like the critically ill patients that they are. Such casualties should not be required to exert themselves to assist with their own rescue. For the same cardiovascular-related reasons, it is sensible to transport hypothermic casualties in a slightly head-down attitude with the head towards the stern of a fast rescue craft or the front of a helicopter.

If the airway of a casualty is under threat, that person should be removed from the water as soon as possible. A vertical lift is permissible if it is just for the brief period necessary to get a casualty over the sponson of a fast rescue craft.

POST-RESCUE COLLAPSE

The most important cause of post-rescue collapse is hypoxia, secondary to the aspiration of water. Therefore, it is critical that following rescue a suitably qualified individual should check an immersion victim to determine whether water has been aspirated and if hospital screening is necessary. A less common cause of post-rescue death is inappropriate rewarming, also referred to as *rewarming collapse*. It is caused by the collapse of arterial blood pressure and poor coronary perfusion if aggressive external rewarming of cold, hypovolaemic or dehydrated casualties is undertaken. It results in peripheral vasodilatation before the body has regained the responses and blood volume necessary to compensate for the redistribution of blood

---

* In this context, *hypothermic* refers to someone who has been in the water long enough (>30 minutes) to have a significantly lowered deep body temperature (<35°C) and profound shifts/loss of body fluid. They are likely to be semi-conscious.

flow. Prehospital treatment of hypothermic victims should not be too aggressive and should be complemented by the provision of warm IV fluid and warm oxygen.

Prolonged survival following submersion (head under) in cold water

On very rare occasions individuals, usually children (67% of cases) or small adults, survive prolonged submersion (>30 minutes) in fresh, very cold water (<6°C) [33]. Although the prognostic indicators of a poor outcome following submersion include a period underwater of longer than 5–10 minutes [34,35], the longest submersion in water at 5°C without sequelae is 66 minutes [36]. Any similarity between this time and the so-called golden hour for the resuscitation of casualties in air is coincidental.

Tipton and Golden [33] reported 44 cases of prolonged submerged survival. Although extremely rare in comparison with poor outcomes, the fact that such survival is possible has influenced the search and rescue 'psyche'. It complicates and confuses the decision about when a rescue should change to body recovery; this decision is essentially a balance between increasing risk to rescuers and decreasing likelihood of being able to resuscitate a casualty.

A number of factors suggest that prolonged submerged survival may be due to rapid and selective brain cooling that extends the hypoxic survival time of the brain by reducing metabolism and thus the tissue oxygen requirements. At normal body temperature (37°C), 10 minutes of acute cerebral hypoxia is associated with significant and lasting cerebral damage. Brain cooling slows this process: a 7°C fall in brain temperature doubles hypoxic survival time, while below 22°C brain activity almost ceases and hypoxic survival time is extended considerably [37].

With regard to the mechanism for selective brain cooling, it has been reported that respiratory movements continue for around 70 seconds following submersion [38]. Falls of 7.5°C–8.5°C in the temperature of blood flowing in the carotid artery during the first two minutes of submersion, with much smaller falls in temperature occurring subsequently when breathing and cardiac activity

have stopped, have also been reported [39]. Thus, it is proposed that the flushing of water in and out of the lung during the process of drowning cools the heart and thereby the carotid artery blood supply to the brain and the brain itself. The fact that it is *selective* brain cooling means that other deep body temperatures are not likely to reflect brain temperature and, therefore, have limited prognostic value. The reason why 67% of the cases of prolonged submerged survival involve children is likely to be due, in part, to the fact that once selective brain cooling ceases additional cooling must then be from the surface of the body, and children and smaller adults have a surface area to mass ratio advantage in this regard compared to larger individuals.

Prolonged survival, and with it the potential for successful resuscitation, is therefore dependent on the brain temperature achieved at the time respiratory and cardiac functions cease. In theory, and it appears in practice, for a given period of time (e.g. 70 seconds), respiratory rate, cardiac output and cerebral blood flow, there will be an upper limit above which insufficient cooling will occur to provide protection against cerebral hypoxia. It seems that this temperature is about 6°C. The existence of this temperature 'threshold', plus the small number of cases, helps to explain the absence of a correlation between submerged survival time and water temperature. On the basis of a review of cases that could be substantiated, Tipton and Golden [33] produced the decision-making guide presented in Figure 6.5.

The recommendation to start the clock upon arrival at the scene removes the necessity to rely on eyewitness accounts, often from very emotional people, on the passage of time.

Note that Figure 6.5 is only a guide, and local circumstances and/or clinical signs may dictate an alternative course of action to the senior medic at the scene. It is likely to be of more use when rescuers are themselves placed at high risk by continuing a search, that is, when the likelihood of saving the life of a casualty is far outweighed by that of losing a rescuer.

PREVENTION AND PROTECTION

An understanding of the physiological hazards to be confronted on immersion in cold water should shape policies for prevention, protection and rescue, as well as highlight the most likely pathologies

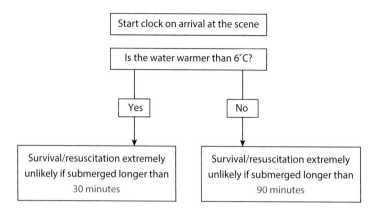

Figure 6.5 Decision-making guide for submersion (head under) incidents where the casualty has not been found.

to be confronted. Legislators and designers of survival equipment should also recognize and understand the physiological incapacitation associated with cooling when considering their safety standards and design criteria.

We now know that the end point of many of the physiological responses to cold water immersion is drowning rather than hypothermia. The physiological 'pathways' to drowning are presented in Figure 6.4 with some possible physiological and technological interventions for partial mitigation.

The technological interventions include the use of the following:

- Lifejackets with splash guards and retaining systems (e.g. crotch straps) [40].
- Immersion drysuits or wetsuits as appropriate.
- Emergency breathing aids (EBAs) in special situations where escape from a submerged craft may be required. A rebreather EBA can help reduce the hypocapnia (lowered CO_2 levels in the blood) associated with the hyperventilation of cold shock.

The physiological and behavioural interventions include the following:

- Do not enter the water unless absolutely necessary. If necessary, enter slowly to minimize cold shock.
- Avoid immersion of the face, which should reduce the likelihood of arrhythmias on immersion.

- Survival may depend on an immersion casualty appreciating that their physical abilities (e.g. swimming, manual function), however good, will quickly diminish following immersion in cold water. Essential survival actions should be undertaken as soon as possible after the attenuation of the cold shock response.
- Subcutaneous body fat protects against hypothermia, and insulation over the upper arms may help maintain swimming ability.
- Because individuals cool four to five times faster in water compared to air at the same temperature, the buoyancy provided by upturned hulls, large pieces of driftwood and so on offers the opportunity for the survivor to get partially or completely out of the water. Despite the fact that it often feels colder out of the water than in it, a survivor will always be better out of the water.
- Assume that those who need rescue could be physically incapacitated.
- The rapid deterioration seen in cold casualties during rescue suggests a cardiovascular rather than thermal problem. Therefore, victims who are very cold, have been immersed or have been in a life raft for a long time, and whose airway is not under threat, should be treated as potentially critically ill. If possible, they should be removed from the water carefully and horizontally, and kept horizontal. Victims should not have to assist in their rescue. However, if the airway is under threat, the victim should be removed from the water as soon as possible.

- As few as five 3-minute immersions in cold water can reduce the cold shock response by 50% through habituation; 25% of the reduction lasts at least 14 months.
- Higher levels of physical fitness are associated with a smaller cold shock response, delayed fatigue and increased ability to generate metabolic heat through shivering on immersion.

CONCLUSION

Immersion remains a major cause of accidental death in most countries of the world. Immersion in cold waters evokes a range of physiological responses associated with significant health risks including drowning, hypothermia and cardiovascular problems. An understanding of the physiological precursors to these hazards and pathologies is essential to provide appropriate training and equipment to the lifesaving and search and rescue community and to deliver optimal interventions and treatments to those at risk of immersion and immersion casualties.

REFERENCES

1. Home Office. *Report of the Working Party on Water Safety*. London: HMSO; 1977.
2. Tipton MJ, McCormack E, Turner C. An international data registration for accidental and immersion hypothermia: The UK National Immersion Incident Survey revisited. In Bierens J (ed.). *Drowning, Prevention, Rescue, Treatment*. Berlin: Springer-Verlag; 2015.
3. Falk F. Versuche uber beziebung der hantnerven zur athmung. *Arch Anat Physiol.* 1884; 8: 455.
4. Alexander L. *The Treatment of Shock from Prolonged Exposure to Cold, Especially Water*. London: Combined Intelligence Objectives Sub-Committee APO 413 C105, Item No. 24, Her Majesty's Stationary Office; 1945.
5. Golden F, Hervey GR. The "afterdrop" and death after rescue from immersion in cold water. In Adam JA (ed.). *Hypothermia Ashore and Afloat*. Aberdeen: Aberdeen University Press; 1981.
6. Tipton MJ. The initial responses to cold-water immersion in man. *Clin Sci.* 1989; 77: 581–8.
7. Keatinge WR, Evans M. The respiratory and cardiovascular response to immersion in cold and warm water. *Q J Exp Physiol.* 1961; 46: 83–94.
8. Keatinge WR, McIlroy MB, Goldfien A. Cardiovascular responses to ice-cold showers. *J Appl Physiol.* 1964; 19: 1145–50.
9. Keatinge WR, Nadel JA. Immediate respiratory response to sudden cooling of the skin. *J Appl Physiol.* 1965; 20: 65–9.
10. Cooper KE, Martin S, Riben P. Respiratory and other responses in subjects immersed in cold water. *J Appl Physiol.* 1976; 40: 903–10.
11. Goode RC, Duffin J, Miller R, Romet TT, Chant W, Ackles A. Sudden cold water immersion. *Respir Physiol.* 1975; 23: 301–10.
12. Tipton MJ, Stubbs DA, Elliott DH. The effect of clothing on the initial responses to cold water immersion in man. *J R Nav Med Serv.* 1990; 76(2): 89–95.
13. Tipton MJ, Stubbs DA, Elliott DH. Human initial responses to immersion in cold water at 3 temperatures and following hyperventilation. *J Appl Physiol.* 1991; 70(1): 317–22.
14. Tipton MJ. Immersion fatalities: Hazardous responses and dangerous discrepancies. *J R Nav Med Serv.* 1995; 81: 101–7.
15. Modell JH. *Pathophysiology and Treatment of Drowning*. Springfield, IL: Charles C. Thomas; 1971.
16. Datta A, Tipton MJ. Respiratory responses to cold water immersion: Neural pathways, interactions and clinical consequences. *J Appl Physiol.* 2006; 100(6): 2057–64.
17. Tipton MJ, Kelleher P, Golden F. Supraventricular arrhythmias following breath-hold submersions in cold water. *Undersea Hyperb Med.* 1994; 21(3): 305–13.
18. Tipton MJ, Gibbs P, Brooks C, Roiz de Sa D, Reilly T. ECG during helicopter underwater escape training. *Aviat Space Environ Med.* 2010; 81: 399–404.
19. Shattock M, Tipton MJ. "Autonomic conflict": A different way to die on immersion in cold water? *J Physiol.* 2012; 590(Pt 14): 3219–30.

20. de Burgh Daly M, Angell-James JE. The 'diving response' and its possible clinical implications. *Int Med.* 1979; 1: 12–19.
21. Douglas WW, Malcolm JL. The effect of localized cooling on conduction in cat nerves. *J Physiol.* 1955; 130: 53–71.
22. Clarke SJ, Hellon RF, Lind AR. The duration of sustained contractions of the human forearm at different muscle temperatures. *J Physiol.* 1958; 143: 454–73.
23. Basbaum CB. Induced hypothermia in peripheral nerve: Electron microscopic and electrophysiological observations. *J Neurocytol.* 1973; 2: 171–87.
24. Vincent MJ, Tipton MJ. The effects of cold immersion and hand protection on grip strength. *Aviat Space Environ Med.* 1988; 59: 738–41.
25. Burton AC, Edholm OG. *Man in a Cold Environment.* London: Edward Arnold; 1955.
26. Golden F. Recognition and treatment of immersion hypothermia. *Proc R Soc Med.* 1973; 66(10): 1058–61.
27. Tipton M, Golden F. The physiology of cooling in cold water. In Bierens J (ed.). *Drowning, Prevention, Rescue, Treatment.* Berlin: Springer-Verlag; 2015.
28. Tipton MJ, Mekjavic IB, Golden F. Hypothermia. In Bove AA (ed.). *Bove & Davis' Diving Medicine.* Philadelphia, PA: Saunders; 2004.
29. Golden F, Hervey GR, Tipton MJ. Circum-rescue collapse: Collapse, sometimes fatal, associated with rescue of immersion victims. *S Pac Underwater Med Soc J.* 1994; 24(3): 171–9.
30. Golden F, Tipton M. *Essentials of Sea Survival.* Champaign, IL: Human Kinetics; 2002.
31. Lin YC, Hong SK. Physiology of water immersion. *Undersea Biomed Res.* 1984; 11: 109–11.
32. Risch WD, Koubenec HJ, Beckmann U, Lange S, Gauer OH. The effect of graded immersion on heart volume, central venous pressure, pulmonary blood distribution, and heart rate in man. *Pflugers Arch.* 1978; 374(2): 115–18.
33. Tipton M, Golden F. Decision-making guide for the search, rescue and resuscitation of submerged (head under) victims. *Resuscitation.* 2011; 82: 819–24.
34. Orlowski JP. Drowning, near-drowning, and ice-water submersions. *Pediatr Clin North Am.* 1987; 34: 75–92.
35. Bierens JJ, van der Velde EA, van Berkel M, van Zanten JJ. Submersion in the Netherlands: Prognostic indicators and results of resuscitation. *Ann Emerg Med.* 1990; 19: 1390–5.
36. Bolte RG, Black PG, Bowers RS, Thorne JK, Corneli HM. The use of extracorporeal rewarming in a child submerged for 66 minutes. *JAMA.* 1988; 260: 377–9.
37. Adams RD, Victor M. Hypoxic hypotensive encephalopathy. In Adams RD, Victor M (eds.). *Principles in Neurology.* New York: McGraw-Hill; 1977.
38. Fainer DC, Martin CG, Ivy AC. Resuscitation of dogs from fresh water drowning. *J Appl Physiol.* 1951; 3: 417–26.
39. Conn AW, Miyasaka K, Katayama M, Fujita M, Orima H, Barker G, Bohn D. A canine study of cold water drowning in fresh versus salt water. *Crit Care Med.* 1995; 12: 2029–37.
40. Lunt H, White D, Long G, Tipton M. Wearing a crotch strap on a correctly fitted lifejacket improves lifejacket performance. *Ergonomics.* 2014; 57(8): 1256–64.

Medical Aspects

7

Injuries and risks while lifeguarding

PETER WERNICKI AND CHRISTY NORTHFIELD

INTRODUCTION

Lifeguarding is a rewarding and challenging occupation. The ultimate aim of the profession is saving lives and preventing aquatic injuries to the general public. To accomplish these goals, lifeguards must meet and maintain significant physical and mental requirements. Lifeguards serve in varied environments with constantly changing conditions. If lifeguards can't perform their duties flawlessly, not only are they putting their own lives in danger, but also the lives of the public that they are employed to protect. These factors make the profession quite unusual. The only other occupations with similar demands are public safety employees such as police, firefighters and the military. The same requirements, working conditions and challenges that make the profession unique can also lead to injury, illness, disability and even death.

The high level of fitness necessary for lifeguarding requires constant training. Lifeguards train in swimming, rowing, paddling and running. This training often leads to sports-type injuries and problems. The nature of the repetitive actions performed in these activities can lead to overuse syndromes. To increase the level of performance and camaraderie, lifeguards often compete in local, regional, national and international rescue competitions. While certainly beneficial, these activities do expose lifeguards to additional risks. The widely varying ages and subsequent physical, intellectual and maturational abilities of lifeguards must be taken into account by any agency.

Although lifeguards strive to keep their work areas clear of hazards, this is never completely possible. Surf conditions, sand irregularities, water quality, weather, marine life and victim behaviour are all factors that cannot be fully controlled by lifeguards. Any of these factors can lead to lifeguard injuries and illnesses. Chris Brewster, president of the United States Lifeguarding Association, has described beach lifeguarding as 'human being vs the power of nature' [1].

Routine medical interventions apply when lifeguards are injured or ill. Usually, there is very little 'light duty' available on the beach. Therefore, when lifeguards are in less than full health, it usually leads to time out of work. Studies, surveys and occupational data have provided information on how, when and where lifeguards are injured. Less data are available on the efficacy of various preventative measures. Nonetheless, agencies should work to optimize training and beach environments with the goal of lowering the overall injury and illness rate in lifeguards.

DAILY HAZARDS

The routine work environment of beach lifeguards presents numerous hazards before they even head out to make a rescue. These hazards include weather, sun, sand and water conditions, lifeguard stands and equipment and the beach-going public. Lifeguards put themselves in harm's way each day. They are subject to clear morbidity and also mortality. Although rare, lifeguards do die in the line of duty [2]. We owe them our best efforts to try and prevent any of these negative events.

Sun

The sun is an obvious component of all beach environments. It is one of the reasons the public comes to the beach. The sun is usually stronger in the summer season when more lifeguards are employed. Although pleasant, the sun presents significant dangers for those on the beach, including the lifeguards [3].

Sun exposure is the number one cause of skin cancer [4]. UV rays have been shown to damage skin cells and to lead to cellular changes resulting in cancer. Research shows that sun exposure at an early age is particularly dangerous. Childhood sunburns may be the single most predictive factor for future skin cancer [5]. Exposure later in life is also harmful. Most lifeguards have spent their youth around water with extensive exposure to the sun. Therefore, they may already be at high risk for skin cancer. Studies of lifeguards in San Diego showed a relatively high rate of skin cancer, including 11 lifeguards in 1989 alone requiring skin cancer–related medical care [6].

All lifeguards should be checked annually by a dermatologist for signs of skin cancer. Skin cancer survival rates are much higher with early detection. Melanoma is the most serious of all skin cancers. It has a significantly worse prognosis than the more common basal cell or squamous cell cancers. The five-year survival rate of melanoma is 91% [7]. This survival rate decreases greatly if the cancer has already spread prior to detection [8]. The World Health Organization estimates that more than 65,000 people a year worldwide die from melanoma [4]. The signs of a skin cancer include a mole that is changing, a spot that is increasing in size, a lesion that bleeds, an irregular spot or a purple, black or red lesion. A dermatologist should check any questionable lesion. Minor (basal, squamous) skin cancers usually require only local removal. Melanoma may need significant surgery and possibly chemotherapy. Individuals with one skin cancer are at a higher subsequent risk for other skin cancers [9,10]. Lifeguards with melanoma are usually advised to seek other less sun-exposed employment. These work-related, life-changing conditions are not only emotionally tough but they also result in significant financial exposure to the employing agency [6].

The prudent way for lifeguards to lower their skin cancer risk is to avoid direct sun exposure whenever possible [11]. All beach lifeguards should be issued uniforms with appropriate sun protection (SPF) including long-sleeved shirts, hats and sunglasses. Their agencies should require that they be worn. When the San Diego lifeguarding agency adopted such policies in the 1970s, the rate of skin cancer in their lifeguards declined dramatically. A side benefit of the uniform policy is an improved perception of professionalism by the public [6]. All employing agencies should also provide appropriate shade for all lifeguards, either in the tower design or with umbrellas. Sunscreen rated SPF 30 or higher should be available for all beach lifeguards. In 2010, new research found that daily sunscreen use cut the incidence of melanoma in half, although it did not completely eliminate the risk [12].

Hours-long exposure to the sun and wind, especially on warmer days, can lead to dehydration [13]. Although rare, heat illnesses such as heat cramps, heat exhaustion and sun stroke can also occur in lifeguards. Heat cramps can prevent lifeguards from performing rescue operations. Heat exhaustion may lead to decreased vigilance and heat stroke can cause death. Signs of heat illness are irritability, headache, weakness, dizziness, chills, heartburn and nausea. Thirst is typically a poor indicator of hydration because it is a delayed response and people are not fully hydrated when their thirst is quenched [14]. Increased physical activity can lead to increased loss of fluid through sweating. All agencies should have adequate water and/or sports drinks readily available to lifeguards at all times to prevent heat-related illnesses [15]. The Australian Lifeguard Service recommends drinking at least 200 mL of water within 30 minutes of any energetic activity. Proper shade should be provided. Agency policy should require that lifeguards rotate frequently on extremely hot days, with breaks taken in air-conditioned locations. Anytime lifeguards feel overheated or are cramping, they should be removed from duty and taken to a cool area for rehydration. Overheated lifeguards will have decreased mental and physical performance. If their conditions do not improve, they must receive further medical care.

The sun can also cause damage to the eyes. UV ray exposure from the sun has been shown to cause several conditions such as pterygium, pinguecula and cataracts [16]. The most common is pterygium. In a recent Miami Beach survey, numerous lifeguards exhibited this condition [17]. The inflammation of the sclera characteristic of pterygium can lead to a loss of vision and may require surgery [3]. Any changes in the appearance of the eye or any changes in vision should be evaluated and treated by an ophthalmologist. Most of these ocular conditions can be successfully treated without any permanent loss of vision, but they often require significant days out of work for recovery [18]. Salt water and blowing sand can also be factors in eye injuries; however, the number one cause is UV exposure. Requiring all beach lifeguards to wear sunglasses with 100% UV screening significantly reduces eye injury. Use should be required even on cloudy days when the UV exposure is still high.

Weather

The weather certainly cannot be controlled. Wind, temperature, lightning and air quality are all possible causes for concern.

Beach locations can experience sudden and severe weather changes resulting in tornadoes, severe thunderstorms, waterspouts, microbursts etc. These storms often result in high winds leading to injury from blowing sand or objects, or directly from the weather itself. Agencies should continuously monitor local weather. When required by weather conditions, agencies should mandate beach evacuations to safe areas. As the last to leave the beach in dangerous weather, lifeguards have the highest risk of weather-related injury. If beach umbrellas are present, lifeguards must monitor even light to moderate winds. Umbrellas should be appropriately anchored in light winds. In moderate or high winds, lifeguards should mandate that umbrellas be taken down.

In certain beach locations, cold temperatures can also be a problem for lifeguards. If lifeguards are required to be on the stand in cold or inclement weather, they can suffer from hypothermia. This condition can decrease performance and cloud judgment. If lifeguards complain of cold, are shivering or appear confused, they should be taken to a warm area, wrapped in blankets and given warm fluids. Hypothermia can lead to confusion, errors of judgment, diminished mental and physical performance and arrhythmias [19]. If lifeguards' conditions do not improve, they should be transported to further medical care. Prevention of cold injuries would include adequate shelter in lifeguard stands, appropriate warm clothing, frequent shift changes and closure of beaches if the weather conditions become too harsh. Wetsuits should be prescribed, where appropriate, to prevent hypothermia when required to enter cold water.

Lightning is always a danger during any outside recreational activity. Lifeguards have been injured and even killed by lightning strikes while on duty [20]. Lifeguards are at increased risk due to the use of elevated stands, which often contain metal. Lightning injuries should be treated with cardiopulmonary resuscitation (CPR) and if required, application of an AED and rapid transport. Prevention of injury by lightning requires that all agencies have a clear, comprehensive lightning protocol and an emergency operation plan (EOP). In addition to the use of the 'flash-to-bang rule', there should be real-time active weather monitoring. The flash-to-bang rule is a way of estimating the distance between your location and a lightning strike. When the lightning flashes, count the seconds to the bang of thunder, then divide the number of seconds by five (sound travels one mile in five seconds) to give the distance in miles from you to the lightning [21]. Monitoring could include local radar, radio and/or phone warnings and possibly a lightning tracking device. Once the EOP is triggered, lifeguards should have equipment (e.g. loud speakers, bull horns, flags) to warn the public and move them to appropriate, protected areas as soon as possible. Swiftly and efficiently carrying out these actions will allow the lifeguards themselves to exit the beach faster and reach safety sooner. Plans should include protocols for dealing with non-compliant patrons and for safe return to the beach [22].

Air quality

Lifeguards are exposed to outside air conditions throughout their day. Extended exposure to high pollution is assumed to be harmful. A study in Galveston, Texas, showed reduced lung function in lifeguards exposed to elevated levels of air pollutants and ozone – up to an 8% decrease in Forced Vital Capacity (FVC) [23]. These changes were usually transient, but they may have decreased pulmonary function during lifeguard training or rescues. As a result of this study, Galveston beaches now fly orange flags when poor air quality may present a health hazard. Frequent indoor rotations and/or appropriate respirators for lifeguards may be beneficial. Algae blooms in coastal waters can produce toxins such as 'red tides'. Lifeguards working in environments with these toxic blooms have shown decreased lung function [24]. A study in the Gulf of Mexico showed that brevetoxins formed by fish-killing dinoflagellates can be transferred from water to air by wind-powered waves. Increased aerosolization of these toxins correlated with increased upper airway symptoms in local lifeguards but was not associated with any acute adverse effects [25].

Sand

Contact with the sand can have negative consequences. It can be extremely hot and cause first- or even second-degree burns to the feet [26]. Beach sand can also house other dangers, including sharp objects, some of which are natural, like shells and rocks. Others are not natural, for example trash such as glass, metal, fish hooks and used hypodermic needles. Beyond simple puncture or laceration, needles can hold even greater health risks. They are a medical waste hazard with possible exposure to bacterial infection, hepatitis and HIV. One study indicated that 79% of lifeguards reported foot injuries from sharp foreign objects [26]. A second study showed that 25% of overall lifeguard injuries were sustained to the foot [27]. Lacerations and burns should be appropriately treated. Return to

duty will depend on the severity of the injury. When medical waste is involved, immediate care by a physician is required. Prevention should include proper footwear, when possible, and routine patrol/scanning of the sand for dangerous items. Fletemeyer's [26] study showed positive responses to use of protective socks while on duty. Other risk management organizations have recommended footwear with non-slip bottoms without laces [28].

Water

The water has the obvious dangers of drowning and surf-related injuries which are inherent to a lifeguard's duties. Some are sensational, such as injuries from sharks, but there are numerous other, less prominent water risks.

Although rare, lifeguards have been seriously injured [29,30] and even killed [31] by shark attacks around the world. In areas where sharks are common, emergency protocols should be in place. When necessary, agencies should activate these protocols, remove the public from the water and therefore limit lifeguards' exposure. When swimmers become victims of shark attacks in guarded areas, lifeguards often have to enter the shark-infested, now bloody, water to perform the rescue [32]. Some areas with significant risks from sharks such as New South Wales, Australia, have installed 'shark nets'. While not meant to be complete barriers, these shark nets can reduce the risk of sharks entering bathing areas. Lifeguards assigned to beaches with shark nets need to carefully monitor the nets' conditions and patrol the protected areas for any unwanted marine intrusion [33].

All of the various open bodies of water that beach lifeguards oversee have hazards from marine life. These vary by location and cannot be discussed in detail in this chapter; however, here are a few additional examples. Jellyfish can be extremely dangerous; in endemic areas, agencies place jellyfish nets to protect swimmers and lifeguards. A sting from a box jellyfish, which inhabits many different waters, can lead to death within minutes [34]. Stings from Portuguese man-of-war jellyfish, while non-lethal, can have serious health consequences. Even stings from less toxic jellyfish can lead to temporary morbidity [17]. In areas with jellyfish nets, lifeguards should patrol the interiors for jellyfish that breach the nets. In areas endemic with serious envenomations, skin suits may be allowed or even required for lifeguards. When lifeguards are seriously injured by marine life, agencies should activate the existing EOP protocols.

Besides jellyfish, other envenomations encountered at beaches throughout the world include octopi, rockfish, skates, rays, sea snakes, alligators, crocodiles. [35]. Each agency should train their lifeguards for the possible local dangers, how to avoid injuries and how to treat them. For more information please refer to the International Lifesaving Federation position statement on marine envenomation at www.ilsf.org.

All water carries various organisms. Many of these organisms can be harmful to marine creatures, the public and lifeguards. The water at beaches in populated areas can have infectious disease contamination from various sources such as sewage discharge, rainwater runoff and animal contamination from livestock, dogs, birds, sea lions and other animals. The public is at increased risk from illness when swimming in contaminated water [36], as are lifeguards. Studies show an increased incidence of lifeguard illness when the lifeguards serve at beaches with higher levels of bacterial water contamination. Los Angeles County, California, has documented this trend mainly in an elevated number of upper respiratory infections among their lifeguards. These cases were diagnosed by physicians and reported as workers' compensation conditions [37]. Studies at Bondi in Australia showed similar findings [38]. When contamination is known or suspected, public access and therefore lifeguard access to the water should be suspended until water quality improves. If any public health concerns are present, lifeguards should avoid swallowing water and entering the water with any open skin lesions. Water quality in areas known to have an increased risk of bacterial contamination should have constant monitoring programs [39].

Work environment

The man-made physical work environment for lifeguards has a significant effect on occupational injuries. A review of Miami Beach lifeguard injuries highlighted the rate of injuries caused by the lifeguard tower alone (14.4%), such as hand injuries from putting up and taking down protective window covers [17]. This review prompted several suggestions to improve the way towers are constructed

with the goal of reducing injuries. With this information, Miami Beach spent $1 million modifying their new lifeguard towers. By necessity, the stands are elevated to provide better surveillance of the water, sand and the public. Lifeguards need training in safe, appropriate ways to get down from these heights to the sand, which is where the rescue begins. Lifeguards often injure themselves during transitions. Sometimes the injuries are mild, sometimes quite serious [17]; studies show that stairs are safer than ramps [18]. Other health concerns include exposure to asbestos in older towers (Figure 7.1) [40].

Lifeguards also suffer work-related injuries from lifting or moving equipment. Studies have indicated the lower back is the number one anatomic location of lifeguard injuries [17,18]. When possible, agencies should install mechanisms to prevent excessive lifting. These could include appropriate rollers or skids for boats, personal watercraft (PWCs) and other equipment; policies to require a minimum number of guards to move certain equipment like lifeguard stands; and training in the proper ergonomics for lifting and moving equipment.

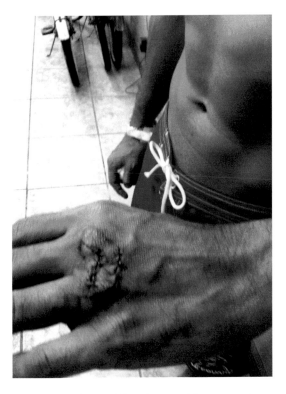

Figure 7.1 Lifeguard hand injury. (Courtesy of Jo Wagenhals, Pompano Beach, Florida. With permission.)

Equipment

The lifeguarding profession requires various technical, situation-specific equipment. The equipment can include rescue buoys, paddleboards, surf skis, rowed boats, PWCs, inflatable rescue boats (IRBs), all-terrain vehicles (ATVs) and motor vehicles. Each piece of equipment is geared to the specific beach location and rescue situation, yet the equipment can have its own dangers. A study of lifeguard injuries among the City and County of Honolulu lifeguards showed that paddleboards were the number one source of trauma. Lifeguards sustained the majority of these injuries while performing rescues. Certain handle designs were associated with finger injuries, even partial amputations. All rescue boards should be checked to assure that they do not contain problematic designs. The second most prevalent injuries were from the lifeguard stands and PWCs [18]. The use of surf skis have resulted in significant injuries, even lifeguard deaths [41]. Rowing has been shown to lead to an increased incidence of injuries, especially to the lower back [42].

IRBs are known to cause significant injury to lifeguards, especially to the feet and ankles. A study in 2000 by the Australian Surf Lifesaving Association showed numerous serious foot and ankle injuries from IRB use [43]. A follow-up study showed that impact forces and foot straps presented a significant hazard [44]. Subsequent modifications were suggested to improve the design and safety of the IRBs [45]. Proper training, required certifications, equipment modifications and use only when appropriate may help to decrease these injuries. Similar advice applies for ATVs and PWCs. While using this motorized equipment, all lifeguard personnel should be required to wear personal flotation devices (PFDs) and helmets. Motor vehicles can obviously have a risk of injury to the public and the lifeguard. Lifeguards should be trained in the proper use of these vehicles to prevent injury.

The public

Lifeguards have a duty to protect the public. In doing so, they must enforce the rules and regulations of their individual locations. Agencies where there are significant peacekeeping duties are required to train their lifeguards to the level of police. Examples are Daytona Beach, Florida, and the California State parks. Lifeguards may be required to carry firearms to protect themselves and the public. Even in other areas where lifeguards have only regular, non-peacekeeping duties, they have been injured in altercations with patrons [18]. In locations where confrontations may occur, lifeguards should be trained in how to avoid violent situations, how to defuse them and how to respond appropriately [46–48].

RESCUE HAZARDS

The original US Lifesaving Service's motto was 'You have to go out; you don't have to come back'. This sums up what lifesavers face in their daily jobs. The universal training goal is for all lifeguards to be well trained so that they will be able to come back. Not all lifeguards do. We should be honoured to be part of a profession where so many risk their lives for the public. Life-threatening risks as well as possible exposure to blood and bodily fluids qualify lifeguarding as a high-risk occupation. This designation may afford lifeguards higher pay and better benefits if injured or ill due to job-related circumstances. All agencies, where appropriate, should work to achieve this designation of high-risk occupation for their lifeguard staff [49].

Open water and surf present a challenging work environment. The Honolulu survey reported that most injuries were sustained during rescues [18]. Each individual portion of a rescue has its unique hazards. A stretch and warm up are not possible in a rescue situation. The 'cold' start characteristic of most rescues can result in cramps or other injuries. For example, an inadvertent run or jump from a tower can lead to injury to the gastrocnemius/soleus in the posterior calf. The term 'lifeguard calf' has been coined for this condition [42]. The sand and terrain can pose hazards to feet and knees from lacerations or lower extremity joint injuries from hidden sand bars or holes. The water can be cold; contain envenomation; have rip currents, pollution and waves; and hold many other dangers that can lead to serious injury or illness. And of course most drowning victims' actions are unpredictable [50]. Will the victim endanger the lifeguard? Was the victim trying to commit suicide and might therefore be uncooperative? Is the victim intoxicated? Does the victim have a related or undiagnosed medical condition? All lifeguards will need to make split-second decisions to save themselves and the victim. Only proper, rigorous and recurrent training will allow lifeguards to develop the skills to assess situations successfully and respond appropriately.

Lifeguards should always have the best, safest, most up-to-date equipment for their jobs. Regardless of location, the basic equipment should include swim fins, rescue buoys and other propulsion devices such as paddleboards. Lifeguards should always have adequate backup to ensure the success of their rescues and their own safety.

Bodily fluids with possible infectious diseases are an unequivocal danger to lifeguards. Most other health care and public safety professionals can take the necessary steps to prevent any contact with potentially infectious bodily fluids [51]. This is not always so for lifeguards. Lifeguards may need to enter water that has been contaminated with blood or other bodily fluids. Lifeguards may also be in a situation where mouth-to-mouth may be required without the availability of a barrier device. Fortunately, there is no known case of a lifeguard having contracted a serious infectious disease from a victim [17]. Experts have indicated that there is an extremely low probability of a lifeguard contracting AIDS from contact with a victim [52]. Despite these facts, lifeguards should always be taught the proper blood and bodily fluid procedures, and they should always be required to have and use a barrier device for CPR. Hepatitis, especially hepatitis B and C, is a hazard for lifeguards exposed to bodily fluids. Medical authorities recommended that all lifeguards be required to have a complete hepatitis B vaccine series paid for by the employer [53]. Hepatitis A vaccines should also be offered for lifeguards in endemic areas [54]. Tetanus immunizations should be up to date [53]. The necessary supplies for fluid containment, clean-up and decontamination must be readily available, e.g. gloves, mask, disinfectant, biohazard containers. Manikins and other equipment always need to be disinfected after use.

Lifeguards are of widely varying ages. This spectrum of ages encompasses a variety of maturities and life experiences, which can present several concerns. Studies have shown that younger employees, such as teenagers, are at a higher risk of injury. These younger lifeguards also underreport their injuries in an effort to appear more mature [55]. The hazing of younger guards has been reported and must be condemned by all employers. Older employees may exhibit a decrease in their performance and have a higher risk of age-related conditions such as arthritis and heart disease. Some studies showed an increase of serious injuries in lifeguards between the ages of 36 and 45 [17]. Many lifeguards are employed on a seasonal basis. Their training and fitness, or lack thereof, in the off-season may place them at an increased risk of injury when the new season starts. These guards often go from little activity to six- or seven-day work activity [42]. Year-round fitness should be encouraged.

Certain beach lifeguard agencies such as that in San Diego, California, perform special types of rescues in addition to their regular beach duties. These include swift water rescue, cliff rescue and operating fireboats. Lifeguards performing these additional duties must be properly trained and skilled. All necessary equipment should be available and maintained. Further information beyond these recommendations is not within the scope of this chapter.

TRAINING HAZARDS

Lifeguard training hazards are similar to those faced by any other professional athlete; lifeguarding is essentially a sport and there are often training errors. These errors include too much, too soon, too often, too hard and too new – causes of standard overuse injuries [56]. One study showed that physical training was the most common cause of lifeguard injuries [17]. A planned, gradual progression of increased activity is the best way to try to avoid injury. All training activity should be monitored and not increased by more than 10% per week. A study of elite lifeguard ironman competitors showed that overtraining was the main cause of injury [57].

All lifeguarding athletes should undergo an appropriate pre-employment physical assessment conducted by a qualified medical professional to assure that each employee can carry out the necessary duties of a lifeguard. Some agencies do not allow lifeguards to be assigned beach duty until they have at least 80 hours of training [1].

Learning proper technique should allow for better use of equipment and less injury. Training itself can result in injury or even death [58]. When training new and/or junior lifeguards, proper oversight and safety protocols must be in place. Appropriate liability releases should be required for all participants [54].

There are obviously many sports that have their associated injuries – swimming, paddling, surf skiing and rowing all have overuse injuries similar to lifeguarding. One study based in Honolulu, Hawaii, showed that the shoulder, after the foot, is the second most injured body part for lifeguards [18]. Training in several of these upper body sports is not cross-training (giving some muscles a rest) because they involve many of the same muscles and joints. As a result, this can actually compound injuries [59]. Lifeguards often suffer shoulder impingement syndrome, which is an inflammation of the rotator cuff. Beach lifeguards can also have higher rates of shoulder injuries from the additional effort of battling waves and currents while managing the additional weight of a victim. Proper adjunctive muscle strengthening programs can help to prevent these injuries. The use of fins can also mediate these risks by decreasing the amount of work required by the upper body during rescues [42].

Paddling injuries include shoulder overuse, neck strains, lateral elbow epicondylitis (tennis elbow) and 'knee knobbies' (bursitis). These conditions are exacerbated by the larger rescue boards, the longer distances and the extra weight of victims.

Running on the beach sand can lead to injuries. Running without footwear decreases biomechanical support. Running on soft sand can cause the heel to sink deeper into the sand, putting increased stress on the Achilles tendon and plantar fascia. Achilles tendonitis and plantar fasciitis are the common result. Patellar tendonitis and shin splints also result from frequent beach running.

Up to 44% of rowers experience low back injuries [41]. Other rowing injuries include different muscular strains, wrist tendonitis, coccyx irritation, blisters and even lower extremity fractures. Rowers have been shown to sustain a significant incidence of chest injuries including rib stress fractures. Lifeguard rowers sit in a fixed seat instead of the sliding mount that scullers use. This setup can lead to increased injuries to the upper torso because the rowers' legs do not provide any significant power [60]. Up to 20% of rowing injuries may sideline lifeguards for the season [42].

All lifeguard athletes should make sure they are preconditioned for their required activities. This measure should lead to a decrease in injuries; however, there are no data to support this presumption.

COMPETITION HAZARDS

Many lifeguards participate in lifesaving competitions; the competitions are held at local, regional, national and international levels. Training and practising for these competitions should enhance lifeguards' skills, performance and comradery, but these competitions can also lead to injuries. Debate continues as to whether lifeguard competition injuries are eligible for workers' compensation. A proper injury reporting system can improve the quality and accuracy of the injury reports [61]. The Australian national championships include over 5000 competitors. Data have shown over 100 injuries per competition day as well as several tragic deaths [41]. The majority of these injuries are musculoskeletal and can be treated at first aid stations. Of the injuries, 22% were referred to a higher level medical practitioner for further treatment. The physician-staffed stations treat the more significant injuries (10%) including fractures, dislocations, lacerations, MIs, asthma, heat stress and dehydration. Each year 5% of patients require transport for a higher level of care. The IRB (29.9%), beach flag (13.8%) and surf boat (11.3%) competitions caused the most injuries (Figure 7.2).

Male and female competitors have equal injury rates and older lifeguards have increased rates of injury [62]. Several modifications have been made to national and international competitions in an attempt to avoid injuries that have serious consequences. The Australian and US national competitions have implemented extensive new multi-modal safety measures. 'Safety is now paramount' [41]. All competitors are now required to wear fluorescent

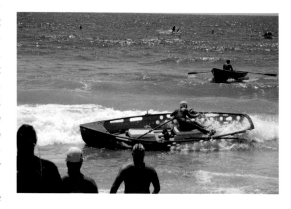

Figure 7.2 Surf boat competition. (Courtesy of Jo Wagenhals, Pompano Beach, Florida. With permission.)

rash guards for better visibility in case the competitors sustain an injury and need to be rescued. New policies stipulate that the competition safety officers have no other conflicting duties [40]. They monitor conditions and have the authority to halt or cancel events when dangerous surf, weather or other conditions warrant it. Protective equipment, including PFDs and head protection, are being evaluated by Surf Life Saving Australia for use by competitors in all watercraft events [40]. Some of this equipment is already required for IRB events and certain rowing events. The use may expand to other craft events if future research shows benefits.

One of the unique competitions at beach lifeguard tournaments involves beach flags. This event usually has a high incidence of injuries, including wrist and leg fractures, shoulder dislocations and concussions. Strict training in technique and enforcement of rules may help reduce these competition injuries (Figure 7.3).

Any craft event can result in trauma. Competitors can be hit by their own or another competitor's board, ski or boat. The result may be bruises, fractures, lacerations, eye injuries or neck or closed-head injuries. High surf elevates the level of danger, especially when craft are overturned by the rough waves.

Ironman events can also result in several injuries to competitors. When multiple types of craft are being used in the same venue, there may be an increased number of injuries in competitors.

Any lifeguard competition should be halted if the surf or any other environmental condition becomes dangerous. There should be dedicated lifeguards at any competitive event. Their only job should be to monitor the competition area for competitors in distress or danger. Adequate first aid personnel and equipment should be on-site. An EOP should be in place for more serious injuries. The event should have adequate organizational personnel to make sure the event is run in a safe and professional manner. The event area should be clear of all hazards. The terrain, including the beach and the water, should be monitored for any sudden drop-offs or holes which could lead to falls or cervical spine or knee injuries. Adequate shade and hydration should be available. Finally, all competitors should demonstrate good sportsmanship and be proficient in their events, especially if crafts are involved, so that they do not endanger others with undue lack of skill and/or care (Figure 7.4) [63].

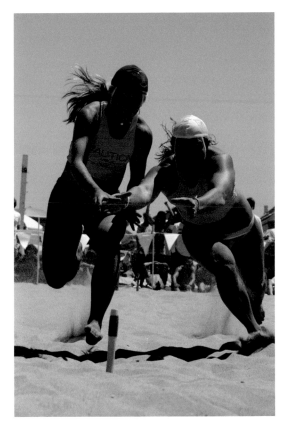

Figure 7.3 Beach flags competition. (Courtesy of Jo Wagenhals, Pompano Beach, Florida. With permission.)

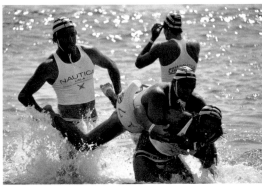

Figure 7.4 Lifeguards showing proficiency and teamwork in a rescue competition. (Courtesy of Jo Wagenhals, Pompano Beach, Florida. With permission.)

TREATMENT

The actual treatment of all possible lifeguard job-related conditions is beyond the scope of this chapter, but several generalities can be made during a discussion of several unique aspects of the job.

Many of the lifeguard on-the-job injuries can initially be treated with the first aid knowledge expected of all lifeguards. For example: Remove the injured guard to a safe location. If a serious injury has occurred, call 911 or the emergency response number in your area. Begin CPR if necessary. Use a defibrillator if indicated. Control bleeding. Immobilize the spine as per local protocol if required. Splint all possible fractures. Transport when feasible for further advanced care.

For lesser injuries, which are usually musculoskeletal, the standard Rest, Ice, Compression, Elevation (RICE) protocol can be applied. If the injuries are minor, this treatment may be all that is required. For more serious injuries, a physician should conduct a full medical evaluation. Further work up – x-rays, MRIs, and blood work – may be required. Specialized treatment may then be prescribed, such as physical therapy, medication, braces, even surgery. On-the-job injuries can result in significant workers' compensation claims and costs [64].

After any serious injury or illness, lifeguards should be required to obtain clearance from their physicians for return to full duty. All lifeguard agencies should have standard guidelines and forms for reporting injuries and returning the injured lifeguards to their duties after treatment [65]. These recorded data can show injury trends and lead to systemic changes that may reduce future injuries [42]. The treating physician should be familiar with the requirements of lifeguarding. Prior to return to full duty, if modified duty is available, lifeguards should be offered this alternative. In instances where the time off was prolonged, lifeguards may be required to requalify or retest for the position. Any full-duty lifeguards must be able to perform all of the athletic and intellectual duties of the job at 100%. A lower standard of competence will put lifeguards and the public in danger. If lifeguards cannot return to full capacity, alternate employment should be sought.

If lifeguards are under the influence of drugs or alcohol, they obviously cannot perform their duties at the highest level. Even lifeguards who are 'hung over' are not at their best. Any lifeguard agency employment programme should feature education, substance abuse policies and a code of ethics to prevent these problems. Drug or alcohol testing protocols should be in place to prevent danger to the public and other lifeguards and to help with the rehabilitation of anyone involved.

PREVENTION

Well-documented evidence about the injuries and illnesses sustained by lifeguards can be found in the literature [21]. Various actions to prevent injury, illness and disability to lifeguards have been addressed earlier in this chapter. Below is a summary of these important and necessary preventative steps for agencies and their lifeguards. The actual science behind these recommendations is often inferred and based on expert opinion.

1. Apply appropriate pre-employment medical screening to all lifeguard applicants.
2. Require all beach lifeguards to meet and maintain at least annually the fitness levels required for their positions.
3. Provide the proper training and testing to assure that all employed lifeguards have the necessary, detailed professional knowledge and skills to perform their duties.
4. Always provide a safe work environment.
5. Require all lifeguards to be fully knowledgeable of the local environmental hazards.
6. Assure adequate shade and other protection from weather and the environment for all lifeguards.
7. Always require lifeguards to wear appropriate uniforms including sun protection (shirts, hats etc.).
8. Always require the use of UV protective sunglasses.
9. Have SPF 30 or greater sunscreen readily available for all lifeguards.
10. Make adequate hydration available at all times for all lifeguards with appropriate procedures and shift rotations to prevent overheating and dehydration.
11. Provide appropriate shelter, clothing and procedures to prevent hypothermia in cold conditions.
12. Require yearly dermatological checks for all lifeguards.

13. Monitor air quality and notify lifeguards and the public when the beaches are unsafe. Have procedures in place to protect lifeguards from hazardous air exposure.

14. Monitor water quality and close the waterfront as necessary to protect the public and lifeguards.

15. Monitor the weather and have procedures in place to protect the public and lifeguards from lightning and other severe weather.

16. Conduct regular and appropriate training on marine envenomations. Ensure that necessary protocols and equipment are present to treat these conditions.

17. Monitor the local marine life for danger and have protocols in place to close the water when hazardous conditions exist.

18. In unsafe surf conditions, have protocols in place to close the waterfront.

19. Keep the sand free of sharp objects and other hazards that can cause lacerations and other injuries.

20. Allow lifeguards to wear appropriate protective clothing as required, e.g. footwear, skin suits and wetsuits.

21. Assure that lifeguard stands are constructed and maintained in a manner that reduces injuries. Make provisions for safe transition to the sand in a rescue.

22. Instruct lifeguards in proper ergonomics, especially avoiding low back and other injuries. If necessary, provide mechanisms to assist with the movement of heavy objects.

23. Require that all lifeguards using equipment are well trained on its proper use.

24. Purchase and use only the safest equipment possible and maintain it to the appropriate standards.

25. Require all lifeguard users of powered equipment (vehicles, PWCs, IRBs, ATVs) to be fully trained and certified.

26. Provide biohazard training for all lifeguards and ensure that they have equipment applicable to their locations. Proper medical protocols should be in place and activated if exposure occurs. All lifeguards should have a complete hepatitis B vaccine course, hepatitis A series where endemic and up-to-date tetanus immunization.

27. Ensure that proper decontamination supplies are available and standards in place for mani-kins and other equipment.

28. All lifeguards need training to appropriately handle unruly patrons. Assure that lifeguards know how to manage altercations. If lifeguards have additional law enforcement responsibilities assure that they are properly trained and have appropriate backup.

29. Require an appropriate level of training and testing to assure that any lifeguard can perform at the highest possible level, but also have programs in place to discourage over-training. Train lifeguards in proper technique. Encourage cross-training.

30. Have clear policies and procedures to deal with injured lifeguards. These should include access to medical evaluation and treatment, time off and duty modification as required and assessments for return to full duty.

31. Have comprehensive policies in place to deal with, monitor and test for lifeguards with possible substance abuse.

COMPETITION PREVENTATIVE ACTIONS

1. Ensure that all participating lifeguards have the proper skills, training and sportsmanship to perform in a safe manner.

2. Ensure that the venue has no visible or hidden hazards on the sand or in the water.

3. Provide a dedicated safety officer who can halt the competition at any time due to unsafe conditions.

4. Consider mandating that all competitors wear highly visible rash guards.

5. Staff events at all times with dedicated safety and first aid personnel who are qualified to support lifeguarding competitions.

6. Adequate shade and hydration should be available for all competitors and officials.

7. Consider PFDs and helmets for all craft competitors.

CONCLUSION

Beach lifeguards dedicate their lives to a unique and heroic profession. The nature of their occupation involves an outdoor, ever-changing environment that includes marine and land hazards and an unpredictable public. This environment results in certain dangers for lifeguards every time they take the stand. Lifeguards are subject to various sports-related injuries during their training, competitions and work. Knowledge about where and how these injuries occur can help lifeguards avoid them. Implementing numerous preventative steps will increase safety for the lifeguards and ultimately improve protection for the public. We will never be able to eliminate all medical, environmental and interpersonal risks to our lifeguards. We should strive to provide them with the highest levels of protection and prevention possible during performance of their lifesaving duties.

REFERENCES

1. Madden K. Lifeguards: Taking a Dive. Available at http://consumer.com/encyclopedia/work-and-health-41/occupational-health-news-507/lifeguards-taking-a-dive-646724.html

2. Gidman J. Utter Tragedy: Swimmer Survives, Lifeguard Dies. 7 July 2014. Available at http://www.usatoday.com/story/news/nation/2014/07/07/newser-lifeguard-dies-swimmer-survives/12288621/

3. Scruggs D. Lifeguards Face Health Hazards. *The Orlando Sentinel*, 29 April 1988. Available at http://articles.orlandosentinel.com/1988-04-29/news/0030400117_1_pterygium-lifeguards-skin-cancer

4. World Health Organization. *Solar Ultraviolet Radiation: Global Burden of Disease from Solar Ultraviolet Radiation*. Environmental Burden of Disease Series, N.13. WHO, Switzerland; 2006.

5. Lin JS, Eder M, Weinmann S. Behavioral counseling to prevent skin cancer: A systematic review for the U.S. Preventive Services Task Force. *Ann Intern Med*. 2011; 154(3): 190–201.

6. Brewster BC. Lifeguard skin cancer protection. *Presented to the International Lifesaving Federation Medical/Rescue Conference*, San Diego, CA, September, 1997.

7. Guidman. American Academy of Dermatology, Draft Research Plan on Screening for Skin Cancer, 2014. Available at http://www.aad.org/media-resources/stats-and-facts/conditions/skin-cancer

8. American Cancer Society. Cancer Facts and Figures. Available at http://www.cancer.org/cancer/skincancer-melanoma/index

9. Bradford PT, Freedman DM, Goldstein AM, Tucker MA. Increased risk of second primary cancers after a diagnosis of melanoma. *Arch Dermatol*. 2010; 146(3): 265–72.

10. Song F, Qureshi AA, Giovannucci EL, et al. Risk of a second primary cancer after non-melanoma skin cancer in white men and women: A prospective cohort study. *PLoS Med*. 2013; 10(4): e1001433. doi:10.1371/journal.pmed.1001433.

11. Hall DM, et al. Effectiveness of a targeted, peer-driven skin cancer prevention programme for lifeguards. *Int J Aquat Res Educ*. 2008; 2(4): 287–97.

12. Green AC, Williams GM, Logan V, Strutton GM. Reduced melanoma after regular sunscreen use: Randomized trial follow-up. *J Clin Oncol*. 2011; 29: 257–63.

13. Lifeguard Hydration. Available at http://www.cultureofsafety.com/aquatics/lifeguard-hydration/

14. Inter-Association Task Force on Exertion Heat Illness Consensus Statement. Available at http://www.nata.org/sites/default/files/Heat-Illness-Task-Force-Consensus-Statement.pdf

15. Gustafson S. The Physical Hazards of Lifeguarding. Available at http://voices.yahoo.com/the-physical-hazards-lifeguarding/content_date_07_05_2009_11.html

16. Vavrek J, Holle RL, Allsopp J. Flash to bang. *Earth Scientist*. 1993; 10: 3–8.

17. Taylor DM, Ashby K, Winkel KD. An analysis of marine animal injuries presenting to emergency departments in Victoria, Australia. *Wilderness Environ Med*. 2002; 13(2): 106–12.

18. Ryan K. Lifeguard injuries in the city and county of Honolulu. *Presented to the USLA Fall Board of Directors Meeting*, Hyanis, 2013.

19. Weinberg AD. Hypothermia. *Ann Emerg Med*. 1993; 22(Pt 2): 370–7.

20. The China Post News Staff with CAN. Lightning Strike Kills Lifeguard, Injures 3 Others. 15 July 2013. Available at http://www.chinapost.comtw/print/383795.htm

21. Bierens JJLM. (ed.). *Handbook on Drowning Prevention, Rescue, Treatment*. Springer, Heidelberg, pp. 515–19.

22. US Life Saving Association. Available at http://www.usla.org/?page=lightning.

23. Thaller EI, et al. Moderate increases in ambient PM2.5 and ozone are associated with lung function decreases in beach lifeguards. *J Occup Environ Med*. 2008; 50(2): 202–11.

24. Backer LC, et al. Occupational exposure to aerosolized brevetoxins during Florida red tide events: Effects on a healthy worker population. *Environ Health Perspect*. 2005; 113(5): 644–9.

25. Chang YS, et al. Characterization of marine aerosol for assessment of human exposure to brevetoxins. *Environ Health Perspect*. 2005; 113(5): 638–43.

26. Fletemeyer J, Roche B. Lifeguard foot injuries occurring in the beach environment. *Presented to the US Lifesaving Association Southeast Region*, San Diego, California, 1 November 1989.

27. US Life Saving Association, San Diego Lifeguard Service Injury Report (1996–1998), San Diego, California.

28. The Redwoods Group. Preventing Lifeguard Slips and Falls. The Redwoods Group Insurance Programs for YMCAs Risk Management Topic, 26 July 2011.

29. Naplesnews.com. Lifeguard Bitten by Shark in Florida. 17 December 2009. Available at http://www.naplesnews.com/news/2009/nov/17/lifeguard-bitten-shark-florida/

30. KATU.com. Hero lifeguard was victim of shark attack. 5 February 2010. Available at http://www.katu.com/news/national/83641372.html; http://surf.transworld.net/1000077882/news/tiger-shark-attacks-and-kills-south-african-lifeguard/

31. Bierschenk E. Vero Beach lifeguard, rescue personnel honored for rescue of shark bite victim. Available at http://www.tcpalm.com/news/vero-beach-lifeguard-rescue-personnel-honored-of

32. Green M, et al. *Report into the NSW Shark Meshing (Bather Protection) Program*. NSW DPI Fisheries Conservation and Aquaculture Branch; 2009; New South Wales, Australia.

33. Tibbals, J., Australian venomous jellyfish, envenomation syndromes, toxins and therapy, *Toxicon*. 2006; 48(7): 830–59.

34. Morizot L. When, where and how ocean rescue lifeguards are suffering occupational injuries? *Paper presented at the USLA Spring Board of Directors Meeting*, Miami, FL, 2012.

35. Corbett SJ, et al. The health effects of swimming at Sydney beaches. The Sydney Beach Users Study Advisory Group. *Am J Public Health*. 1993; 83(12): 1701–6.

36. Sullivan CSB. Acute illnesses among Los Angeles County lifeguards according to worksite exposures. *Am J Public Health*. 1989; 79: 1561–3.

37. Kueh CS, Grohmann GS. Recovery of viruses and bacteria in waters off Bondi beach: A pilot study. *Med J Aust*. 1989; 151: 632–8.

38. Schiff KC, Weisberg SB, Dorsey JH. Microbiological monitoring of marine recreational waters in southern California. *Environ Manag*. 2001; 27: 149–57.

39. Wortman B. Testing for asbestos closes tower. 9 July 2012. Available at http://www.sunshinecoastdaily.com.au/news/testing-for-asbestos-closes-patrol-tower-sunshine-/1445637/

40. Available at http://sls.com.au/content/australian-championships-inquiries-update

41. Wernicki P, Glorioso J. Lifeguarding: The sport, the profession, the hazards. *Physician Sports Med*. 1991; 19(4): 84–95.

42. Bigby K, McClure R, Green A. The incidence of inflatable rescue boat injuries in Queensland surf lifesavers. *Med J Aust*. 2000; 172: 485–8.

43. Ludcke J, Pearcy M, Evans J, et al. Impact data for the investigation of injuries in inflatable rescue boats (IRBs). *Aust Phys Eng Sci Med*. 2001; 24: 95–101.

44. Ashton L, Grujic L. Foot and ankle injuries occurring during inflatable rescue boats (IRB) during surf lifesaving activities. *J Orthop Surg*. 2001; 9: 39–43.

45. Available at au/news/national/man-charged-over-lifeguard-assault/2005/12/07/11338

46. Available at http://www.mauinews.com/page/content.detail/id/507183/Man--31--faces-charges-in-assault-on-lifeguard.html

47. Available at http://www.pressofatlanticcity.com/news/press/atlantic_city/article_d800ed64-a7e7-11df-99d8-001cc4c002e0.html

48. Eve Samples. Martin County ocean lifeguards deserve high risk designation. *TCPalm*, 8 February 2010. Available at http://www.tcpalm.com/news/columnists/eve-samples-ocean-lifeguards-deserve-high-risk

49. Dahl AM, Miller DI. Body contact swimming rescues—What are the risks? *Am J Public Health*. 1979; 69: 150–2.

50. Occupational Health and Safety Administration. *Occupational Exposure to Bloodborne Pathogens. 29 CFR Part 1910.1030.* Occupational Health and Safety Administration, US Department of Labor, Washington DC; 1991.

51. Dobbins JG. Communicable disease avoidance for lifeguards. *Presented at the International Lifesaving Medical/Rescue Conference*, San Diego, CA, 1997.

52. United States department of Labor, Occupational Safety and Health Administration. *Occupational Exposure to Bloodborne Pathogens*, US Dept. of Labor. Washington, DC, 1992.

53. Kozlowski J. Junior Lifeguard Competition Participant Assumes Risk of Injury. 2000. Available at http://cehdclass.gmu.edu/jkozlows/lawarts/07JUL00.pdf

54. Breslin FC, et al. Workplace injury or "part of the job?" Towards a gendered understanding of injuries and complaints among young workers. *Soc Sci Med*. 2007; 64(4): 782–93.

55. Van Mechelen W, Hlobil H, Kemper H. Incidence, severity, a etiology and prevention of sports injuries. A review of concepts. *Sports Med*. 1992; 14: 8.

56. Pen LJ, et al. An injury profile of elite ironman competitors. *Aust J Med Sport*. 1996; 28(1): 7–11

57. Parsons D. Junior Lifeguard's death devastates Huntington Beach. Available at http://articles.latimes.com/2009/jul/16/local/me-junior-lifeguard16

58. McFarland EG, Wasik M. Injuries in female collegiate swimmers due to swimming and cross training. *Clin J Sport Med*. 1996; 6: 178–82.

59. Hickey GJ, Fricker PA, McDonald WA. Injuries to elite rowers over a 10-yr period. *Med Sci Sports Exerc*. 1997; 29: 1567–72.

60. Erby R, Heard R, O'Loughlin K. Trial of an injury reporting system for surf lifesavers in Australia. *Work*. 2010; 36: 181–92.

61. Mitchell R, Brighton B, Sherker S. The epidemiology of competition and training-based surf sport-related injury in Australia, 2003–2011. *J Sci Med Sport*. 2012; 16: 18–21. doi:10.1016/j.jsams.2012.05.009.

62. Surf Life Saving Australia. *Australian Surf Sports Manual. No. 3.* 33rd ed. Sydney: Surf Life Saving Australia; 2008.

63. Atlantic County New Jersey, US Municipal Joint Insurance Fund. Analysis of lifeguard accidents. *Presented at the Annual Risk Management Seminar*, Ocean City, NJ, 2000.

64. Australian Lifeguard Service. Health and Safety. Available at http://www.lifeguards.com.au/My_Lifeguard_Service/Health

65. Neale RE, Purdie JL, Hirst LW, Green AC. Sun exposure as a risk factor for nuclear cataract. *Epidemiology*. 2003; 14(6): 707–12.

8

Beach lifeguard first aid

KEVIN MORAN AND JUSTIN SEMPSROTT

INTRODUCTION

Throughout history the beach has been identified as a popular site of recreation and community leisure [1]. While a visit to the beach is generally viewed as indicative of a healthy lifestyle, it does have its attendant risks – the omnipresent threat of drowning being the most obvious. A modern phenomenon in many countries has been the provision of lifeguard services primarily charged with the role of preventing drowning. A study of lifesaving experts agreed that the lifeguard service was the single most important component on a beach that could prevent injuries and accidents [2]. While this role remains the *raison d'être* for such provision, a secondary role related to the provision of non-drowning, primary medical care has emerged as an adjunct to the task of drowning prevention. For example, in the five years from 2007 to 2012, Surf Life Saving New Zealand (SLSNZ) reported that lifeguards provided first aid treatment to almost 9000 beachgoers, an average of 1772 cases per annum – more than the average number of rescues (*n* = 1343) performed each year [3]. In spite of this emergent, and in some cases, increasing responsibility of beach lifeguards, little is known

about the nature of beach injuries or medical conditions necessitating first aid at the beach. It is the purpose of this chapter to review what is known about lifeguard first aid by using available evidence from selected countries where first aid knowledge and practice is a part of everyday lifeguarding and where there is a public expectation that such a role be performed on the front line at the beach.

This chapter follows a slightly different format in that it provides the best epidemiologic data about the conditions encountered by lifeguards throughout the world and a compendium of the treatment of common non-drowning medical problems presented to beach lifeguards. There is also an up-to-date reference list, which constitutes the evidence for the advice offered and recommendations made. As is normally the case at the forefront of medical science, many areas are lacking in definitive evidence, the evidence is contested or the approaches adopted vary by region. Beach environments around the world vary greatly both in their physical geography, water currents, potential risks and injuries encountered. For example, more traumatic injuries may occur in areas with steep cliffs or rocky outcroppings, while more jellyfish stings and heat illness may occur at a flat, sandy beach with year-round warm water.

Thus, while it is the intention that the advice offered be a useful guide, beach lifeguards should consult their local medical advisors and guidelines where appropriate.

EPIDEMIOLOGICAL STUDY

New Zealand

Leisure-related injuries and other conditions requiring first aid attention by lifeguards patrolling New Zealand surf beaches from 2007 to 2012 were evaluated to determine the nature and extent of non-drowning-related incidents [4]. The frequency and diversity of non-drowning-related injury/illness incidents necessitating first aid treatment ($n = 8,547$) found in this study suggests that risk of beach-related injury is omnipresent, even though many of the incidents were minor, and most victims (82%) left the scene in a stable condition. More injuries were sustained by males (57%).

In a study on childhood beach injuries using the same database, Moran and Webber [5] noted that children aged less than 16 accounted for one-half (52%) of all injuries; of these 55% were male, and incidence peaked in the 11 to 15 year age group (24%). Most incidents (90%) required minor treatment, with lacerations (44%) the most common injury. Marine stings accounted for one-quarter (24%) of injuries and were most frequent among younger children (<10 years). Injuries to the extremities were frequently noted in the incident reports, the feet (33%) and hands (8%) being common sites.

Volunteer lifeguards who patrol the beaches on summer weekends and public holidays were the most frequent type of lifeguard service provider ($n = 4508$; 53%), with regional lifeguards employed during the weekdays during busy summer months (from December through February) providing 42% of first aid responses ($n = 3580$) [4]. Call out lifeguards (usually engaged in after-hours emergencies) and special events lifeguards (used in aquatic sports such as triathlons) also contributed to the provision of first aid ($n = 145$; 2%). Almost one-fifth of injuries were to members of surf life-saving clubs ($n = 1503$; 18%).

Table 8.1 shows that soft tissue injuries including lacerations and bruising accounted for more than half (59%) of all injuries requiring lifeguard first aid. Marine and insect stings were responsible for one-fifth (21%) of cases.

More than half (54%) of the injuries were sustained in the water, one-third (35%) of these being swimming related. Almost one-third (32%) of all injuries from 2007 to 2012 were attributed to walking/running activity. In a separate study of surfing-related injuries, Moran and Webber found that surfing injuries accounted for 16% of all first aid cases [6]. More males than females were treated for surfing injuries (68% male, 31% female). Lacerations (59%) and bruising (15%) accounted for most of the injuries. The head was the most common site of surfing injury (32%), and most injuries were caused by contact with the victim's own board (50%).

Figure 8.1 shows that almost half (43%) of the injuries were to the lower limbs, with one-quarter (26%) of these confined to the feet. The upper limbs accounted for almost one-fifth (17%) of beach injuries, with soft tissue injuries to the hand, fingers and wrists (11%) being the most frequent. Head and neck injuries (13%) consisted mainly of lacerations, with nose bleeds ($n = 80$; 2%) also identified as a specific injury.

Figure 8.2 shows that most incidents (71%) required the use of first aid disposables (such as

Table 8.1 New Zealand beach first aid incidents (SLSNZ), 2007–2012

Nature of injury	n	%
Laceration	3986	47.2
Bruising	1005	11.9
Marine sting	1376	16.3
Breathing difficulties	228	2.7
Cramp	71	0.8
Insect sting	367	4.4
Sunburn/burns	64	0.8
Other (feeling unwell)	389	4.6
Other (unspecified)	960	11.4
Total	8446	100.0

Source: SLSNZ Patrol Statistics 2007–2012. Surf Life Saving New Zealand. Available at www.surflifesaving.org.nz/lifeguarding/patrolled-beaches/patrol-statistics/

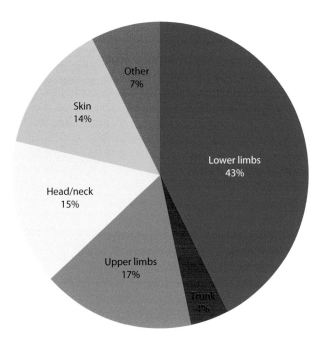

Figure 8.1 New Zealand beach first aid incidents by location of injury, 2007–2012. (From SLSNZ Patrol Statistics 2007–2012, Surf Life Saving, New Zealand, p. 116.)

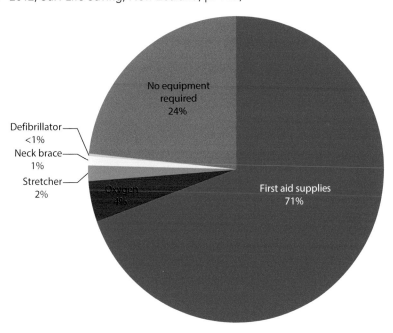

Figure 8.2 Equipment used by lifeguards in treating first aid casualties, SLSNZ 2007–2012. (From SLSNZ Patrol Statistics 2007–2012, Surf Life Saving, New Zealand, p. 116.)

wound dressings, surgical tape, adhesive plasters and medi-wipes). One-quarter (24%) of incidents required no equipment, and a small proportion required oxygen therapy (4%), stretcher (2%), neck brace (1%) or defibrillation (<1%).

Most first aid treatments (82%) were minor and patients left the scene in a stable condition after treatment. That one-fifth (18%) of incidents were sufficiently severe for further medical intervention to be recommended or required suggests that some injuries incurred at beaches are potentially serious. The use of advanced equipment including defibrillation for cardiac arrest (n = 22), immobilization via stretcher/neck braces (n = 226) or oxygen therapy (n = 372) further suggests that some cases may also be life-threatening. The seriousness of incidents is compounded by the diversity of pre-existing conditions (n = 129) that beachgoers bring to the beach. These conditions may be exacerbated when an individual is active at the beach. Some examples of conditions that would be worsened include exercised-induced asthma, hypoglycaemia in diabetics, seizures among epilepsy sufferers, cardiorespiratory conditions (for example, heart and circulatory in older beachgoers engaged in water- or land-based recreation) and extreme temperature-related conditions (n = 60) such as hypothermia, hyperthermia and dehydration.

Australia

In Australia, several sources of data, including admissions to emergency departments and lifeguard incident statistics, provide an indication of the nature and extent of beach injury and the need for lifeguard first aid. A pilot study of injuries sustained on a Victorian resort beach during the Australian summer holiday period of 1991 found that, of 211 injuries recorded, 37% were lacerations/cuts and 18% were rescues [7]. Of the listed causes of injury, 20% were from surfboards and 19% were from beach litter. In a study of admissions to the emergency departments of nine Queensland hospitals, Hockey [8]

reported that, of 1587 water-related injuries presented, drowning-related injuries formed a relatively small proportion of injuries (7%) compared with injuries resulting from being struck by an object or other persons (30%), low falls (17%) and cutting/piercing objects (11%). Swimming was the activity being undertaken prior to injury for more than a quarter (28%) of cases. Marine stings accounted for 62% of cases reported in emergency departments in Victorian hospitals from 1995 to 2000 [9]. A survey by Taylor and colleagues in 2004 found that a quarter (26%) of 646 surfers surveyed at eight Victorian beaches had sustained acute injuries, which included lacerations (46%), sprains (29%), dislocations (11%) and fractures (9%). The lower limbs (46%) and the head (26%) were the most frequently reported sites of injury [10].

Data from incident report forms reported in the annual statistics of Surf Life Saving Australia (SLSA) in their 2012 Annual Report indicate that surf lifeguards treated more than a quarter of a million beachgoers in the five years from 2008 to 2012, an average of over 50,000 patients per annum, which represents an increase of 24% in that time (Table 8.2) [11].

Analysis of the 2012 Annual Report of SLSA provides clear indication of the nature and extent of first aid incidents. Figure 8.3 shows that marine stings accounted for more than three-quarters (77%) of all first aid incidents, followed by minor cuts/abrasions (14%).

As is the case with New Zealand, Australian lifeguards now attend almost three times as many first aid incidents as they do rescue incidents.

Table 8.2 Australian first aid incidents (SLSA), 2008–2012

	2008	2009	2010	2011	2012	Total	Mean
First aid by surf lifesavers[a]	21,844	35,416	45,860	17,652	34,097	154,869	30,973
First aid by ALS lifeguards[b]	12,772	18,383	21,659	17,326	30,548	100,688	20,137
Total	34,616	53,799	67,519	34,978	64,645	255,557	51,110

Note: SLSA, Surf Life Saving Australia; Advanced Life Support (ALS).
[a] Surf lifesavers are volunteer members of SLSA.
[b] Surf lifeguards are employed members of SLSA.

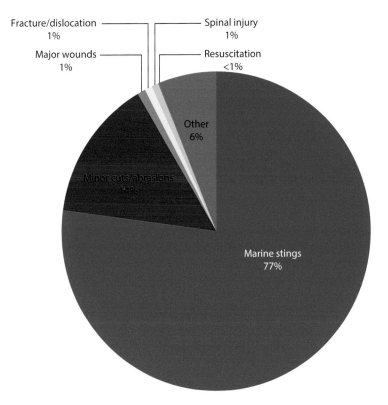

Figure 8.3 Australia beach injury type requiring lifeguard first aid, SLSA 2012. (From SLSA, sls.com. au/publications, SLSA, Roseberg, Sydney, NSW.)

Table 8.3 United Kingdom first aid incidents (RNLI), 2008–2013

	2008	2009	2010	2011	2012	2013	Total	Mean
Major first aid	612	776	972	862	870	1041	5133	856
Minor first aid	6301	8888	12,063	11,198	9584	14,297	62,331	10,389
Total	6913	9664	13,035	12,060	10,454	15,338	67,464	11,245

Source: Royal National Lifeboat Institution (RNLI); Annual Operational Statistics Reports, 2013.
Note: RNLI, Royal National Lifeboat Institution, Poole, UK.

From July 2013 to June 2014, SLSA reported 31,332 first aid responses compared with 11,055 rescue responses.*

United Kingdom

In the six years from 2008 to 2013, Royal National Lifeboat Institution (RNLI) beach lifeguards attended more than 50,000 first aid incidents, an average of 10,425 per annum (Table 8.3).

* http://sls.com.au/publications

An overview of lifeguard statistics for 2008–2013 found that 856 cases per annum were classified as major first aid incidents where the outcome was considered serious enough to warrant further medical attention [12]. In addition, they undertook an average of 10,389 minor first aid incidents per annum where the risk was low and no further treatment was required. In the same six-year period, UK lifeguards attended more first aid incidents than rescues (n = 1602 per annum), a situation similar to that of Australia and New Zealand reported above.

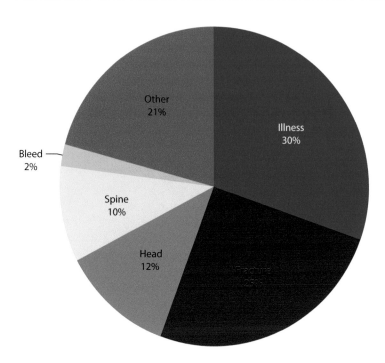

Figure 8.4 United Kingdom major beach first aid incidents (RNLI) 2012. (From Royal National Lifeboat Institution; Annual Operational Statistics Reports 2012, Royal National Life board Institution, Poole, UK.)

Analysis of the 2012 incident report forms indicates the nature of the major and minor first aid cases attended. Figure 8.4 shows that, of the non-drowning-related incidents (*n* = 857) in 2012, illnesses such as epilepsy (*n* = 33; 3.5%), chest pain (*n* = 26; 2.7%), allergy (*n* = 20; 2.1%), asthma (*n* = 16; 1.7%) and diabetes (*n* = 14; 1.5%) accounted for almost one-third (30%) of incidents. Fractures accounted for one-quarter (25%) of all major incidents, followed by head injuries (12%), spinal injuries (10%) and major bleeding (2%). Other incidents such as loss of consciousness (3.3%), hypothermia (4.6%) and hyperthermia (4.3%) accounted for a further one-fifth (21%) of major first aid cases treated by beach lifeguards. In most instances, the casualty handover for further medical treatment was to the ambulance service (56.8%) or to a relative/caregiver (23.6%).

Table 8.4 shows the more frequently occurring minor first aid incidents that necessitated treatment but no further intervention. Marine stings (primarily from contact with the poisonous dorsal spines and gills of the weever fish, which buries itself in the sand) accounted for half (50%) of the minor first aid incidents in 2012. Small lacerations and puncture wounds accounted for more than a quarter (27%) of

Table 8.4 United Kingdom minor first aid incidents (RNLI), 2012

Nature of injury	n	%
Marine sting	4752	49.6
Laceration/puncture	2607	27.2
Abrasion/bruising	1050	11.0
Eye injury	287	3.0
Insect bite/sting	113	1.2
Sprain/strain	102	1.1
Unknown	88	0.9
Other	585	6.0
Total	9584	100.0

Note: RNLI, Royal National Lifeboat Institution.

minor incidents. Among the less frequently occurring first aid incidents reported, but indicative of the variety of incident types that challenge beach lifeguards' knowledge and training, were nosebleeds, dog bites, panic attacks, cramps, splinters, burns, sunburn and fish hook entrapment [12].

RNLI operational statistics for 2012 also indicate that, for minor first aid cases, hot water was the most frequent treatment (26%), not surprising since half of all minor incidents were attributed to weever fish sting (where irrigation of the sting site with hot water is the standard treatment). Other equipment used in the treatment of superficial wounds include the use of medi-wipes (17%); adhesive plasters (16%); wound closure dressings such as surgical tape, gauze and crepe bandages (6%); eyewash (5%); and cold compresses (2%).

United States

Some research evidence is available to indicate the nature of beach injuries in the United States. An early study of paediatric water-related injuries in Hawaii found that, of 133 paediatric cases reported in a 12-month period, most incidents occurred at beaches (75%), involved males (70%) and were sustained when playing, swimming or surfing [13]. Injuries included head and neck trauma (7.5%), external injuries (66.2%) and 34 other injuries (25.6%). A more recent paediatric study in the Norfolk/Virginia Beach area found that the most common types of injuries were lacerations/puncture wounds (32%), followed by musculoskeletal injuries (26%), marine stings (13%), abrasions/contusions (13%), head injury (3%) and sunburn (3%) [14]. Some evidence is available on surfing injuries via descriptive data obtained from a web-based survey of 1348 surfers that reported lacerations accounted for 42% of all acute injuries, followed by contusions (13%), sprains/strains (12%) and fractures (8%) [15].

National statistics on the nature and extent of first aid interventions are solicited annually (there is no statutory requirement to report) from all public and private beach lifeguard organizations by the United States Lifesaving Association (USLA), though surf beaches are not differentiated from other sites of lifeguard activity such as lakes and inland waterways [16]. Over 100 organizations have reported in recent years. Table 8.5 identifies first aid incidents in terms of major and minor incidents. Major first aid cases require further

Table 8.5 United States first aid incidents (USLA), 2007–2013

Nature of injury	n	%
Minor	1,883,199	94.5
Major	109,673	5.5
Total	1,992,872	100.0

Note: USLA, US Lifesaving Association.

attention from higher levels of medical care such as paramedics, emergency transport or specialized medical response. Minor first aid incidents do not require a higher level of medical care beyond that provided by the lifeguard.

While the nature and cause of beach injuries treated by lifeguards are not routinely analyzed and published, the incident report forms used by some US lifeguard organizations require the reporting of information including the nature of the injury (such as abrasion, laceration, burn, fracture and 'other' injury) the activity prior to treatment (such as swimming, surfing walking/running, beach activity and jumping/diving) as well as the treatment outcome (such as released, released to parent, advised to see physician, ambulance or police). Copies of the USLA recommended incident report forms are available in *Open Water Lifesaving – The USLA Manual* [17].

Further indication of the integral part that first aid response plays in US lifeguarding is evidenced in the requirements for lifeguard qualification. For a beach lifeguard organization to achieve USLA certification (accreditation), all lifeguards employed on a seasonal basis are required at minimum to undergo a 21-hour first aid course (with CPR in addition). Lifeguards employed full time, year-round must at minimum complete a 43.5-hour First Responder course. The USLA encourages all beach lifeguard employers to require the First Responder course for their seasonal lifeguards and the Emergency Medical Technician course (120–150 hours) for their year-round lifeguards. This level of training is the norm in California, for example (Chris Brewster, personal communication, 6 June 2014). Some agencies, most notably Los Angeles County, have some paramedic lifeguards who provide the full range of paramedic services (Figure 8.5).

Brazil

Statistics on first aid responses at beaches in Brazil are not routinely published even though beach lifeguards perform many such services at patrolled beaches along the almost 7000 km of coastline. Some evidence of the nature of this provision is available from case study research conducted along the beaches of Rio de Janeiro. In the capital city, the Lifeguard Service (GMar-CBMERJ) is responsible for beach safety along a 90-km coastline that employs 1200 lifeguards and includes specialized medical teams in two different

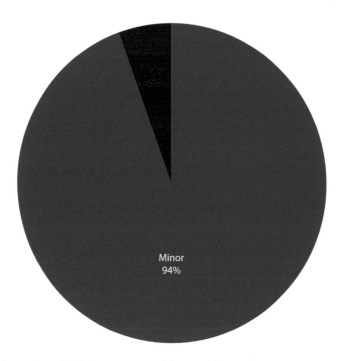

Figure 8.5 United States beach injuries requiring lifeguard first aid, USLA 2011–2012. (From US Lifesaving Association, San Diego, US, Available at arc.usla.org/statistics/public.asp)

medical-care centres, called *drowning resuscitation centres* (DRC). The centres provide pre-hospital emergency facilities at the beach and have been specifically developed to deal with aquatic emergencies. A retrospective study of all rescues and medical emergencies dispatched or at the DRC from 1991 to 2000 in one centre (which is responsible for a 32-mile-long coastline) was presented at the World Congress on Drowning in Amsterdam in 2002 by Szpilman et al. [18]. In addition to reporting on drowning emergencies ($n = 930$), the study also reported on 3480 non-drowning-related cases. These included 1590 clinical cases (dehydration, alcohol/drug overdose, convulsion, hypothermia, flu), 1404 traumas (e.g. related to cars, bikes, watercraft, paragliders, being swept off rocks, scuba diving, dog bites, surfing, cervical spine injury, fish hooks, fights, spearfishing, shoulder dislocation), 375 marine envenomations (jellyfish, hydroid) and 111 cases with missing data that could not be categorized. Of these cases, there were 12 fatalities. For all drowning and non-drowning incidents ($n = 4410$ patients), the average age was 22.4 years (SD ± 11.4), the average time in attendance at the centre was 1.12 hours (SD ± 0.23) and the average time of day when treated was 13:45 hours. Males were

Table 8.6 Brazil (Rio de Janeiro) first aid incidents (GMar-CBMERJ), 1991–2000

Nature of injury	n	%
Clinical	1590	45.7
Trauma	1404	40.3
Marine stings	375	10.8
Other (missing data)	111	3.2
Total	3480	100.0

Note: GMar-CBMERJ, Rio de Janeiro Lifeguard Service.

assisted twice as often as females, and 468(10.6%) were referred to a hospital (142 drowning-related and 319 non-drowning-related cases) (Table 8.6).

The authors concluded that the creation of a DRC at the beach was worthwhile because it reduced dispatch time, reduced the need to refer a patient to a hospital and provided excellent support for the lifeguards on the beach.

Further indication of the commitment to first aid provision by Brazil's lifeguard organisation (Sobrasa – Sociedade Brasileira de Salvamento Aquatico) is evidenced in the training and certification programme in place for beach lifeguards [19]. In its Beach Lifeguard Certificate course of

110 hours, lifeguards are trained to implement basic life support at the beach, perform a secondary examination including head-to-toe palpation, treat suspected cervical trauma in a rescue situation, learn how to proceed in both clinical and traumatic emergencies and know how to plan for civil disaster and major emergencies. Further information on lifeguarding courses is available on the Sobrasa website.*

PRACTICAL IMPLICATIONS

On the basis of the research findings reported here, it is recommended that beach lifeguards and their organizations adopt and promote the following to treat beach injuries:

1. Continued refinement of lifeguard first aid training to address frequently occurring specific injuries (for example, soft tissue injuries of the foot and ankle).
2. Close attention to ways of tending to children and paediatric first aid cases during lifeguard training.
3. Increase in research and publication on first aid incidents internationally.
4. Adoption of evidence-based practice guidelines for treatment of injuries. A compendium of common injuries encountered by beach lifeguards is presented below.

Basic soft tissue injuries (haemorrhage control) [20–94]

Lifeguards often encounter bleeding wounds ranging from minor scrapes and abrasions to major lacerations and amputations. There are no studies on haemorrhage control in the lifeguard environment and guidelines are extrapolated from other prehospital and operating theatre experience. Direct pressure remains the primary means of stopping bleeding. Elevating the wound and compression of proximal pressure points have little evidence and are not shown to be effective. Application of a pressure bandage utilizing gauze and an elastic bandage can supplement direct pressure.

There are numerous commercially available haemostatic gauze agents with varied mechanisms of action. No product has been found to

* http://www.sobrasa.org/cursos/cursos.htm

be superior to any other haemostatic gauze, but all have been found superior to cotton gauze for stopping moderate to severe bleeding. Their use should be considered in the treatment of moderate to severe bleeding as an adjunct to direct pressure.

As a result of experience from recent armed conflicts worldwide, the use of tourniquets has increased exponentially. Numerous military studies show that stopping severe extremity haemorrhage with tourniquets has saved lives. Civilian use has followed this trend and tourniquets are now utilized by emergency medical service agencies and by many non-medical law enforcement and first response personnel. With appropriate training, tourniquets can be safely used in the lifeguard setting for life-threatening extremity haemorrhage. Despite conventional teaching that tourniquet application will universally result in limb amputation, two hours is a conservative amount of time that a limb can be ischaemic without adverse consequences, although there are numerous case reports of tourniquet application ranging from 4 to 16 hours without resultant loss of limb. Commercially available tourniquets have fewer complications and better efficacy than improvised tourniquets. A properly applied tourniquet will be painful and requires training specific to the device used. Tourniquet use must be accompanied by appropriate training, as improper application can exacerbate pain and bleeding.

Wounds and abrasions [95–129]

Lifeguards are often tasked with cleaning minor wounds that may or may not require further treatment at a healthcare facility. There are no studies specific to wound care in the lifeguard environment and recommendations are based on extrapolation from pre-hospital, emergency department, outpatient and inpatient studies. There is considerable evidence that wound infection rates are similar for wounds irrigated with tap water or sterile saline. Hydrogen peroxide and isopropyl alcohol are potent antiseptics, but also damage healthy tissue and have been shown to delay wound healing. In areas where antibiotic ointments are available without prescription, they have been shown to be superior to petroleum jelly alone and to no treatment. It is recommended that lifeguards cleanse wounds with sterile saline or tap water under pressure, then apply antibiotic ointment, if available, and protective gauze dressing as indicated. All wounds that penetrate deeper than the subcutaneous fat should be referred to a doctor for further evaluation and treatment.

Basic orthopaedic injuries [130–148]

No published studies were identified for the treatment of suspected fractures, sprains or strains of extremities in the lifeguard setting, and guidelines are extrapolated from pre-hospital, outpatient and emergency department data. Any injury to an extremity with swelling, pain, inability to bear weight or loss of normal function should be assumed to have an underlying fracture to the bone. Initial assessment should include documentation of pulse, motor and sensory function distal to the injury. Treatment should involve application of ice and splinting in the position found. For lifeguards with advanced medical training operating in remote areas with prolonged access to definitive healthcare, partial reduction of angulated fractures in pulse-less extremity should be considered.

Hyperthermia [149–202]

No studies were identified specific to the treatment of hyperthermia (heat cramps, heat exhaustion, heat stroke) in the lifeguard setting. Guidelines are extrapolated from pre-hospital and emergency department data. Heat illness can be caused by exposure to elevated environmental temperatures, especially with coexistent exertion. Consideration should be given to medical causes such as diabetes, heart disease and medication side effects in patients with non-exertional heat illness. All patients considered to have any heat-related illness should be removed from the exposure to a cooler environment. Patients with heat cramps will require only additional support from salt-containing beverages for oral rehydration. Heat exhaustion should additionally be treated with cooling fans, misting devices or ice packs and transfer to emergency medical services. Heatstroke, as characterized by heat illness with altered mental status or other neurologic deficit, is a life-threatening emergency and should be aggressively treated by any means possible. If the heatstroke is associated with a collapse in peripheral blood flow, cooling will have to be via conductive cooling by immersion in a bath of cold water. Patients with a viable peripheral circulation can be cooled by wetting with misting devices or copious amounts of water and evaporative cooling with fans.

Hypothermia [203–222]

No studies were identified specific to the treatment of hypothermia by lifeguards. Guidelines are extrapolated from case reports, manikins and limited healthy human volunteer studies.

Normal human body temperature is 36°C–38°C. Hypothermia is arbitrarily divided into mild (32°C–35°C), moderate (28°C–32°C) and severe (<28°C). Water is thermoneutral at 35°C, which means that any water temperature below this point will cause a naked immersed person to lose body heat and eventually become hypothermic. Drowning patients and rescued persons can become hypothermic, even if the air and water temperature seem warm. In the absence of a thermometer, all rescued persons should be assumed to have mild hypothermia if they are shivering after rescue, and moderate to severe hypothermia if they are not shivering, unconscious, in cardiac arrest or have any other neurologic symptoms after rescue. Neurologic symptoms include ataxia, decreased coordination, confusion and slurred speech. Moderate and severely hypothermic casualties (identified by their level of consciousness) should be handled carefully and as critically ill patients; rough handling (including manual handling and removing clothing) can precipitate ventricular fibrillation. The presence or absence of shivering is a rough guide and not a definitive diagnostic criterion. Acutely hypothermic persons can shiver at lower temperatures, and shivering may be absent entirely in persons with chronic medical conditions, regardless of temperature.

Techniques for rewarming can be separated into passive, active external and active internal. Passive rewarming techniques with proven benefit include removal of wet clothing, moving into areas protected from cold and wind and the use of a vapour barrier against the skin with an insulating outer layer. Studies are limited in their ability to identify a single, best insulating material. Such methods result in slow rewarming, but in situations where the casualty has been cold for a long period ('chronic' hypothermia, not the norm in beach rescues) slow rewarming (<1°C.hour^{-1}) is advocated. Active external warming can be applied to all 'acutely' hypothermic patients with moderate or severe hypothermia. Techniques with proven benefit include the application of chemical heating pads, hot water bags, hot air blowers, charcoal heaters and electric blankets. Care should be taken to avoid causing burns to the patient and not to overheat the patient, thereby causing a rewarming collapse of blood pressure as the peripheral vasculature opens before the cold-induced reduction in circulating blood volume is restored. Active internal heating is beyond the scope of pre-hospital lifeguard treatment of hypothermia.

Of special note are hypothermia and drowning in the context of prognosis. Despite numerous case reports of neurologically intact survival in patients who have drowned in very cold (<6°C) water, prognosis is worse if the drowning occurs in cold water. This is further complicated because the profoundly hypothermic person may appear dead, but still have a chance to survive. Unless obvious signs of death are present or submersion time is known to be greater than 90 minutes, lifeguards should attempt resuscitation on all drowning patients regardless of water temperature. Termination of resuscitation and prognostication should be deferred to advanced practitioners and local protocol.

Spinal injury management [223–250]

Routine cervical spine immobilization with cervical collars and long spine backboards have long been components of lifeguard practice. Cervical spine injuries are rare in drowning patients, except where a mechanism of injury is expected. Patients who have experienced high-velocity ejections from watercraft, diving into shallow waters, head injury occurring in the water or focal neurologic deficits should be considered to have cervical spine injuries and restriction of spinal movement should be the mainstay of treatment. Immobilization should be accomplished by manual stabilization of the cervical spine by placing the hands on the patient's bilateral trapezius muscles and applying pressure to the head with the forearms.

Cervical collars and long spine backboards have been shown to cause harm and are of equivocal benefit in patients with known and suspected cervical spine injuries. They should only be applied by trained providers with clear indications from medical direction.

Marine envenomations [251–286]

Contact with venomous marine animals is common in the open water lifeguard environment. While the majority of these envenomations are mild, some require additional consideration. Well-controlled clinical trials and high-quality evidence are lacking, and guidelines are primarily derived from case reports, animal studies and expert opinion. The available evidence is conflicting and lacks consensus. A full discussion on management and pathophysiology of marine envenomations in all regions of the world is beyond the scope of this chapter.

Regardless of the offending organism, the patient should be safely removed from the water and acute life threats, such as bleeding or airway compromise, should be managed. Consideration should be given to anaphylaxis, which should be treated according to the scope of practice of the lifeguard. Patients with severe pain or systemic symptoms may require additional treatment at a medical facility.

For stingrays, stonefish, lionfish, Portuguese man-of-war (*Physalia physalis*), weever fish and sea urchins, immersion in hot water can provide pain relief. All tropical Australian jellyfish, including the box jellyfish (*Chironex fleckeri*), should be treated with decontamination from cold seawater, followed by 5% acetic acid (vinegar). If acetic acid is unavailable, then a slurry of baking soda and water can be used. There is some conflicting literature that acetic acid may increase the amount of venom released by some species; however, more rigorous evidence exists that it stops the stinging process. There are conflicting studies on hot water immersion versus application of cold packs and cold water. A reasonable approach for all other jellyfish is to attempt hot water immersion for 20 minutes after application of 5% acetic acid (vinegar), or application of cold if more readily available. Decontamination by removing tentacles should be performed while wearing gloves to prevent injury to the lifeguard. Pressure bandages should be avoided and may increase the amount of venom released.

PREVENTING BEACH AND SURFING INJURIES

The following should be employed to prevent beach injuries occurring in the first place:

1. Close supervision of children by parents/ caregivers during beach play should be promoted – it is as necessary on land as it is during water-based activity.
2. Beachgoers should be encouraged to include a first aid kit on their visit to the beach, especially where such hazards as rocks and litter are likely to be present.
3. To minimize the risk of foot injuries, beach-goers should wear reef shoes or lightweight sandals at the beach, especially where hazards are known to be present. In addition, local authorities should undertake appropriate beach grooming to reduce potentially danger-ous beach litter.
4. To minimize risk of marine stings, lightweight protective clothing such as Lycra rash guards or suits should be used in the water.
5. The parents of children with a known his-tory of asthma or allergies should bring their child's medication to the beach.
6. Lifeguards and local authorities should warn beachgoers of the presence of jellyfish via news media and beach signage.
7. Further research should be undertaken on optional or mandatory helmet use to pre-vent head injuries when engaging in surfing activities.
8. To help prevent laceration and puncture wounds when surfing, further efforts should be made to make manufacturers and users aware of the danger of sharp surfboard fins and noses. Equipment modifications (such as blunt fin edges and protective guards on pointed surfboard noses) should help.
9. Surfing activity should be monitored and managed by lifeguards, the public should be educated about risks and risk management should be practised when surfing; all of these measures are likely to reduce surfing injury incidence.
10. Swimmer and surfer zones should continue to be separated on patrolled beaches; universal signage should be adopted, with illustrations to indicate swimmer/surfer zones.

SUMMARY

The statistics and case studies reported in this chapter clearly indicate the diversity and mag-nitude of first aid incidents on patrolled beaches, and they highlight the critical role that the beach lifeguard plays as a first responder in a physi-cally demanding environment. While most of these incidents are minor and victims are released without the need for further medical attention, some incidents are life-threatening and require immediate pre-hospital medical treatment. While the prevention of drowning remains the pri-mary goal of beach lifeguards, the increasingly frequent demands on their time and skills for non-drowning-related injuries and illnesses sug-gest that first aid training will continue to be an important and increasingly more complex part of the skillset of modern beach lifeguards. The chal-lenge for beach lifeguard organizations is to use the evidence provided by research and their own statistics to target first aid training to address the correct treatment of frequently reported causes of injury (such as soft tissue injuries of the foot and ankle). In addition, it is incumbent on these orga-nizations to promote beach injury prevention and beach safety, especially among high-risk beachgo-ers (such as males, children and surfers). An enjoy-able and safe day at the beach for all is too good a goal to be left to chance.

ACKNOWLEDGEMENTS

Our thanks to lifeguard friends and colleagues who contributed to this section; without their guidance and knowledge, information on such a critical part of our lifeguard work would not have been available to share with our lifeguarding col-leagues worldwide.

REFERENCES

1. Lencek L, Bosker G. *The Beach. The History of Paradise on Earth.* London: Pimlico; 1999.
2. Abraldes JA, Pérez-Gómez J. Assessment of risk factors for injuries on beaches. *Int J Aquat Res Educ.* 2009; 3: 272–83.
3. Surf Life Saving New Zealand (SLSNZ). *Patrol Statistics.* 2012. Available at http:// www.slsnz.org.nz/Article.aspx?ID = 870

4. Moran K, Webber J. Leisure-related injuries at the beach: An analysis of lifeguard incident report forms in New Zealand, 2007–12. *Int J Inj Contr Saf Promot.* 2014; 21(1): 68–74. doi: 10.1080/17457300.2012.760611.

5. Moran K, Webber J. Surf, sand, scrapes, and stings: A study of first aid incidents involving children at New Zealand Beaches, 2007–12. *J Paediatr Child Health.* 2014; 50: 221–5. doi: 10.1111/jpc.12467.

6. Moran K, Webber J. Surfing injuries requiring first aid in New Zealand, 2007–12. *Int J Aquat Res Educ.* 2013; 7(3): 192–203.

7. Grenfell RD, Ross KN. How dangerous is that visit to the beach? A pilot study of beach injuries. *Aust Fam Phys.* 1992; 21(8): 1145–8.

8. Hockey R. Recreational water injuries. Queensland Injury Surveillance Unit. *Inj Bull.* 1998; 51: 1–4. doi: 10.1080/17457300. 2012.760611.

9. Taylor DM, Ashby K, Winkel KD. An analysis of marine animal injuries presenting to emergency departments in Victoria, Australia. *Wilderness Environ Med.* 2002; 13: 106–12.

10. Taylor DM, Bennett D, Carter M, Garewal D, Finch CF. Acute injury and chronic disability resulting from surfboard riding. *J Sci Med Sport.* 2004; 7(4): 429–37.

11. SLSA (Surf Life Saving Australia). *Annual Report, 2012.* Available at http://sls.com.au/publications

12. RNLI (Royal National Lifeboat Institution). *Annual Operational Statistics Report 2012.* 2012. Available at http://rnli.org/SiteCollectionDocuments/13_345%20RNLI%20Operational%20Statistics%202012%20LR.pdf

13. Yamamoto LG, Yee AB, Mathews WJ, Wiebe RA. A one-year series of pediatric ED water-related injuries: The Hawaii EMS-C project. *Pediatr Emerg Care.* 1992; 8: 129–33.

14. Petronis KA, Welch JC, Pruitt CW. Independent risk factors for beach-related injuries in children. *Clin Pediatr.* 2009; 48(5): 534–8.

15. Nathanson A, Haynes P, Galanis D. Surfing injuries. *Am J Emerg Med.* 2002; 20: 155–60.

16. USLA (United States Lifesaving Association). Statistics. Available from: arc.usla.org/statistics/public.asp

17. Brewster BC (ed.). *Open Water Lifesaving.* The United States Lifesaving Association Manual. Upper Saddle River, NJ: Prentice-Hall; 2003.

18. Szpilman D, Elmann J, Cruz Filho FES. Drowning Resuscitation Center – Ten years of medical beach attendance in Rio de Janeiro, Brazil. *Paper Presented at the World Congress on Drowning*, Amsterdam, 26–28 June 2002. Book of Abstracts, p. 167.

19. Sobrasa – Socidade Brasileira de Salvamento Aquatico. Courses lifesaving. Available at http://www.sobrasa.org/cursos/cursos.htm

20. Pillgram-Larsen J, Mellesmo S. [Not a tourniquet, but compressive dressing. Experience from 68 traumatic amputations after injuries from mines]. *Tidsskr Laegeforen.* 1992; 112(17): 2188–90. Norwegian.

21. Larson MJ, Bowersox JC, Lim RC Jr, Hess JR. Efficacy of a fibrin hemostatic bandage in controlling hemorrhage from experimental arterial injuries. *Arch Surg.* 1995; 130(4): 420–2.

22. Landi A, Saracino A, Pinelli M, Caserta G, Facchini MC. Tourniquet paralysis in microsurgery. *Ann Acad Med Singapore.* 1995; 24(4 Suppl): 89–93.

23. Jackson MR, Friedman SA, Carter AJ, Bayer V, Burge JR, MacPhee MJ, Drohan WN, Alving BM. Hemostatic efficacy of a fibrin sealant-based topical agent in a femoral artery injury model: A randomized, blinded, placebo-controlled study. *J Vasc Surg.* 1997; 26(2): 274–80.

24. Holcomb J, MacPhee M, Hetz S, Harris R, Pusateri A, Hess J. Efficacy of a dry fibrin sealant dressing for hemorrhage control after ballistic injury. *Arch Surg.* 1998; 133(1): 32–5.

25. Kokki H, Väätäinen U, Penttilä I. Metabolic effects of a low-pressure tourniquet system compared with a high-pressure tourniquet system in arthroscopic anterior crucial ligament reconstruction. *Acta Anaesthesiol Scand.* 1998; 42(4): 418–24.

26. Simon A, Bumgarner B, Clark K, Israel S. Manual versus mechanical compression for femoral artery hemostasis after cardiac catheterization. *Am J Crit Care*. 1998; 7(4): 308–13.

27. Mohler LR, Pedowitz RA, Lopez MA, Gershuni DH. Effects of tourniquet compression on neuromuscular function. *Clin Orthop Relat Res*. 1999; 359: 213–20.

28. Savvidis E, Parsch K. Prolonged transitory paralysis after pneumatic tourniquet use on the upper arm. *Unfallchirurg*. 1999; 102(2): 141–4. German.

29. Lehmann KG, Heath-Lange SJ, Ferris ST. Randomized comparison of hemostasis techniques after invasive cardiovascular procedures. *Am Heart J*. 1999; 138(6 Pt 1): 1118–25.

30. Calkins D, Snow C, Costello M, Bentley TB. Evaluation of possible battlefield tourniquet systems for the far-forward setting. *Mil Med*. 2000; 165(5): 379–84.

31. Naimer SA, Chemla F. Elastic adhesive dressing treatment of bleeding wounds in trauma victims. *Am J Emerg Med*. 2000; 18(7): 816–19.

32. Wakai A, Wang JH, Winter DC, Street JT, O'Sullivan RG, Redmond HP. Tourniquet-induced systemic inflammatory response in extremity surgery. *J Trauma*. 2001; 51(5): 922–6.

33. Walker SB, Cleary S, Higgins M. Comparison of the FemoStop device and manual pressure in reducing groin puncture site complications following coronary angioplasty and coronary stent placement. *Int J Nurs Pract*. 2001; 7(6): 366–75.

34. Lakstein D, Blumenfeld A, Sokolov T, Lin G, Bssorai R, Lynn M, Ben-Abraham R. Tourniquets for hemorrhage control on the battlefield: A 4-year accumulated experience. *J Trauma*. 2003; 54(5 Suppl): S221–5.

35. Yadav JS, Ziada KM, Almany S, Davis TP, Castaneda F. Comparison of the QuickSeal Femoral Arterial Closure System with manual compression following diagnostic and interventional catheterization procedures. *Am J Cardiol*. 2003; 91(12): 1463–6, A6.

36. Kornbluth ID, Freedman MK, Sher L, Frederick RW. Femoral, saphenous nerve palsy after tourniquet use: A case report. *Arch Phys Med Rehabil*. 2003; 84(6): 909–11.

37. Alam HB, Uy GB, Miller D, Koustova E, Hancock T, Inocencio R, Anderson D, Llorente O, Rhee P. Comparative analysis of hemostatic agents in a swine model of lethal groin injury. *J Trauma*. 2003; 54(6): 1077–82.

38. Koreny M, Riedmüller E, Nikfardjam M, Siostrzonek P, Müllner M. Arterial puncture closing devices compared with standard manual compression after cardiac catheterization: Systematic review and meta-analysis. *JAMA*. 2004; 291(3): 350–7.

39. Alam HB, Chen Z, Jaskille A, Querol RI, Koustova E, Inocencio R, Conran R, et al. Application of a zeolite hemostatic agent achieves 100% survival in a lethal model of complex groin injury in Swine. *J Trauma*. 2004; 56(5): 974–83.

40. Naimer SA, Anat N, Katif G, Rescue Team. Evaluation of techniques for treating the bleeding wound. *Injury*. 2004; 35(10): 974–9.

41. Naimer SA, Nash M, Niv A, Lapid O. Control of massive bleeding from facial gunshot wound with a compact elastic adhesive compression dressing. *Am J Emerg Med*. 2004; 22(7): 586–8.

42. Wenke JC, Walters TJ, Greydanus DJ, Pusateri AE, Convertino VA. Physiological evaluation of the U.S. Army one-handed tourniquet. *Mil Med*. 2005; 170(9): 776–81.

43. Walters TJ, Wenke JC, Kauvar DS, McManus JG, Holcomb JB, Baer DG. Effectiveness of self-applied tourniquets in human volunteers. *Prehosp Emerg Care*. 2005; 9(4): 416–22.

44. Acheson EM, Kheirabadi BS, Deguzman R, Dick EJ Jr, Holcomb JB. Comparison of hemorrhage control agents applied to lethal extremity arterial hemorrhages in swine. *J Trauma*. 2005; 59(4): 865–74; discussion 874–5.

45. Mlekusch W, Dick P, Haumer M, Sabeti S, Minar E, Schillinger M. Arterial puncture site management after percutaneous transluminal procedures using a hemostatic wound dressing (Clo-Sur P.A.D.) versus conventional manual compression: A randomized controlled trial. *J Endovasc Ther*. 2006; 13(1): 23–31.

46. Wedmore I, McManus JG, Pusateri AE, Holcomb JB. A special report on the chitosan-based hemostatic dressing: Experience in current combat operations. *J Trauma*. 2006; 60(3): 655–8.

47. King RB, Filips D, Blitz S, Logsetty S. Evaluation of possible tourniquet systems for use in the Canadian Forces. *J Trauma*. 2006; 60(5): 1061–71.

48. Upponi SS, Ganeshan AG, Warakaulle DR, Phillips-Hughes J, Boardman P, Uberoi R. Angioseal versus manual compression for haemostasis following peripheral vascular diagnostic and interventional procedures—A randomized controlled trial. *Eur J Radiol*. 2007; 61(2): 332–4.

49. Ahuja N, Ostomel TA, Rhee P, Stucky GD, Conran R, Chen Z, Al-Mubarak GA, Velmahos G, Demoya M, Alam HB. Testing of modified zeolite hemostatic dressings in a large animal model of lethal groin injury. *J Trauma*. 2006; 61(6): 1312–20.

50. McManus J, Hurtado T, Pusateri A, Knoop KJ. A case series describing thermal injury resulting from zeolite use for hemorrhage control in combat operations. *Prehosp Emerg Care*. 2007; 11(1): 67–71.

51. Gustafson SB, Fulkerson P, Bildfell R, Aguilera L, Hazzard TM. Chitosan dressing provides hemostasis in swine femoral arterial injury model. *Prehosp Emerg Care*. 2007; 11(2): 172–8.

52. Ersoy G, Kaynak MF, Yilmaz O, Rodoplu U, Maltepe F, Gokmen N. Hemostatic effects of microporous polysaccharide hemosphere in a rat model with severe femoral artery bleeding. *Adv Ther*. 2007; 24(3): 485–92.

53. Ward KR, Tiba MH, Holbert WH, Blocher CR, Draucker GT, Proffitt EK, Bowlin GL, Ivatury RR, Diegelmann RF. Comparison of a new hemostatic agent to current combat hemostatic agents in a Swine model of lethal extremity arterial hemorrhage. *J Trauma*. 2007; 63(2): 276–83; discussion 283–4.

54. Brown MA, Daya MR, Worley JA. Experience with chitosan dressings in a civilian EMS system. *J Emerg Med*. 2009; 37(1): 1–7.

55. Arnaud F, Tomori T, Saito R, McKeague A, Prusaczyk WK, McCarron RM. Comparative efficacy of granular and bagged formulations of the hemostatic agent QuikClot. *J Trauma*. 2007; 63(4): 775–82.

56. Fan Y, Sun H, Pei G, Ruan C. Haemostatic efficacy of an ethyl-2-cyanoacrylate-based aerosol in combination with tourniquet application in a large wound model with an arterial injury. *Injury*. 2008; 39(1): 61–6.

57. Kozen BG, Kircher SJ, Henao J, Godinez FS, Johnson AS. An alternative hemostatic dressing: Comparison of CELOX, HemCon, and QuikClot. *Acad Emerg Med*. 2008; 15(1): 74–81. doi: 10.1111/j.1553-2712.2007.00009.x.

58. Beekley AC, Sebesta JA, Blackbourne LH, Herbert GS, Kauvar DS, Baer DG, Walters TJ, Mullenix PS, Holcomb JB, 31st Combat Support Hospital Research Group. Prehospital tourniquet use in Operation Iraqi Freedom: Effect on hemorrhage control and outcomes. *J Trauma*. 2008; 64(2 Suppl): S28–37; discussion S37. doi: 10.1097/TA.0b013e318160937e.

59. Kragh JF Jr, Walters TJ, Baer DG, Fox CJ, Wade CE, Salinas J, Holcomb JB. Practical use of emergency tourniquets to stop bleeding in major limb trauma. *J Trauma*. 2008; 64(2 Suppl): S38–49; discussion S49–50. doi: 10.1097/TA.0b013e31816086b1.

60. Rhee P, Brown C, Martin M, Salim A, Plurad D, Green D, Chambers L, Demetriades D, Velmahos G, Alam H. QuikClot use in trauma for hemorrhage control: Case series of 103 documented uses. *J Trauma*. 2008; 64(4): 1093–9. doi: 10.1097/TA.0b013e31812f6dbc.

61. Carraway JW, Kent D, Young K, Cole A, Friedman R, Ward KR. Comparison of a new mineral based hemostatic agent to a commercially available granular zeolite agent for hemostasis in a swine model of lethal extremity arterial hemorrhage. *Resuscitation*. 2008; 78(2): 230–5. doi: 10.1016/j.resuscitation.2008.02.019.

62. Kalish J, Burke P, Feldman J, Agarwal S, Glantz A, Moyer P, Serino R, Hirsch E. The return of tourniquets.

Original research evaluates the effectiveness of prehospital tourniquets for civilian penetrating extremity injuries. *JEMS*. 2008; 33(8): 44–6, 49–50, 52, 54. doi: 10.1016/S0197-2510(08)70289-4.

63. Kheirabadi BS, Edens JW, Terrazas IB, Estep JS, Klemcke HG, Dubick MA, Holcomb JB. Comparison of new hemostatic granules/powders with currently deployed hemostatic products in a lethal model of extremity arterial hemorrhage in swine. *J Trauma*. 2009; 66(2): 316–26; discussion 327–8. doi: 10.1097/ TA.0b013e31819634a1.

64. Swan KG Jr, Wright DS, Barbagiovanni SS, Swan BC, Swan KG. Tourniquets revisited. *J Trauma*. 2009; 66(3): 672–5. doi: 10.1097/ TA.0b013e3181986959.

65. Li J, Yan W, Jing L, Xueyong L, Yuejun L, Wangzhou L, Shaozong C. Addition of an alginate to a modified zeolite improves hemostatic performance in a swine model of lethal groin injury. *J Trauma*. 2009; 66(3): 612–20. doi: 10.1097/ TA.0b013e318160ff4d.

66. Velmahos GC, Tabbara M, Spaniolas K, Duggan M, Alam HB, Serra M, Sun L, de Luis J. Self-expanding hemostatic polymer for control of exsanguinating extremity bleeding. *J Trauma*. 2009; 66(4): 984–8. doi: 10.1097/ TA.0b013e31819ce457.

67. Sambasivan CN, Cho SD, Zink KA, Differding JA, Schreiber MA. A highly porous silica and chitosan-based hemostatic dressing is superior in controlling hemorrhage in a severe groin injury model in swine. *Am J Surg*. 2009; 197(5): 576–80; discussion 580. doi: 10.1016/j. amjsurg.2008.12.011.

68. Arnaud F, Teranishi K, Tomori T, Carr W, McCarron R. Comparison of 10 hemostatic dressings in a groin puncture model in swine. *J Vasc Surg*. 2009; 50(3): 632–9, 639.e1. doi: 10.1016/j. jvs.2009.06.010.

69. Arnaud F, Parreño-Sadalan D, Tomori T, Delima MG, Teranishi K, Carr W, McNamee G, et al. Comparison of 10 hemostatic dressings in a groin

transection model in swine. *J Trauma*. 2009; 67(4): 848–55. doi: 10.1097/ TA.0b013e3181b2897f.

70. Gegel BT, Burgert JM, Lockhart C, Austin R 3rd, Davila A, Deeds J, Hodges L, et al. Effects of Celox and TraumaDEX on hemorrhage control in a porcine model. *AANA J*. 2010; 78(2): 115–20.

71. Gegel B, Burgert J, Cooley B, MacGregor J, Myers J, Calder S, Luellen R, Loughren M, Johnson D. The effects of BleedArrest, Celox, and TraumaDex on hemorrhage control in a porcine model. *J Surg Res*. 2010; 164(1): e125–9. doi: 10.1016/j. jss.2010.07.060.

72. Ran Y, Hadad E, Daher S, Ganor O, Kohn J, Yegorov Y, Bartal C, Ash N, Hirschhorn G. QuikClot Combat Gauze use for hemorrhage control in military trauma: January 2009 Israel Defense Force experience in the Gaza Strip—A preliminary report of 14 cases. *Prehosp Disaster Med*. 2010; 25(6): 584–8.

73. MacIntyre AD, Quick JA, Barnes SL. Hemostatic dressings reduce tourniquet time while maintaining hemorrhage control. *Am Surg*. 2011; 77(2): 162–5.

74. Kragh JF, O Neill ML, Beebe DF, Fox CJ, Beekley AC, Cain JS, Parsons DL, Mabry RL, Blackbourne LH. Survey of the indications for use of emergency tourniquets. *J Spec Oper Med*. 2011; 11(1): 30–8.

75. Guo JY, Liu Y, Ma YL, Pi HY, Wang JR. Evaluation of emergency tourniquets for prehospital use in China. *Chin J Traumatol*. 2011; 14(3): 151–5.

76. Taylor DM, Vater GM, Parker PJ. An evaluation of two tourniquet systems for the control of prehospital lower limb hemorrhage. *J Trauma*. 2011; 71(3): 591–5. doi: 10.1097/ TA.0b013e31820e0e41.

77. Parker P, Limb Trauma Working Group. Consensus statement on decision making in junctional trauma care. *J R Army Med Corps*. 2011; 157(3 Suppl 1): S293–5.

78. King DR, van der Wilden G, Kragh JF Jr, Blackbourne LH. Forward assessment of 79 prehospital battlefield tourniquets used in the current war. *J Spec Oper Med*. 2012; 12(4): 33–8.

79. Rush RM Jr, Arrington ED, Hsu JR. Management of complex extremity injuries: Tourniquets, compartment syndrome detection, fasciotomy, and amputation care. *Surg Clin North Am.* 2012; 92(4): 987–1007, ix. doi: 10.1016/j. suc.2012.06.003.

80. Johnson D, Agee S, Reed A, Gegel B, Burgert J, Gasko J, Loughren M. The effects of QuikClot Combat Gauze on hemorrhage control in the presence of hemodilution. *US Army Med Dep J.* 2012: 36–9.

81. Lairet JR, Bebarta VS, Burns CJ, Lairet KF, Rasmussen TE, Renz EM, King BT, et al. Prehospital interventions performed in a combat zone: A prospective multicenter study of 1,003 combat wounded. *J Trauma Acute Care Surg.* 2012; 73(2 Suppl 1): S38–42.

82. Satterly S, Nelson D, Zwintscher N, Oguntoye M, Causey W, Theis B, Huang R, et al. Hemostasis in a noncompressible hemorrhage model: An end-user evaluation of hemostatic agents in a proximal arterial injury. *J Surg Educ.* 2013; 70(2): 206–11. doi: 10.1016/j. jsurg.2012.11.001.

83. Burnett LR, Richter JG, Rahmany MB, Soler R, Steen JA, Orlando G, Abouswareb T, Van Dyke ME. Novel keratin (KeraStat™) and polyurethane (Nanosan(R)-Sorb) biomaterials are hemostatic in a porcine lethal extremity hemorrhage model. *J Biomater Appl.* 2014; 28(6): 869–79. doi: 10.1177/0885328213484975.

84. Rall JM, Cox JM, Songer AG, Cestero RF, Ross JD. Comparison of novel hemostatic dressings with QuikClot combat gauze in a standardized swine model of uncontrolled hemorrhage. *J Trauma Acute Care Surg.* 2013; 75(2 Suppl 2): S150–6. doi: 10.1097/ TA.0b013e318299d909.

85. Passos E, Dingley B, Smith A, Engels PT, Ball CG, Faidi S, Nathens A, Tien H, Canadian Trauma Trials Collaborative. Tourniquet use for peripheral vascular injuries in the civilian setting. *Injury.* 2014; 45(3): 573–7. doi: 10.1016/ j.injury.2013.11.031.

86. Robertson J, McCahill P, Riddle A, Callaway D. Another civilian life saved by law enforcement-applied tourniquets. *J Spec Oper Med.* 2014; 14(3): 7–11.

87. Bennett BL, Littlejohn LF, Kheirabadi BS, Butler FK, Kotwal RS, Dubick MA, Bailey JA. Management of external hemorrhage in tactical combat casualty care: Chitosan-based hemostatic gauze dressings—TCCC guidelines-change 13-05. *J Spec Oper Med.* 2014; 14(3): 40–57.

88. Callaway DW, Robertson J, Sztajnkrycer MD. Law enforcement-applied tourniquets: A case series of life-saving interventions. *Prehosp Emerg Care.* 2015; 19(2): 320–7. doi: 10.3109/10903127.2014.964893.

89. Kirkpatrick AW, McKee JL. Tactical hemorrhage control case studies using a point-of-care mechanical direct pressure device. *J Spec Oper Med.* 2014; 14(4): 7–10.

90. Kue RC, Temin ES, Weiner SG, Gates J, Coleman MH, Fisher J, Dyer S. Tourniquet use in a civilian emergency medical services setting: A descriptive analysis of the Boston EMS experience. *Prehosp Emerg Care.* 2015; 19: 399–404.

91. Grissom TE, Fang R. Topical hemostatic agents and dressings in the prehospital setting. *Curr Opin Anaesthesiol.* 2015; 28(2): 210–16. doi: 10.1097/ ACO.0000000000000166.

92. Littlejohn L, Bennett BL, Drew B. Application of current hemorrhage control techniques for backcountry care: Part two, hemostatic dressings and other adjuncts. *Wilderness Environ Med.* 2015; 26: 246–54. doi: 10.1016/j. wem.2014.08.018.

93. Drew B, Bennett BL, Littlejohn L. Application of current hemorrhage control techniques for backcountry care: Part one, tourniquets and hemorrhage control adjuncts. *Wilderness Environ Med.* 2015; 26: 236–45. doi: 10.1016/ j.wem.2014.08.016.

94. King DR, Larentzakis A, Ramly EP, Boston Trauma Collaborative. Tourniquet use

at the Boston Marathon bombing: Lost in translation. *J Trauma Acute Care Surg.* 2015; 78(3): 594–9. doi: 10.1097/ TA.0000000000000561.

95. Worster B, Zawora MQ, Hsieh C. Common questions about wound care. *Am Fam Physician.* 2015; 91(2): 86–92.

96. Wilkins RG, Unverdorben M. Wound cleaning and wound healing: A concise review. *Adv Skin Wound Care.* 2013; 26(4): 160–3. doi: 10.1097/01. ASW.0000428861.26671.41.

97. Weiss EA, Oldham G, Lin M, Foster T, Quinn JV. Water is a safe and effective alternative to sterile normal saline for wound irrigation prior to suturing: A prospective, double-blind, randomised, controlled clinical trial. *BMJ Open.* 2013; 3(1). pii: e001504. doi: 10.1136/ bmjopen-2012-001504.

98. Henton J, Jain A. Cochrane corner: Water for wound cleansing. *J Hand Surg Eur Vol.* 2012; 37(4): 375–6. doi: 10.1177/1753193412443640.

99. Li TS, Choong MY, Wu SF, Chen KJ. Irrigating methicillin-resistant *Staphylococcus aureus*-colonised and - infected chronic wounds with tap water. *Int Wound J.* 2013; 10(3): 359. doi: 10.1111/j.1742-481X.2011.00934.x.

100. Fernandez R, Griffiths R. Water for wound cleansing. *Cochrane Database Syst Rev.* 2012; 15(2): CD003861. doi: 10.1002/14651858.CD003861.pub3.

101. Breen JO. Skin and soft tissue infections in immunocompetent patients. *Am Fam Physician.* 2010; 81(7): 893–9.

102. Heal CF, Buettner PG, Cruickshank R, Graham D, Browning S, Pendergast J, Drobetz H, Gluer R, Lisec C. Does single application of topical chloramphenicol to high risk sutured wounds reduce incidence of wound infection after minor surgery? Prospective randomised placebo controlled double blind trial. *BMJ.* 2009; 338: a2812. doi: 10.1136/bmj.a2812.

103. Beam JW. Occlusive dressings and the healing of standardized abrasions. *J Athl Train.* 2008; 43(6): 600–7. doi: 10.4085/1062-6050-43.6.600.

104. Edmonds M. Irrigation of simple lacerations with tap water or sterile saline in the emergency department did not differ for wound infections. *Evid Based Med.* 2007; 12(6): 181.

105. Moscati RM, Mayrose J, Reardon RF, Janicke DM, Jehle DV. A multicenter comparison of tap water versus sterile saline for wound irrigation. *Acad Emerg Med.* 2007; 14(5): 404–9.

106. Claus EE, Fusco CF, Ingram T, Ingersoll CD, Edwards JE, Melham TJ. Comparison of the effects of selected dressings on the healing of standardized abrasions. *J Athl Train.* 1998; 33(2): 145–9.

107. Wilson JR, Mills JG, Prather ID, Dimitrijevich SD. A toxicity index of skin and wound cleansers used on in vitro fibroblasts and keratinocytes. *Adv Skin Wound Care.* 2005; 18(7): 373–8.

108. Griffiths RD, Fernandez RS, Ussia CA. Is tap water a safe alternative to normal saline for wound irrigation in the community setting? *J Wound Care.* 2001; 10(10): 407–11.

109. Valente JH, Forti RJ, Freundlich LF, Zandieh SO, Crain EF. Wound irrigation in children: Saline solution or tap water? *Ann Emerg Med.* 2003; 41(5): 609–16.

110. Bansal BC, Wiebe RA, Perkins SD, Abramo TJ. Tap water for irrigation of lacerations. *Am J Emerg Med.* 2002; 20(5): 469–72.

111. Atiyeh BS, Ioannovich J, Magliacani G, Masellis M, Costagliola M, Dham R, Al-Farhan M. Efficacy of moist exposed burn ointment in the management of cutaneous wounds and ulcers: A multicenter pilot study. *Ann Plast Surg.* 2002; 48(2): 226–7.

112. Davis SC, Eaglstein WH, Cazzaniga AL, Mertz PM. An octyl-2-cyanoacrylate formulation speeds healing of partial-thickness wounds. *Dermatol Surg.* 2001; 27(9): 783–8.

113. Berger RS, Pappert AS, Van Zile PS, Cetnarowski WE. A newly formulated topical triple-antibiotic ointment minimizes scarring. *Cutis.* 2000; 65(6): 401–4. Erratum in: *Cutis.* 2000; 66(5): 382.

114. Moscati R, Mayrose J, Fincher L, Jehle D. Comparison of normal saline with tap water for wound irrigation. *Am J Emerg Med.* 1998; 16(4): 379–81.

115. Hollander JE, Singer AJ, Valentine S. Comparison of wound care practices in pediatric and adult lacerations repaired in the emergency department. *Pediatr Emerg Care.* 1998; 14(1): 15–18.

116. Langford JH, Artemi P, Benrimoj SI. Topical antimicrobial prophylaxis in minor wounds. *Ann Pharmacother.* 1997; 31(5): 559–63.

117. Smack DP, Harrington AC, Dunn C, Howard RS, Szkutnik AJ, Krivda SJ, Caldwell JB, James WD. Infection and allergy incidence in ambulatory surgery patients using white petrolatum vs bacitracin ointment. A randomized controlled trial. *JAMA.* 1996; 276(12): 972–7.

118. Anglen J, Apostoles PS, Christensen G, Gainor B, Lane J. Removal of surface bacteria by irrigation. *J Orthop Res.* 1996; 14(2): 251–4.

119. Dire DJ, Coppola M, Dwyer DA, Lorette JJ, Karr JL. Prospective evaluation of topical antibiotics for preventing infections in uncomplicated soft-tissue wounds repaired in the ED. *Acad Emerg Med.* 1995; 2(1): 4–10.

120. Bencini PL, Galimberti M, Signorini M, Crosti C. Antibiotic prophylaxis of wound infections in skin surgery. *Arch Dermatol.* 1991; 127(9): 1357–60.

121. Hendley JO, Ashe KM. Effect of topical antimicrobial treatment on aerobic bacteria in the stratum corneum of human skin. *Antimicrob Agents Chemother.* 1991; 35(4): 627–31.

122. Dire DJ, Welsh AP. A comparison of wound irrigation solutions used in the emergency department. *Ann Emerg Med.* 1990; 19(6): 704–8.

123. Eaglstein WH, Davis SC, Mehle AL, Mertz PM. Optimal use of an occlusive dressing to enhance healing. Effect of delayed application and early removal on wound healing. *Arch Dermatol.* 1988; 124(3): 392–5.

124. Leyden JJ, Bartelt NM. Comparison of topical antibiotic ointments, a wound protectant, and antiseptics for the treatment of human blister wounds contaminated with *Staphylococcus aureus. J Fam Pract.* 1987; 24(6): 601–4.

125. Longmire AW, Broom LA, Burch J. Wound infection following high-pressure syringe and needle irrigation. *Am J Emerg Med.* 1987; 5(2): 179–81.

126. Lindsey D, Nava C, Marti M. Effectiveness of penicillin irrigation in control of infection in sutured lacerations. *J Trauma.* 1982; 22(3): 186–9.

127. Caro D, Reynolds KW, De Smith J. An investigation to evaluate a topical antibiotic in the prevention of wound sepsis in a casualty department. *Br J Clin Pract.* 1967; 21(12): 605–7.

128. Hinman CD, Maibach H. Effect of air exposure and occlusion on experimental human skin wounds. *Nature.* 1963; 200: 377–8.

129. Winter GD. Formation of the scab and the rate of epithelization of superficial wounds in the skin of the young domestic pig. *Nature.* 1962; 193: 293–4.

130. Dykstra JH, Hill HM, Miller MG, Cheatham CC, Michael TJ, Baker RJ. Comparisons of cubed ice, crushed ice, and wetted ice on intramuscular and surface temperature changes. *J Athl Train.* 2009; 44(2): 136–41. doi: 10.4085/1062-6050-44.2.136.

131. Ficke JR, Pollak AN. Extremity war injuries: Development of clinical treatment principles. *J Am Acad Orthop Surg.* 2007; 15(10): 590–5.

132. Melamed E, Blumenfeld A, Kalmovich B, Kosashvili Y, Lin G, Israel Defense Forces Medical Corps Consensus Group on Prehospital Care of Orthopedic Injuries. Prehospital care of orthopedic injuries. *Prehosp Disaster Med.* 2007; 22(1): 22–5.

133. Perkins TJ. Fracture management. Effective prehospital splinting techniques. *Emerg Med Serv.* 2007; 36(4): 35–7, 39.

134. Bleakley CM, McDonough SM, MacAuley DC, Bjordal J. Cryotherapy for acute ankle sprains: A randomised controlled study of two different icing protocols. *Br J Sports Med.* 2006; 40(8): 700–5; discussion 705.

135. Lee C, Porter KM. Prehospital management of lower limb fractures. *Emerg Med J.* 2005; 22(9): 660–3.

136. Kanlayanaphotporn R, Janwantanakul P. Comparison of skin surface temperature during the application of various cryotherapy modalities. *Arch Phys Med Rehabil.* 2005; 86(7): 1411–15.

137. Airaksinen OV, Kyrklund N, Latvala K, Kouri JP, Grönblad M, Kolari P. Efficacy of cold gel for soft tissue injuries: A prospective randomized double-blinded trial. *Am J Sports Med.* 2003; 31(5): 680–4.

138. Merrick MA, Jutte LS, Smith ME. Cold modalities with different thermodynamic properties produce different surface and intramuscular temperatures. *J Athl Train.* 2003; 38(1): 28–33.

139. Chesterton LS, Foster NE, Ross L. Skin temperature response to cryotherapy. *Arch Phys Med Rehabil.* 2002; 83(4): 543–9.

140. Graham CA, Stevenson J. Frozen chips: An unusual cause of severe frostbite injury. *Br J Sports Med.* 2000; 34(5): 382–3.

141. Moeller JL, Monroe J, McKeag DB. Cryotherapy-induced common peroneal nerve palsy. *Clin J Sport Med.* 1997; 7(3): 212–16.

142. Bassett FH 3rd, Kirkpatrick JS, Engelhardt DL, Malone TR. Cryotherapy-induced nerve injury. *Am J Sports Med.* 1992; 20(5): 516–18.

143. Coté DJ, Prentice WE Jr, Hooker DN, Shields EW. Comparison of three treatment procedures for minimizing ankle sprain swelling. *Phys Ther.* 1988; 68(7): 1072–6.

144. Meeusen R, Lievens P. The use of cryotherapy in sports injuries. *Sports Med.* 1986; 3(6): 398–414.

145. Auerbach PS, Geehr EC, Ryu RK. The reel splint: Experience with a new traction splint apparatus in the prehospital setting. *Ann Emerg Med.* 1984; 13(6): 419–22.

146. Hocutt JE Jr, Jaffe R, Rylander CR, Beebe JK. Cryotherapy in ankle sprains. *Am J Sports Med.* 1982; 10(5): 316–19.

147. McMaster WC, Liddle S, Waugh TR. Laboratory evaluation of various cold therapy modalities. *Am J Sports Med.* 1978; 6(5): 291–4.

148. Basur RL, Shephard E, Mouzas GL. A cooling method in the treatment of ankle sprains. *Practitioner.* 1976; 216(1296): 708–11.

149. Santelli J, Sullivan JM, Czarnik A, Bedolla J. Heat illness in the emergency department: Keeping your cool. *Emerg Med Pract.* 2014; 16(8): 1–21; quiz 21–2.

150. Hostler D, Rittenberger JC, Schillo G, Lawery M. Identification and treatment of heat stroke in the prehospital setting. *Wilderness Environ Med.* 2013; 24(2): 175–7. doi: 10.1016/j.wem.2012.10.006.

151. Marom T, Itskoviz D, Lavon H, Ostfeld I. Acute care for exercise-induced hyperthermia to avoid adverse outcome from exertional heat stroke. *J Sport Rehabil.* 2011; 20(2): 219–27.

152. Zeller L, Novack V, Barski L, Jotkowitz A, Almog Y. Exertional heatstroke: Clinical characteristics, diagnostic and therapeutic considerations. *Eur J Intern Med.* 2011; 22(3): 296–9. doi: 10.1016/j.ejim.2010.12.013.

153. Evans GH, Shirreffs SM, Maughan RJ. Postexercise rehydration in man: The effects of osmolality and carbohydrate content of ingested drinks. *Nutrition.* 2009; 25(9): 905–13. doi: 10.1016/j.nut.2008.12.014.

154. Jeukendrup AE, Currell K, Clarke J, Cole J, Blannin AK. Effect of beverage glucose and sodium content on fluid delivery. *Nutr Metab (Lond).* 2009; 6: 9. doi: 10.1186/1743-7075-6-9.

155. Merson SJ, Maughan RJ, Shirreffs SM. Rehydration with drinks differing in sodium concentration and recovery from moderate exercise-induced hypohydration in man. *Eur J Appl Physiol.* 2008; 103(5): 585–94. doi: 10.1007/s00421-008-0748-0.

156. Gagnon D, Jay O, Reardon FD, Journeay WS, Kenny GP. Hyperthermia modifies the nonthermal contribution to postexercise heat loss responses. *Med Sci Sports Exerc.* 2008; 40(3): 513–22. doi: 10.1249/MSS.0b013e31815eb7b8.

157. Bouchama A, Dehbi M, Mohamed G, Matthies F, Shoukri M, Menne B. Prognostic factors in heat wave related deaths: A meta-analysis. *Arch Intern Med.* 2007; 167(20): 2170–6.

158. Kenefick RW, Maresh CM, Armstrong LE, Riebe D, Echegaray ME, Castellani JW. Rehydration with fluid of varying

tonicities: Effects on fluid regulatory hormones and exercise performance in the heat. *J Appl Physiol (1985)*. 2007; 102(5): 1899–905.

159. Kenefick RW, O'Moore KM, Mahood NV, Castellani JW. Rapid IV versus oral rehydration: Responses to subsequent exercise heat stress. *Med Sci Sports Exerc*. 2006; 38(12): 2125–31.

160. Michell MW, Oliveira HM, Kinsky MP, Vaid SU, Herndon DN, Kramer GC. Enteral resuscitation of burn shock using World Health Organization oral rehydration solution: A potential solution for mass casualty care. *J Burn Care Res*. 2006; 27(6): 819–25.

161. Stofan JR, Zachwieja JJ, Horswill CA, Murray R, Anderson SA, Eichner ER. Sweat and sodium losses in NCAA football players: A precursor to heat cramps? *Int J Sport Nutr Exerc Metab*. 2005; 15(6): 641–52.

162. Jung AP, Bishop PA, Al-Nawwas A, Dale RB. Influence of hydration and electrolyte supplementation on incidence and time to onset of exercise-associated muscle cramps. *J Athl Train*. 2005; 40(2): 71–5.

163. Scott CG, Ducharme MB, Haman F, Kenny GP. Warming by immersion or exercise affects initial cooling rate during subsequent cold water immersion. *Aviat Space Environ Med*. 2004; 75(11): 956–63.

164. Rav-Acha M, Hadad E, Epstein Y, Heled Y, Moran DS. Fatal exertional heat stroke: A case series. *Am J Med Sci*. 2004; 328(2): 84–7.

165. Hadad E, Rav-Acha M, Heled Y, Epstein Y, Moran DS. Heat stroke: A review of cooling methods. *Sports Med*. 2004; 34(8): 501–11.

166. Clements JM, Casa DJ, Knight J, McClung JM, Blake AS, Meenen PM, Gilmer AM, Caldwell KA. Ice-water immersion and cold-water immersion provide similar cooling rates in runners with exercise-induced hyperthermia. *J Athl Train*. 2002; 37(2): 146–50.

167. Bergeron MF. Heat cramps: Fluid and electrolyte challenges during tennis in the heat. *J Sci Med Sport*. 2003; 6(1): 19–27.

168. Proulx CI, Ducharme MB, Kenny GP. Effect of water temperature on cooling efficiency during hyperthermia in humans. *J Appl Physiol (1985)*. 2003; 94(4): 1317–23.

169. Barclay RL, Depew WT, Vanner SJ. Carbohydrate-electrolyte rehydration protects against intravascular volume contraction during colonic cleansing with orally administered sodium phosphate. *Gastrointest Endosc*. 2002; 56(5): 633–8.

170. Mitchell JB, Schiller ER, Miller JR, Dugas JP. The influence of different external cooling methods on thermoregulatory responses before and after intense intermittent exercise in the heat. *J Strength Cond Res*. 2001; 15(2): 247–54.

171. Clapp AJ, Bishop PA, Muir I, Walker JL. Rapid cooling techniques in joggers experiencing heat strain. *J Sci Med Sport*. 2001; 4(2): 160–7.

172. Kenefick RW, Maresh CM, Armstrong LE, Castellani JW, Riebe D, Echegaray ME, Kavorous SA. Plasma vasopressin and aldosterone responses to oral and intravenous saline rehydration. *J Appl Physiol (1985)*. 2000; 89(6): 2117–22.

173. Donoghue AM, Bates GP. The risk of heat exhaustion at a deep underground metalliferous mine in relation to body-mass index and predicted VO2max. *Occup Med (Lond)*. 2000; 50(4): 259–63.

174. Donoghue AM, Sinclair MJ, Bates GP. Heat exhaustion in a deep underground metalliferous mine. *Occup Environ Med*. 2000; 57(3): 165–74.

175. Shahid MS, Hatle L, Mansour H, Mimish L. Echocardiographic and Doppler study of patients with heatstroke and heat exhaustion. *Int J Card Imaging*. 1999; 15(4): 279–85.

176. Greenleaf JE, Jackson CG, Geelen G, Keil LC, Hinghofer-Szalkay H, Whittam JH. Plasma volume expansion with oral fluids in hypohydrated men at rest and during exercise. *Aviat Space Environ Med*. 1998; 69(9): 837–44.

177. Shirreffs SM, Maughan RJ. Volume repletion after exercise-induced volume depletion in humans: Replacement of water and sodium losses. *Am J Physiol*. 1998; 274(5 Pt 2): F868–75.

178. Armstrong LE, Maresh CM, Gabaree CV, Hoffman JR, Kavouras SA, Kenefick RW, Castellani JW, Ahlquist LE. Thermal and circulatory responses during exercise: Effects of hypohydration, dehydration, and water intake. *J Appl Physiol (1985)*. 1997; 82(6): 2028–35.

179. Castellani JW, Maresh CM, Armstrong LE, Kenefick RW, Riebe D, Echegaray M, Casa D, Castracane VD. Intravenous vs. oral rehydration: Effects on subsequent exercise-heat stress. *J Appl Physiol (1985)*. 1997; 82(3): 799–806.

180. Riebe D, Maresh CM, Armstrong LE, Kenefick RW, Castellani JW, Echegaray ME, Clark BA, Camaione DN. Effects of oral and intravenous rehydration on ratings of perceived exertion and thirst. *Med Sci Sports Exerc*. 1997; 29(1): 117–24.

181. Shirreffs SM, Taylor AJ, Leiper JB, Maughan RJ. Post-exercise rehydration in man: Effects of volume consumed and drink sodium content. *Med Sci Sports Exerc*. 1996; 28(10): 1260–71.

182. Armstrong LE, Crago AE, Adams R, Roberts WO, Maresh CM. Whole-body cooling of hyperthermic runners: Comparison of two field therapies. *Am J Emerg Med*. 1996; 14(4): 355–8.

183. Bergeron MF. Heat cramps during tennis: A case report. *Int J Sport Nutr*. 1996; 6(1): 62–8.

184. Ross BH, Thomas CK. Human motor unit activity during induced muscle cramp. *Brain*. 1995; 118(Pt 4): 983–93.

185. Maughan RJ, Leiper JB. Sodium intake and post-exercise rehydration in man. *Eur J Appl Physiol Occup Physiol*. 1995; 71(4): 311–19.

186. Holtzhausen LM, Noakes TD, Kroning B, de Klerk M, Roberts M, Emsley R. Clinical and biochemical characteristics of collapsed ultra-marathon runners. *Med Sci Sports Exerc*. 1994; 26(9): 1095–101.

187. Bertolasi L, De Grandis D, Bongiovanni LG, Zanette GP, Gasperini M. The influence of muscular lengthening on cramps. *Ann Neurol*. 1993; 33(2): 176–80.

188. Costrini A. Emergency treatment of exertional heatstroke and comparison of whole body cooling techniques. *Med Sci Sports Exerc*. 1990; 22(1): 15–18.

189. Shearer S. Dehydration and serum electrolyte changes in South African gold miners with heat disorders. *Am J Ind Med*. 1990; 17(2): 225–39.

190. Brodeur VB, Dennett SR, Griffin LS. Exertional hyperthermia, ice baths, and emergency care at the Falmouth Road Race. *J Emerg Nurs*. 1989; 15(4): 304–12.

191. Vaernes RJ, Hammerborg D. Evoked potential and other CNS reactions during a heliox dive to 360 msw. *Aviat Space Environ Med*. 1989; 60(6): 550–7.

192. Armstrong LE, Hubbard RW, Szlyk PC, Sils IV, Kraemer WJ. Heat intolerance, heat exhaustion monitored: A case report. *Aviat Space Environ Med*. 1988; 59(3): 262–6.

193. Kielblock AJ, Van Rensburg JP, Franz RM. Body cooling as a method for reducing hyperthermia. An evaluation of techniques. *S Afr Med J*. 1986; 69(6): 378–80.

194. Mills KR, Newham DJ, Edwards RH. Severe muscle cramps relieved by transcutaneous nerve stimulation: A case report. *J Neurol Neurosurg Psychiatry*. 1982; 45(6): 539–42.

195. Hart GR, Anderson RJ, Crumpler CP, Shulkin A, Reed G, Knochel JP. Epidemic classical heat stroke: Clinical characteristics and course of 28 patients. *Medicine (Baltimore)*. 1982; 61(3): 189–97.

196. Weiner JS, Khogali M. A physiological body-cooling unit for treatment of heat stroke. *Lancet*. 1980; 1(8167): 507–9.

197. Richards D, Richards R, Schofield PJ, Ross V, Sutton JR. Management of heat exhaustion in Sydney's the Sun City-to-Surf run runners. *Med J Aust*. 1979; 2(9): 457–61.

198. Costrini AM, Pitt HA, Gustafson AB, Uddin DE. Cardiovascular and metabolic manifestations of heat stroke and severe heat exhaustion. *Am J Med*. 1979; 66(2): 296–302.

199. O'Donnell TF Jr. Acute heat stroke. Epidemiologic, biochemical, renal, and coagulation studies. *JAMA*. 1975; 234(8): 824–8.

200. Beller GA, Boyd AE 3rd. Heat stroke: A report of 13 consecutive cases without mortality despite severe hyperpyrexia and

neurologic dysfunction. *Mil Med.* 1975; 140(7): 464–7.

201. Adolph EF. Tolerance to heat and dehydration in several species of mammals. *Am J Physiol.* 1947; 151(2): 564–75.

202. Talbott JH, Michelsen J. Heat cramps. A clinical and chemical study. *J Clin Invest.* 1933; 12(3): 533–49.

203. Gordon L, Paal P, Ellerton JA, Brugger H, Peek GJ, Zafren K. Delayed and intermittent CPR for severe accidental hypothermia. *Resuscitation.* 2015; 90: 46–9. doi: 10.1016/j.resuscitation.2015.02.017.

204. Henriksson O, Lundgren PJ, Kuklane K, Holmér I, Giesbrecht GG, Naredi P, Bjornstig U. Protection against cold in prehospital care: Wet clothing removal or addition of a vapor barrier. *Wilderness Environ Med.* 2015; 26(1): 11–20. doi: 10.1016/j.wem.2014.07.001.

205. Kieboom JK, Verkade HJ, Burgerhof JG, Bierens JJ, Rheenen PF, Kneyber MC, Albers MJ. Outcome after resuscitation beyond 30 minutes in drowned children with cardiac arrest and hypothermia: Dutch nationwide retrospective cohort study. *BMJ.* 2015; 350: h418. doi: 10.1136/bmj.h418.

206. Jussila K, Rissanen S, Parkkola K, Anttonen Hannu. Evaluating cold, wind, and moisture protection of different coverings for prehospital maritime transportation-a thermal manikin and human study. *Prehosp Disaster Med.* 2014; 29(6): 580–8. doi: 10.1017/S1049023X14001125.

207. Quan L, Mack CD, Schiff MA. Association of water temperature and submersion duration and drowning outcome. *Resuscitation.* 2014; 85(6): 790–4. doi: 10.1016/j.resuscitation.2014.02.024. Erratum in: *Resuscitation.* 2014; 85(9): 1304.

208. Sran BJ, McDonald GK, Steinman AM, Gardiner PF, Giesbrecht GG. Comparison of heat donation through the head or torso on mild hypothermia rewarming. *Wilderness Environ Med.* 2014; 25(1): 4–13. doi: 10.1016/j.wem.2013.10.005.

209. Claret PG, Bobbia X, Dingemans G, Onde O, Sebbane M, de La Coussaye JE. Drowning, hypothermia and cardiac arrest: An 18-year-old woman with an automated external defibrillator recording. *Prehosp Disaster Med.* 2013; 28(5): 517–19. doi: 10.1017/S1049023X13008649.

210. Lundgren P, Henriksson O, Naredi P, Björnstig U. The effect of active warming in prehospital trauma care during road and air ambulance transportation— A clinical randomized trial. *Scand J Trauma Resusc Emerg Med.* 2011; 19: 59. doi: 10.1186/1757-7241-19-59.

211. Thomassen Ø, Færevik H, Østerås Ø, Sunde GA, Zakariassen E, Sandsund M, Heltne JK, Brattebø G. Comparison of three different prehospital wrapping methods for preventing hypothermia— A crossover study in humans. *Scand J Trauma Resusc Emerg Med.* 2011; 19: 41. doi: 10.1186/1757-7241-19-41.

212. Tipton MJ, Golden FS. A proposed decision-making guide for the search, rescue and resuscitation of submersion (head under) victims based on expert opinion. *Resuscitation.* 2011; 82(7): 819–24. doi: 10.1016/j.resuscitation.2011.02.021.

213. Henriksson O, Lundgren JP, Kuklane K, Holmér I, Bjornstig U. Protection against cold in prehospital care-thermal insulation properties of blankets and rescue bags in different wind conditions. *Prehosp Disaster Med.* 2009; 24(5): 408–15.

214. Lundgren JP, Henriksson O, Pretorius T, Cahill F, Bristow G, Chochinov A, Pretorius A, Bjornstig U, Giesbrecht GG. Field torso-warming modalities: A comparative study using a human model. *Prehosp Emerg Care.* 2009; 13(3): 371–8. doi: 10.1080/10903120902935348.

215. Hultzer MV, Xu X, Marrao C, Bristow G, Chochinov A, Giesbrecht GG. Prehospital torso-warming modalities for severe hypothermia: A comparative study using a human model. *CJEM.* 2005; 7(6): 378–86.

216. Paal P, Beikircher W, Brugger H. [Avalanche emergencies. Review of the current situation]. *Anaesthesist.* 2006; 55(3): 314–24. German.

217. Williams AB, Salmon A, Graham P, Galler D, Payton MJ, Bradley M. Rewarming of healthy volunteers after induced mild hypothermia: A healthy volunteer study. *Emerg Med J.* 2005; 22(3): 182–4.

218. Greif R, Rajek A, Laciny S, Bastanmehr H, Sessler DI. Resistive heating is more effective than metallic-foil insulation in an experimental model of accidental hypothermia: A randomized controlled trial. *Ann Emerg Med.* 2000; 35(4): 337–45.

219. Watts DD, Roche M, Tricarico R, Poole F, Brown JJ Jr, Colson GB, Trask AL, Fakhry SM. The utility of traditional prehospital interventions in maintaining thermostasis. *Prehosp Emerg Care.* 1999; 3(2): 115–22.

220. Walpoth BH, Walpoth-Aslan BN, Mattle HP, Radanov BP, Schroth G, Schaeffler L, Fischer AP, von Segesser L, Althaus U. Outcome of survivors of accidental deep hypothermia and circulatory arrest treated with extracorporeal blood warming. *N Engl J Med.* 1997; 337(21): 1500–5.

221. Steele MT, Nelson MJ, Sessler DI, Fraker L, Bunney B, Watson WA, Robinson WA. Forced air speeds rewarming in accidental hypothermia. *Ann Emerg Med.* 1996; 27(4): 479–84.

222. Danzl D. Accidental hypothermia. In Auerbach P (ed.). *Wilderness medicine.* St. Louis: Mosby; 2007, pp. 125–60.

223. Sporer KA. Why we need to rethink C-spine immobilization: We need to reevaluate current practices and develop a saner cervical policy. *EMS World.* 2012; 41(11): 74–6.

224. Hauswald M. A re-conceptualisation of acute spinal care. *Emerg Med J.* 2013; 30(9): 720–3. doi: 10.1136/emermed-2012-201847.

225. Ben-Galim P, Dreiangel N, Mattox KL, Reitman CA, Kalantar SB, Hipp JA. Extrication collars can result in abnormal separation between vertebrae in the presence of a dissociative injury. *J Trauma.* 2010; 69(2): 447–50. doi: 10.1097/TA.0b013e3181be785a.

226. Benger J, Blackham J. Why do we put cervical collars on conscious trauma patients? *Scand J Trauma Resusc Emerg Med.* 2009; 17: 44. doi: 10.1186/1757-7241-17-44.

227. Pieretti-Vanmarcke R, Velmahos GC, Nance ML, Islam S, Falcone RA Jr, Wales PW, Brown RL, et al. Clinical clearance of the cervical spine in blunt trauma patients younger than 3 years: A multicenter study of the American association for the surgery of trauma. *J Trauma.* 2009; 67(3): 543–9; discussion 549–50. doi: 10.1097/TA.0b013e3181b57aa1.

228. Shafer JS, Naunheim RS. Cervical spine motion during extrication: A pilot study. *West J Emerg Med.* 2009; 10(2): 74–8.

229. Sundheim SM, Cruz M. The evidence for spinal immobilization: An estimate of the magnitude of the treatment benefit. *Ann Emerg Med.* 2006; 48(2): 217–18; author reply 218–19.

230. Hwang V, Shofer FS, Durbin DR, Baren JM. Prevalence of traumatic injuries in drowning and near drowning in children and adolescents. *Arch Pediatr Adolesc Med.* 2003; 157(1): 50–3.

231. Touger M, Gennis P, Nathanson N, Lowery DW, Pollack CV Jr, Hoffman JR, Mower WR. Validity of a decision rule to reduce cervical spine radiography in elderly patients with blunt trauma. *Ann Emerg Med.* 2002; 40(3): 287–93.

232. Stiell IG, Wells GA, Vandemheen KL, Clement CM, Lesiuk H, De Maio VJ, Laupacis A, et al. The Canadian C-spine rule for radiography in alert and stable trauma patients. *JAMA.* 2001; 286(15): 1841–8.

233. Hackl W, Hausberger K, Sailer R, Ulmer H, Gassner R. Prevalence of cervical spine injuries in patients with facial trauma. *Oral Surg Oral Med Oral Pathol Oral Radiol Endod.* 2001; 92(4): 370–6.

234. Watson RS, Cummings P, Quan L, Bratton S, Weiss NS. Cervical spine injuries among submersion victims. *J Trauma.* 2001; 51(4): 658–62.

235. Stiell IG, Lesiuk H, Wells GA, Coyle D, McKnight RD, Brison R, Clement C, et al. Canadian CT head rule study for patients with minor head injury: Methodology for phase II (validation and economic analysis). *Ann Emerg Med.* 2001; 38(3): 317–22.

236. Viccellio P, Simon H, Pressman BD, Shah MN, Mower WR, Hoffman JR, NEXUS Group. A prospective multicenter study of cervical spine injury in children. *Pediatrics*. 2001; 108(2): E20.

237. Panacek EA, Mower WR, Holmes JF, Hoffman JR, NEXUS Group. Test performance of the individual NEXUS low-risk clinical screening criteria for cervical spine injury. *Ann Emerg Med*. 2001; 38(1): 22–5.

238. Lowery DW, Wald MM, Browne BJ, Tigges S, Hoffman JR, Mower WR, NEXUS Group. Epidemiology of cervical spine injury victims. *Ann Emerg Med*. 2001; 38(1): 12–16.

239. Brimacombe J, Keller C, Künzel KH, Gaber O, Boehler M, Pühringer F. Cervical spine motion during airway management: A cinefluoroscopic study of the posteriorly destabilized third cervical vertebrae in human cadavers. *Anesth Analg*. 2000; 91(5): 1274–8.

240. Hoffman JR, Mower WR, Wolfson AB, Todd KH, Zucker MI. Validity of a set of clinical criteria to rule out injury to the cervical spine in patients with blunt trauma. National Emergency X-Radiography Utilization Study Group. *N Engl J Med*. 2000; 343(2): 94–9. Erratum in: *N Engl J Med*. 2001; 344(6): 464.

241. Domeier RM, Evans RW, Swor RA, Hancock JB, Fales W, Krohmer J, Frederiksen SM, Shork MA. The reliability of prehospital clinical evaluation for potential spinal injury is not affected by the mechanism of injury. *Prehosp Emerg Care*. 1999; 3(4): 332–7.

242. Hauswald M, Ong G, Tandberg D, Omar Z. Out-of-hospital spinal immobilization: Its effect on neurologic injury. *Acad Emerg Med*. 1998; 5(3): 214–19.

243. Davis JW, Phreaner DL, Hoyt DB, Mackersie RC. The etiology of missed cervical spine injuries. *J Trauma*. 1993; 34(3): 342–6.

244. Bijur PE, Haslum M, Golding J. Cognitive and behavioral sequelae of mild head injury in children. *Pediatrics*. 1990; 86(3): 337–44.

245. Bivins HG, Ford S, Bezmalinovic Z, Price HM, Williams JL. The effect of axial traction during orotracheal intubation of the trauma victim with an unstable cervical spine. *Ann Emerg Med*. 1988; 17(1): 25–9.

246. Reid DC, Henderson R, Saboe L, Miller JD. Etiology and clinical course of missed spine fractures. *J Trauma*. 1987; 27(9): 980–6.

247. Balla JI, Elstein AS. Skull x-ray assessment of head injuries: A decision analytic approach. *Methods Inf Med*. 1984; 23(3): 135–8.

248. Podolsky S, Baraff LJ, Simon RR, Hoffman JR, Larmon B, Ablon W. Efficacy of cervical spine immobilization methods. *J Trauma*. 1983; 23(6): 461–5.

249. Bohlman HH. Acute fractures and dislocations of the cervical spine. An analysis of three hundred hospitalized patients and review of the literature. *J Bone Joint Surg Am*. 1979; 61(8): 1119–42.

250. Kennedy E. *Spinal Cord Injury: The Facts and Figures*. Birmingham: University of Alabama Press; 1986.

251. Lakkis NA, Maalouf GJ, Mahmassani DM. Jellyfish stings: A practical approach. *Wilderness Environ Med*. 2015; 26(3): 422–429.

252. Berling I, Isbister G. Marine envenomations. *Aust Fam Physician*. 2015; 44(1): 28–32.

253. Reese E, Depenbrock P. Water envenomations and stings. *Curr Sports Med Rep*. 2014; 13(2): 126–31. doi: 10.1249/JSR.0000000000000042.

254. Balhara KS, Stolbach A. Marine envenomations. *Emerg Med Clin North Am*. 2014; 32(1): 223–43. doi: 10.1016/j.emc.2013.09.009.

255. Junior VH, Cardoso JL, Neto DG. Injuries by marine and freshwater stingrays: History, clinical aspects of the envenomations and current status of a neglected problem in Brazil. *J Venom Anim Toxins Incl Trop Dis*. 2013; 19(1): 16. doi: 10.1186/1678-9199-19-16.

256. Carrette TJ, Seymour JJ. Long-term analysis of Irukandji stings in Far North Queensland. *Diving Hyperb Med*. 2013; 43(1): 9–15.

257. Carrette TJ, Underwood AH, Seymour JE. Irukandji syndrome: A widely misunderstood and poorly researched tropical marine envenoming. *Diving Hyperb Med*. 2012; 42(4): 214–23.

258. Fernandez I, Valladolid G, Varon J, Sternbach G. Encounters with venomous sea-life. *J Emerg Med.* 2011; 40(1): 103–12. doi: 10.1016/j.jemermed.2009.10.019.

259. Haddad V Jr, Lupi O, Lonza JP, Tyring SK. Tropical dermatology: Marine and aquatic dermatology. *J Am Acad Dermatol.* 2009; 61(5): 733–50; quiz 751–2. doi: 10.1016/j.jaad.2009.01.046.

260. Lakshmi C, Srinivas CR. Type I hypersensitivity to *Parthenium hysterophorus* in patients with *parthenium* dermatitis. *Indian J Dermatol Venereol Leprol.* 2007; 73(2): 103–5.

261. Atkinson PR, Boyle A, Hartin D, McAuley D. Is hot water immersion an effective treatment for marine envenomation? *Emerg Med J.* 2006; 23(7): 503–8.

262. Loten C, Stokes B, Worsley D, Seymour JE, Jiang S, Isbister GK. A randomised controlled trial of hot water (45 degrees C) immersion versus ice packs for pain relief in bluebottle stings. *Med J Aust.* 2006; 184(7): 329–33.

263. Corkeron M, Pereira P, Makrocanis C. Early experience with magnesium administration in Irukandji syndrome. *Anaesth Intensive Care.* 2004; 32(5): 666–9.

264. Lee JY, Teoh LC, Leo SP. Stonefish envenomations of the hand—A local marine hazard: A series of 8 cases and review of the literature. *Ann Acad Med Singapore.* 2004; 33(4): 515–20.

265. Perkins RA, Morgan SS. Poisoning, envenomation, and trauma from marine creatures. *Am Fam Physician.* 2004; 69(4): 885–90.

266. Little M, Pereira P, Mulcahy R, Cullen P, Carrette T, Seymour J. Severe cardiac failure associated with presumed jellyfish sting. Irukandji syndrome? *Anaesth Intensive Care.* 2003; 31(6): 642–7.

267. Corkeron MA. Magnesium infusion to treat Irukandji syndrome. *Med J Aust.* 2003; 178(8): 411.

268. Bailey PM, Little M, Jelinek GA, Wilce JA. Jellyfish envenoming syndromes: Unknown toxic mechanisms and unproven therapies. *Med J Aust.* 2003; 178(1): 34–7.

269. Nomura JT, Sato RL, Ahern RM, Snow JL, Kuwaye TT, Yamamoto LG. A randomized paired comparison trial of cutaneous treatments for acute jellyfish (Carybdea alata) stings. *Am J Emerg Med.* 2002; 20(7): 624–6.

270. Seymour J, Carrette T, Cullen P, Little M, Mulcahy RF, Pereira PL. The use of pressure immobilization bandages in the first aid management of cubozoan envenomings. *Toxicon.* 2002; 40(10): 1503–5.

271. Fenner PJ, Hadok JC. Fatal envenomation by jellyfish causing Irukandji syndrome. *Med J Aust.* 2002; 177(7): 362–3.

272. Yoshimoto CM, Yanagihara AA. Cnidarian (coelenterate) envenomations in Hawai'i improve following heat application. *Trans R Soc Trop Med Hyg.* 2002; 96(3): 300–3.

273. Thomas CS, Scott SA, Galanis DJ, Goto RS. Box jellyfish (*Carybdea alata*) in Waikiki. The analgesic effect of sting-aid, Adolph's meat tenderizer and fresh water on their stings: A double-blinded, randomized, placebo-controlled clinical trial. *Hawaii Med J.* 2001; 60(8): 205–7, 210.

274. Mianzan HW, Fenner PJ, Cornelius PF, Ramírez FC. Vinegar as a disarming agent to prevent further discharge of the nematocysts of the stinging hydromedusa *Olindias sambaquiensis. Cutis.* 2001; 68(1): 45–8.

275. Pereira PL, Carrette T, Cullen P, Mulcahy RF, Little M, Seymour J. Pressure immobilisation bandages in first-aid treatment of jellyfish envenomation: Current recommendations reconsidered. *Med J Aust.* 2000; 173(11–12): 650–2.

276. Burnett JW, Purcell JE, Learn DB, Meyers T. A protocol to investigate the blockade of jellyfish nematocysts by topical agents. *Contact Dermatitis.* 1999; 40(1): 55–6.

277. Currie B. Clinical implications of research on the box-jellyfish *Chironex fleckeri. Toxicon.* 1994; 32(11): 1305–13.

278. Exton DR, Fenner PJ, Williamson JA. Cold packs: Effective topical analgesia in the treatment of painful stings by Physalia and other jellyfish. *Med J Aust.* 1989; 151(11–12): 625–6.

279. Fenner PJ, Williamson JA, Burnett JW, Colquhoun DM, Godfrey S, Gunawardane K, Murtha W. The "Irukandji syndrome" and acute pulmonary oedema. *Med J Aust.* 1988; 149(3): 150–6.

280. Burnett JW, Calton GJ. Jellyfish envenomation syndromes updated. *Ann Emerg Med.* 1987; 16(9): 1000–5.

281. Burnett JW, Rubinstein H, Calton GJ. First aid for jellyfish envenomation. *South Med J.* 1983; 76(7): 870–2.

282. Hartwick R, Callanan V, Williamson J. Disarming the box-jellyfish: Nematocyst inhibition in *Chironex fleckeri. Med J Aust.* 1980; 1(1): 15–20.

283. Williamson JA, Callanan VI, Hartwick RF. Serious envenomation by the Northern Australian box-jellyfish (*Chironex fleckeri*). *Med J Aust.* 1980; 1(1): 13–16.

284. Sutherland SK, Tibballs J. *Australian Animal Toxins.* Melbourne: Oxford University Press; 2001.

285. Williamson JA, Burnett JW, Fenner PJ, Rifkin JF (eds.) *Venomous and Poisonous Marine Animals: A Medical and Biological Handbook.* Sydney, Australia: University of New South Wales Press; 1996.

286. International Life Saving Federation. Policy Statement MPS-05; Marine Envenomation. Medical statement on marine envenomation. Available at http://www.ilsf.org/about/position-statements

Drowning

DAVID SZPILMAN

INTRODUCTION

Drowning is an endemic 'disaster' all over the world usually related to leisure situations affecting mostly the young that turn into a dramatic and unexpected event for the majority of the population. Parents, friends, relatives, babysitters or guardians may feel not only profound loss and grief, but also guilt for a failure to fulfil protection responsibilities, or intense anger at others who did not provide adequate supervision or medical care.

According to the World Health Organization, 0.7% of all deaths worldwide are due to unintentional drowning, resulting in approximately 42 drowning deaths every hour, every day [1]. This number greatly underestimates the real figures, even for high income countries [2]. Estimates suggest that researchers see only 6% of the problem, as dataset measurement is usually based on attendance at hospitals or by counting death certificates, rather than focusing where drowning occurs – at the pre-hospital setting [3]. Almost all drowning victims are able to help themselves or are rescued in time by bystanders or professional rescuers. In areas where a lifeguard service operates fully, less than 6% of all rescued persons need medical attention and 0.5% of those need cardiopulmonary resuscitation (CPR) [4]. In one report of rescues by bystanders, almost 30% of persons rescued from drowning required CPR [5], which may demonstrate a more severe drowning picture than where lifeguards are on duty. Unfortunately, lifeguard or layperson rescues and first aid attendance are rarely considered in national databases, and the result is a distorted drowning burden scenario worldwide. From 1972 to 2002 the Fire Department of Rio de Janeiro–Lifeguard Service made approximately 166,000 rescues on the beaches, and 8500 victims needed to be attended by the medical team in a drowning resuscitation centre. In this scenario of a full lifeguard service operation, approximately 290 rescues were reported for each death (0.34%), and one death for each 10 victims admitted for medical care in a drowning resuscitation centre [4,6]. The bias produced by not counting the real drowning figures not only affects the importance given to the problem, keeping it as a neglected public health problem [7], but also gives the false impression that every drowning demands CPR and consequently the requirement to know how to resuscitate – a reactive action – becomes the most important tool to save people from drowning.

Drowning involves principles and interventions that are rarely, if ever, found in any other medical situation. It occurs in a hostile environment that does not seem dangerous and this by itself poses a significant problem. The exposure-adjusted, person-time estimations for drowning are 200 times higher than road traffic fatalities [8]. Nevertheless, over 85% of drowning deaths can be prevented by a series of intervention actions [9,10]. When preventative measures fail, responders need to be able to perform the necessary steps to interrupt the drowning process. The first challenge is to recognize someone in the water at risk of drowning and appreciate the need for rescue and emergency medical services (EMS or ambulance) appropriately. Early self-rescue or rescue by others may stop the drowning process and prevent the majority of initial and subsequent water aspiration, respiratory distress and medical complications.

The drowning process happens quickly, but it is critical that rescuers take precautions so they do not become another victim by engaging in inappropriate or dangerous rescue responses [5,11]. Removing the victim from this hostile environment has the potential to do harm to the rescuer, especially for those who are not properly trained or for laypeople with no training at all. This operation may represent a high-risk situation to professional medical responders not trained in water safety. Therefore, it is essential not just for lifeguards but for health professionals to be aware of the complete sequence of actions in drowning, especially how to help a victim who is still in the water [12]. Untrained rescuers should be advised to only provide help from out of the water. Safe rescue techniques for untrained rescuers include reaching to the drowning person with an object such as a pole, towel or tree branch or by throwing a buoyant object. These quick, safe responses are often neglected and should be taught as part of water safety education, to health professionals as well. The recently published article 'Creating a drowning chain of survival' [12] refers to a series of water safety interventions that, when put into action, should reduce the mortality associated with drowning and attempted aquatic rescue. The term 'chain of survival' has provided a useful metaphor for the elements of the emergency cardiac care system for sudden cardiac arrest; however, the drowning process interventions and patient management involve principles and actions that are specific to emergency drowning situations. A unique drowning chain of survival can guide the important lifesaving steps for lay and professional rescuers and may significantly improve chances of prevention, survival and recovery for people in potential danger in water [12].

SCIENTIFIC EVIDENCE ON DROWNING

Much has changed in beach lifeguarding from its early origins as a purely voluntary humanitarian service to a professional vocation. But drowning is essentially an out-of-hospital 'disease' involving a high number of physical (water temperature, surf conditions, hazards etc.) and human (lifeguard and victims – physical fitness, preconditions or morbidity, behaviours etc.) variables, the action and interaction of which are largely unknown [13,14]. With the low level of scientific evidence-base, best practice tends to be based on expert opinion formed from experience (level of evidence 4). This situation will only be improved with the completion of more high-quality definitive research.

The expectation of the public to be protected when they visit the beach and the increasingly litigious society in which we live have driven the requirement for high standards. In many cases, these lifeguarding standards need to be properly tested by the application of scientific research. Furthermore, it is imperative not only to include current scientific research but also to consider the practical implications and provide reasonable recommendations for the application of this research and further research that could enhance our understanding and contribute to saving more lives.

Drowning varies in severity and this variation should be recognized; different grades of drowning need specific approaches and stratification to reduce bias. At its worst, the prognosis for a drowning cardiopulmonary arrest, despite the continuing effort to improve resuscitation and post-resuscitation care, remains poor. Although modern CPR has existed for more than 50 years, the majority of old and new interventions, other than stopping the drowning process early and providing ventilation and chest compression, have not been shown to improve survival rates [4,13,15]. More than half of survivors sustain neurological injury to some degree and fewer than 12% show full recovery and are eventually able to return to work [4,6,13,15,16]. If drowning is not stratified appropriately by severity, there is a large variation in survival, implying that these conflicting results are due to differences in the definitions of variables, which creates misleading conclusions and outcomes [4,14,17]. The challenge for researchers is to stratify their cases into subgroups to reduce bias without losing statistical power, especially with cases requiring CPR where there is usually much missing information. Such cases are known as the 'Labiruzzle quiz' [14], a CPR challenge with missing puzzle pieces, where researchers have to collect as many variables as possible and are challenged to select a track based on the best available scientific evidence.

For the proper advance in drowning science, it is essential for researchers to accept and use the 'drowning Utstein Style', a set of guidelines for uniform reporting of drowning and resuscitation [18]. These guidelines include the adoption of uniform definitions and nomenclature, a glossary of key terms, an updated chain of survival, recommendations based on medical evidence and best practice, and uniform classifications and registration systems. By using the Utstein guidelines for reporting drowning cases, researchers should be able to collaborate and share hypotheses. There remains a strong requirement to create a web-based multicentre data management system, a tool that would compare standard data on drowning.

Any research reporting an improvement in lifeguarding intervention or treatment must be treated with great caution, as the lifeguarding world is anxious to put into practice new techniques to save more people. Such claims must be validated properly in a realistic scenario before being introduced and increasing variability and confusion.

As with much published science, drowning study results are mostly positive (publication bias) and the process of research is almost all positive, which suggests that the novelty of having research conducted and the increased attention from such could lead to temporary increases in productivity and improvement in the quality of the service – the Hawthorne effect [19].

The aim of this chapter is to bring together the most up-to-date scientific research on drowning with a commentary on its application to the real world of the beach.

DEFINITION AND TERMINOLOGY

A new definition of drowning was established in 2002 and adopted by the World Health Organization [20]: 'Drowning is the process of experiencing respiratory impairment from submersion or immersion in liquid'.

The drowning process is a continuum, beginning with respiratory impairment as the victim's airway goes below the surface of the liquid (submersion) or when water splashes over the face (immersion). If the victim is rescued at any point, the process of drowning is interrupted, and it is a nonfatal drowning. If the victim dies at any point, it is a fatal drowning. Any submersion or immersion incident without evidence of respiratory impairment should be considered a water rescue and not a drowning. Terms such as 'near-drowning', 'dry or wet drowning', 'secondary drowning', 'active and passive drowning' and 'delayed onset of respiratory distress' should not be used [20]. A uniform way to report data following drowning to allow comparison among different centres is to adopt the Utstein template for reporting drowning deaths [18,21].

PATHOPHYSIOLOGY

When a drowning person can no longer keep his or her airway clear, water entering the mouth is voluntarily spat out or swallowed. The next conscious response is to try and hold the breath, but this lasts for no more than seconds [22]. When the victim is no longer able to protect their airway, some amount of water is aspirated into the airways, and coughing occurs as a reflex response. In less than 2% of cases [23,24], laryngospasm may be present, but the onset of hypoxia will terminate this rapidly. If the person is not rescued, aspiration of water continues and hypoxaemia quickly leads to loss of consciousness and apnea at the same time. A sequence of cardiac rhythm deterioration with a period of tachycardia followed by bradycardia, pulseless electrical activity (PEA) and, finally, asystole has been suggested [25,26]. The whole drowning process, from submersion or immersion to cardiac arrest, usually occurs in seconds to a few minutes, but in unusual situations, such as rapid hypothermia, this process can last for up to an hour [27].

In some cases, even an early and effective rescue will not prevent medical consequences of the drowning process. In those cases, basic life support (BLS) and advanced life support may be needed. When it is safe and appropriate, rescue breathing may need to be initiated while the victim is still in the water [3,28].

If the person is rescued alive, the clinical picture is determined predominantly by the volume of water that has been aspirated and the reactivity of the person's airways to this water, but not to the type of water (salt or fresh). Water in the alveoli can cause surfactant destruction and washout. Salt and fresh water aspiration cause similar degrees of pathology [25] although there are differences in osmotic gradients. In either situation, the effect of the osmotic gradient on the very delicate alveolar-capillary membrane can disrupt the integrity of the membrane, increase its permeability and exacerbate fluid, plasma and electrolyte shifts [25]. The clinical picture of the damage, depending on the amount of water aspirated, the reactivity of the person's airways and damage caused to the alveolar–capillary membrane, is a regional or general pulmonary oedema that may decrease in different proportion the exchange of O_2 and CO_2 [4,25,29].

In animal research, the aspiration of 2.2 mL of water per kilogram of body weight leads to a severe disturbance of the exchange of oxygen, decreasing the arterial oxygen pressure (PaO_2) to approximately 60 mm Hg within three minutes [30]. In humans, it seems that as little as 1–3 mL/kg of water aspiration produces profound alterations in pulmonary gas exchange and decreases pulmonary compliance by 10%–40% [25]. The combined effects of fluid in the lungs, loss of surfactant and increased capillary–alveolar permeability (alveolitis) can result in decreased lung compliance, increased right-to-left shunting in the lungs, atelectasis and bronchospasm [25].

One of the unique features, and a last stage of drowning, is that apnea and hypoxia cause and precede the cardiac arrest by a few seconds or minutes. In most drowning cases, the heart tissue is relatively healthy and stops due to the hypoxia insult, after a period of apnea [4,11]. In those cases, immediate in-water resuscitation provides the greatest benefit, if provided safely and effectively [28].

If the victim needs CPR, neurological damage is similar to other arrest situations but exceptions exist. Hypothermia associated with drowning can provide a protective mechanism that allows victims to survive prolonged submersion episodes [3,27]. Hypothermia can reduce brain oxygen consumption, prolonging the interval until cellular anoxia and adenosine triphosphate (ATP) depletion occur. Hypothermia reduces the electrical and metabolic activity of the brain in a temperature-dependent fashion. The rate of cerebral oxygen consumption is reduced by approximately 5% per degree Celsius reduction in temperature within the range of 37°C–20°C [31].

DROWNING CHAIN OF SURVIVAL – PREVENTION TO HOSPITAL

The drowning chain of survival is a new concept that is presented in Figure 9.1.

Prevent drowning to be safe in and around the water

Prevention is the most effective step in the chain of drowning survival. It has been estimated that the great majority of drownings may be preventable [10,32]. Unintentional drowning incidents have the highest case fatality rates compared to other injuries. In the nations with the highest drowning rates, there are often no rescue systems or EMS/ambulance or

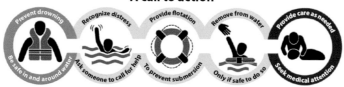

Figure 9.1 Drowning chain of survival. (From Szpilman D, et al., *Resuscitation*, 85(9), 1149–52, 2014.)

hospital intensive care units to manage victims of drowning. In high income nations, only 10%–20% of drowning victims who go into cardiac arrest survive despite receiving the care outlined in each link in the chain of survival, and fewer than 30% of survivors are neurologically intact [21,33–35]. Thus, prevention of drowning is paramount. Drowning requires multiple layers of protection. To be effective, drowning prevention must be used by individuals near, on or around the water and by those who supervise or care for others in water settings.

Recognize distress and ask someone to call for help

The first challenge to the provision of help is to recognize a person in distress in the water and know how to activate the lifeguard and emergency medical services (EMS/ambulance). Frank Pia [36], the first author to hypothesize the 'instinctive drowning response' in a film in 1970s, contradicted the prevailing notions that most victims struggle at the water surface, call or wave for help and actively attempt to attract rescuers. He showed that a person who is struggling and about to drown cannot usually call for help, which consequently proved to be of major importance in recognizing the primitive movement patterns that reflect a potential risk or an actual drowning.

In 1995, Langendorfer and Bruya [37] identified key developmental components of aquatic readiness and water competency, which included the following: body position, from vertical to horizontal; arm actions, from ineffective to effective; leg actions, from ineffective to effective; and combined actions, little/no progress to efficient forward progress. They called this an 'aquatic readiness assessment'. A drowning risk assessment (DRA) was created using the developmental principle of regressive change [38]. The identified recognizable elements of a person at high risk of drowning include the following: near-vertical body position, ineffective downward arm movements, ineffective pedalling or kicking leg actions and little or no forward progress in water. It was also noted that many lifeguarding programs fail to adequately train lifeguards in observational skills. Lanagan-Leitzel [39,40] demonstrated that trained lifeguards and lifeguard instructors were unable to identify drowning victims in video scenarios. A lack of ability to recognize a person at risk of drowning is a high professional risk for any lifeguard to carry. Interestingly, non-lifeguards trained in DRA were equally as likely as lifeguards to identify persons at risk of drowning. This fact may present an opportunity to educate laypeople on the importance of being able to recognize a person drowning and then send someone to call for help.

Sending someone to call for help upon recognizing a person in water distress is a key element in the drowning response chain that ensures early activation of the EMS (ambulance)/rescue services or, if unavailable, a skilled helper. Delays in activating EMS (ambulance)/rescue services increase the risk of fatal drowning.

Provide flotation to stop the process of drowning

In drowning, the first priority or tactical goal is to interrupt the drowning process by providing flotation (buoyancy) to the victim. This is especially important if the victim cannot be immediately removed from the water. Providing flotation as an interim measure to reduce the submersion risk is a strategy not widely employed in aquatic emergencies, despite buying valuable time for emergency services to arrive or for those on the scene to plan rescue efforts. Most rescuers tend to focus on the strategic goal of getting the victim out of the water even if there is a high threat to life or rescuer safety, multiple victims or delays in executing the rescue [41,42]. Devices such as ring buoys (lifebuoys) are purpose-designed to provide flotation; however, they are not always available at the scene of a drowning incident. Therefore, improvised buoyancy aids such as empty plastic bottles/containers, bodyboards, surfboards, driftwood, ice chests and so on should be used [43,44]. It is critical that laypeople take precautions not to become another victim by engaging in inappropriate or dangerous rescue responses [5,11]. Given the number of bystanders who get into difficulty or drown while attempting to rescue others, reaching out with, throwing or dropping a buoyancy aid without entering the water is the preferred method of providing flotation to a drowning victim [45].

A panicked and struggling victim can be dangerous to a would-be rescuer. A victim attempting to cling to life and breathe can drown their would-be rescuer. For this reason, it is always best to approach a struggling victim with an intermediary object. Lifeguards use rescue or torpedo buoys for this purpose, which can also double as thorax and face flotation devices to keep the head out of the water and the airways free [11].

In-water resuscitation if indicated and possible

A conscious victim should be brought to land, and basic life support should be started as soon as possible [4,28].

If not interrupted, the drowning process leads first to unconsciousness and apnea, followed by cardiac arrest within minutes. During this short window of opportunity, immediate in-water resuscitation (ventilation only) provides the greatest benefit if provided safely and effectively.

For an unconscious victim, in-water resuscitation can increase the discharge from hospital without sequelae by more than threefold [28]. In-water resuscitation is only possible if the rescuer is highly trained and if the action consists of ventilation alone. Attempts at chest compression while the rescuer and victim are in deep water are futile, so checking for a pulse does not serve any purpose [28]. Victims with only respiratory arrest usually respond after a few rescue breaths. If there is no response, the victim should be assumed to be in cardiac arrest and should be moved as quickly as possible to dry land where effective CPR can be initiated (Figure 9.2) [28].

Another medical concern is the possibility of cervical spine injury (CSI). Few studies have examined how often in-water CSI occurs. One such study, concerning sand beaches, retrospectively evaluated 46,060 water rescues and demonstrated that the incidence of CSI in this setting is very low (0.009%) [46]. In another retrospective survey of more than 2400 drownings, only 11 (<0.5%) had a CSI and all of these had a history of obvious trauma from diving, falling from a height or a motor vehicle accident [47]. Other water locations may have different rates depending on a wide variety of elements. Furthermore, any time spent immobilizing the cervical spine in unconscious victims with no signs of trauma could lead to a cardiopulmonary deterioration and even death. Considering this low incidence of CSI and the high risk to wasted time in ventilation when needed, routine cervical spine immobilization of water rescues, without reference to whether a traumatic injury was sustained, is not recommended [46–48].

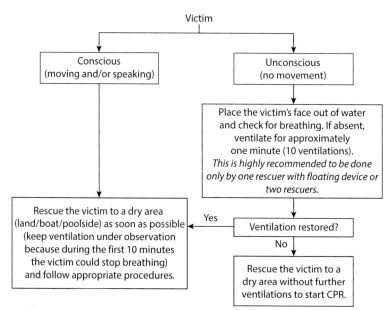

IWR flow chart decision – Szpilman 2015 – Exceptions to attempt IWR include threats to the safety of the rescuer and the victim if immediate rescue is not initiated, in those cases where a dry place (land/boat/poolside) is near enough to get the victim out of the water immediately and cases of *known* submersion over 15 minutes

Figure 9.2 In-water basic life support flow chart decision – only for use by lifeguards and trained providers.

Rescuers who suspect a spinal cord injury should float the victim, supine, into a horizontal position allowing the airways to be out of water and check if there is spontaneous breathing. If not, they should start protocols for in-water resuscitation (mouth-to-mouth) without putting themselves or the victim in the water at greater risk. If there is spontaneous breathing, the rescuer should stabilize the victim's neck by hand in a neutral position; keep floating the victim using, if possible, a back support device before moving the victim; rescue the victim to a dry place, maintaining the neck in a neutral position as much as possible; align and support the head, neck, chest and body if the victim must be moved or turned [49]. Therefore, no attempt to immobilize the spine should be made without a strong indication and certainly not in cases where the victim appears lifeless [50].

Remove from water – Rescue only if safe to do so

Removing the victim from water is essential in order to reduce further aspiration and provide a definitive end to the drowning process [28]. Removal to dry land also allows for better assessment and care of the victim and safety for the rescuer.

Several strategies for removal can be used. For lay/untrained rescuers, attempt to remove the victim without fully entering the water by utilizing rescue techniques such as throwing assist, reaching assist and wading assist with equipment [12]; assist the victim to get out of the water by giving directions, i.e. pointing out to the closest and safest place to get out of the water or how to perform a self-rescue; if everything else fails, the lay rescuer may consider entering the water to attempt to rescue the victim. The entry of an untrained person into the water to rescue someone is very dangerous [5]. According to the New Zealand National Drowning Database [42], 81 would-be rescuers drowned between 1980 and 2012 while attempting to rescue someone. To enter the water is a personal decision theoretically related to the following: relationship with the victim; depth of the water/distance to swim; swimming and rescue skills of the lay responder; level of danger involved; consequences of not providing aid to the victim; age of victim; and other factors.

The attempt to perform a rescue typically involves three phases: approach, contact and stabilizing the

victim. In order to mitigate the risk to the layperson during the contact and stabilization phases, they must bring a source of flotation [45].

Transporting drowning victims from the water and positioning them on land requires unique adaptations described in Table 9.1 [51].

Provide care as needed – Basic life support to hospital

Early basic and advanced life support improves drowning outcomes and should be initiated as soon as possible at the drowning scene [3].

Initial management of a drowning victim on land

As soon as the drowning person is removed from the water, lay and professional rescuers must recognize the drowning severity, especially if there is a life-threatening situation such as an isolated respiratory or full cardiopulmonary arrest, so that immediate care can be provided. If a rescuer is in doubt as to whether the person is alive or not, they should always start CPR as this gives the patient a much greater chance of survival [4].

One of the most difficult medical decisions a lifeguard or an emergency medical technician (EMT) must make is how to treat a drowning victim appropriately. Cardiopulmonary or isolated respiratory arrest comprises approximately 0.5% of all rescues. The questions that arise include the following: Should the rescuer administer oxygen, call an ambulance, transport the person to a hospital or observe for a time at the site? Even hospital emergency physicians may be in doubt as to the most appropriate immediate and continued support, as drowning victims vary in severity of injury. Based on these needs, a classification system was developed in Rio de Janeiro (Brazil) in 1972 and updated in 1997 [4] to assist lifeguards, ambulance personnel and physicians with treatment. It was based on an analysis of 41,279 rescues, of which 2304 (5.5%) needed medical attention. It was revalidated in 2001 by a 10-year study with 46,080 rescues [6]. This classification (Figure 9.3) [4] is stratified into six grades plus a rescue and a non-resuscitation condition encompassing all the support from the site of the accident to the hospital. It recommends the most appropriate intervention/treatment and shows the likelihood

Table 9.1 Recommendations for positioning a drowning victim without suspected spinal injury according to setting and the condition of the victim

Setting	Condition of the drowning victim	
	Conscious victim	**Exhausted, confused or unconscious victim**
In water (during rescue)	Position victim according to the rescue technique chosen.	Whenever possible, rescuers should keep the face of the victim out of the water, extend the neck to open the airway and keep it clear during the rescue process. 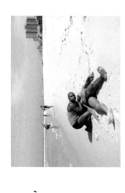
Recovery onto land	Transport vertically with head up. Keep horizontal if immersion was prolonged or in cold water. 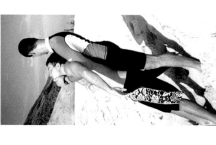	Transport in as near a horizontal position as possible but with the head still maintained above body level. The airway should be kept open and the victim should be kept horizontal if prolonged immersion or cold water is involved. 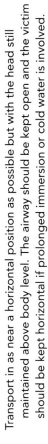
On land	Maintain the victim in a supine position with head up.	If cardiopulmonary resuscitation is required, place victim supine, as horizontal as possible, and parallel with the waterline.

(Continued)

Table 9.1 (*Continued*) Recommendations for positioning a drowning victim without suspected spinal injury according to setting and the condition of the victim

Setting	Condition of the drowning victim	
	Conscious victim	Exhausted, confused or unconscious victim

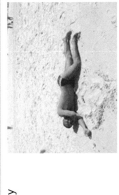

Unconscious but breathing: place in recovery position.

The Basic Life Support Working Group of the International Liaison Committee on Resuscitation has agreed on six principles that should be followed when managing an unconscious, spontaneously breathing victim [52]:

- The victim should be in as near a true lateral position as possible with the head dependent to allow free drainage of fluid.
- The position should be stable.
- Any pressure on the chest that impairs breathing should be avoided.
- It should be possible to turn the victim onto the side and return to the back easily and safely, having particular regard for the possibility of cervical spine injury.
- Good observation of and access to the airway should be possible.
- The position itself should not give rise to any injury to the victim.

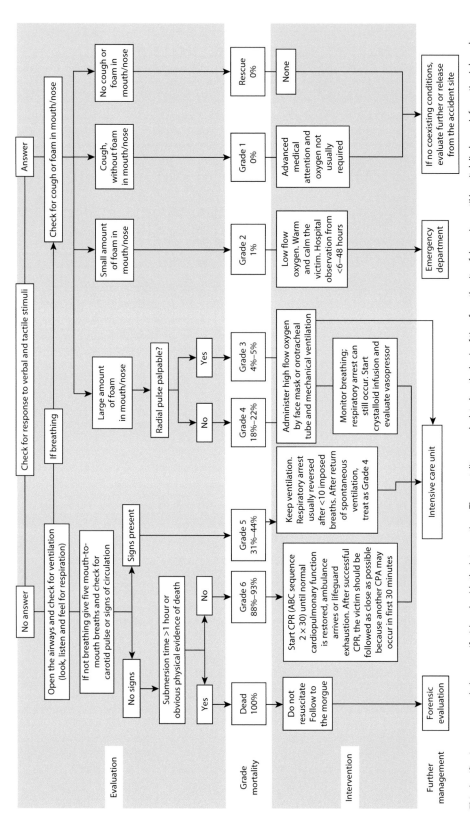

This classification system can help to stratify risk and guide the interventions. The mortality was calculated on the basis of time from the site of drowning until hospital discharge. Information is based on a retrospective review of 41,279 rescues recorded by lifeguards, of which 94% (38,975 cases) were just rescues (no water aspiration) and 6% of these cases involved the receipt of medical attention, but 1% (473) were not reported with sufficient information to classify the grade of presentation [21,34]. Of the 1,831 persons seen by a medical doctor at the Drowning Resuscitation Centre in Rio de Janeiro from 1972 to 1991, 65% were classified as Grade 1 presentations (1189 cases), 18% as Grade 2 (338), 3% as Grade 3 (58), 2% as Grade 4 (36), 1% as Grade 5 (25), and 10% as Grade 6 (185) [21].
ABC, airway–breathing–circulation; CPR, cardiopulmonary resuscitation; CPA, cardiopulmonary arrest.

Figure 9.3 Drowning severity classification for lifeguards.

of death based on the severity of injury. The severity is easily assessed by an on-scene rescuer, EMT or physician using only clinical variables [4].

Once on land, the victim should be placed supine with trunk and head at the same level (in general parallel to the shore line) and the standard checks for responsiveness and breathing should be carried out [28]. If the victim is unconscious but breathing, the recovery position (lateral decubitus) should be used [51]. If the victim is not breathing, rescue ventilation is essential [4,11,50,53].

Cardiac arrest from drowning is due primarily to lack of oxygen, when the usually healthy heart muscle stops beating following a period of apnea [4,11,50,53,54]. For this reason, it is important that CPR should follow the 'traditional' airway–breathing–circulation (ABC) [55] and not the circulation–airway–breathing (CAB) sequence – start with five initial rescue breaths followed by 30 chest compressions, and continue with two rescue breaths to 30 compressions until signs of life re-appear, rescuer exhaustion occurs or advanced life support becomes available. In drowning, the European Resuscitation Council [53] recommend an initial five ventilations instead of two (the American Heart Association's recommendation) [50] as upper airway management is always challenging due to vomiting and the fluid that interferes with airway management, making the initial ventilations and an effective alveolar expansion more difficult [50,56].

Cardiac compression–only CPR, is not advised in drowning [50,53,54].

The most frequent complication during a resuscitation attempt is regurgitation of the stomach contents, which occurs in more than 65% of victims who need rescue breathing alone and in 86% of those who require CPR [57]. The presence of vomitus in the airway can result in further aspiration injury and impairment of oxygenation [28]. Active efforts to expel water from the airway (abdominal thrusts or placing the victim head down) should be avoided as they only delay the initiation of ventilation, increase the risk of vomiting by more than five-fold and lead to a significant increase in mortality [28,51]. If vomiting occurs, turn the victim's mouth to the side, remove the vomitus with a finger sweep or cloth or use suction and continue resuscitation.

It is important to recognize that resuscitation of drowning victims often takes place under very different circumstances. There may be problems recovering the victim to dry land, and the delay until emergency medical system arrival may be longer than usual. On the other hand, victims are generally young, and the rate of success is potentially higher [5,26,35]. These variables influence lifeguards' decisions and the correct course of action.

The cost-effectiveness of providing an automated external defibrillator (AED) at sites of aquatic activity has been debated, as the predominantly cardiac arrest rhythm on drowning is asystole [58]. On the other hand, cardiac arrest at aquatic sites may occur due to causes other than drowning when the presence of an AED may be lifesaving [58].

Recommendations for when to start and stop resuscitation are different from non-drowning-related cardiac arrest (Table 9.2) [3,26].

The majority of people with mild distress may not actually aspirate water and, thus, EMS/ambulance

Table 9.2 Drowning: When to initiate CPR and when to discontinue

Question	Recommendations
On whom to begin CPR?	• Give ventilatory support for respiratory distress/arrest to avoid cardiac arrest. • Start CPR in all victims submerged <60 minutes who do not present obvious physical evidence of death (rigor mortis, body decomposition or dependent lividity).
When to discontinue CPR?	• Basic life support should continue unless signs of life reappear, rescuer becomes exhausted or advanced life support takes over. • Advanced life support should be ongoing until the patient has been rewarmed (if hypothermic) and asystole persists for more than 20 minutes.

Source: Data from Szpilman D, et al., *N Engl J Med*, 366, 2102–10, 2012.

Table 9.3 Description of cases requiring further medical help after rescue from the water (MPS 06)

(a) The following persons should be sent to hospital in most cases:
  - Any patient who lost consciousness even for a brief period.
  - Any patient who required expired air resuscitation (rescue breathing).
  - Any patient who required cardiopulmonary resuscitation.
  - Any patient in whom a serious condition is suspected such as heart attack, spinal injury, other injury, asthma, epilepsy, stinger, intoxication, delirium.

(b) The following persons may be considered for release from care at the scene if, after 10–15 minutes of careful observation, while being warmed with blankets or other coverings as required, the patient has ALL of the following. In such cases, it is unwise for the patient to drive a vehicle and the patient should be so advised. If any of these conditions do not apply or if the lifesaver has any doubt, then the patient should be advised to seek early medical attention.
  - No cough
  - Normal rate of breathing
  - Normal circulation as measured by pulse in strength and rate and blood pressure (if available)
  - Normal colour and skin perfusion
  - No shivering
  - Fully conscious, awake and alert

(c) There is always a risk of delayed lung complications. All immersion victims should therefore be warned that if they later develop cough, breathlessness, fever or any other worrying symptom, they should seek medical advice immediately. It is preferable that these persons not return to a home environment where they are alone for the next 24 hours.

may not be summoned. Therefore, it is important to educate lifeguards and responders about when to call the EMS (ambulance) or to seek medical assistance/hospital care in cases of drowning. Table 9.3 describes who needs further medical help after rescue from the water [59].

Advanced pre-hospital management

In addition to immediate BLS, advanced life support teams should be alerted as soon as possible to attend the incident.

A victim with pulmonary damage may initially be able to maintain adequate oxygenation through an abnormally high respiratory rate and can be managed by administering oxygen by face mask at a rate of 15 litres of oxygen/minute. Early intubation and mechanical ventilation is indicated when the victim shows signs of deterioration or fatigue (Grades 3 and 4) [4]. New airway devices, such as the supraglottis airway, need to be carefully evaluated before incorporation into daily use by lifeguards. The important clinical issue here is not whether it is comfortable or quick for the lifeguards to use, but whether it is fit for the purpose of properly ventilating a drowning victim [56]. Once intubated,

most victims can be oxygenated and ventilated effectively. Despite continuous, copious, pulmonary oedema fluid appearing in the endotracheal tube, suctioning can disturb oxygenation and should be balanced against the need to ventilate and oxygenate [60,61]. Pre-hospital providers should insure adequate oxygenation to maintain arterial saturation between 92% and 96%, while insuring adequate chest rise during ventilation [62]. Positive end-expiratory pressure should be added as soon as it is available to decrease pulmonary arterial shunt and increase oxygenation [60]. If abdominal distention becomes a restriction to ventilation, an orogastric tube can be inserted, after a secure definitive airway is established.

Peripheral venous access is the preferred route for drug administration in the pre-hospital setting. Intraosseous access is an alternative route. Endotracheal administration of drugs is not recommended for drowning [53]. If hypotension is not corrected by oxygenation, a rapid crystalloid infusion should be administered, regardless of whether salt or fresh water has been inhaled [29].

The presenting rhythm in cases of cardiac arrest following drowning (Grade 6) is usually asystole or PEA. Ventricular fibrillation is rarely reported, but may occur if there is a history of coronary artery disease, due to the use of epinephrine, or in the presence of severe hypothermia [26]. During CPR, if ventilation and chest compression do not result in cardiac activity, cumulative doses of epinephrine 1 mg IV (or 0.01 mg/Kg/dose) can be considered. Because of the mechanisms of cardiac arrest secondary to hypoxia and the effects of hypothermia, a higher subsequent dose, although controversial [63], may be considered if the initial doses fail.

Drowning is sometimes precipitated by an injury or medical condition (e.g. trauma, seizure, cardiac arrhythmia etc.) and this co-morbidity should be considered [4,64] especially by professional responders, as it might guide specific approaches to rescue and resuscitation. On Rio de Janeiro beaches, precipitant causes are discernible in 13% of all cases attended by the medical staff: alcohol (37%); convulsion (18%); trauma, including boating accidents (16.3%); cardiopulmonary disease (14.1%); skin diving and scuba diving (3.7%); diving resulting in head or spinal cord injuries; and others, e.g. homicide, suicide, syncope, cramps or immersion syndrome (11.6%) [65].

The majority of drowning victims will have aspirated only small amounts of water, if any, and will recover spontaneously. Only 6% of all who are rescued by lifeguards need medical attention in a hospital [4]. Rescue and Grade 1 victims presenting with good arterial oxygenation (pulse oximetry) without adjuvant therapy and no other associated morbidity can safely be released home.

Emergency department attendance is recommended for all Grades 2–6 patients. Most Grade 2 victims tolerate non-invasive oxygen administration, will normalize their clinical situation within 6–8 hours and can be sent home [4]. Those who deteriorate are admitted to an intermediate care unit for prolonged observation.

Hospital attendance

For Grades 3–6 patients, who usually need intubation and mechanical ventilation support, assistance at an intensive care unit may be required [4]. As the pulmonary lesion is caused by temporary and local injury, pulmonary distress following drowning tends to heal much faster than other diseases, and there is usually no late pulmonary sequelae [60]. Water in the lungs is absorbed (fresh water faster, salt water more slowly) into the blood across the pulmonary capillary membrane and excreted in urine within 24–48 hours. There are very few procedures that may help the lung to heal other than mechanical ventilation and to wait to wean the patient off ventilation until after 24–72 hours. It is common practice to be careful to wean a drowning case from mechanical ventilation before 24 hours, even when they appear to be breathing adequately; it is suggested that the local pulmonary injury has not yet been repaired and this may cause the return of pulmonary oedema with the need for re-intubation, leading to a prolonged hospital stay and further morbidity [66].

At the emergency department, after the airway has been secured, oxygenation has been optimized, the circulation stabilized and a gastric tube has been inserted, thermal insulation of the patient should be instituted. This step is followed by physical examination, measurement of arterial blood gases and chest radiography. Metabolic acidosis occurs in the majority of cases and will be compensated for better minute ventilation [29]. Routine use of sodium bicarbonate is not recommended.

In most drowning cases, the circulation becomes adequate after oxygenation, rapid crystalloid infusion and restoration of normal body temperature [25,60]. Early cardiac dysfunction can occur following severe drowning [25], which adds a cardiogenic component to the non-cardiogenic pulmonary oedema. No evidence supports the use of a specific fluid therapy for salt and fresh water drowning [25], i.e. the use of diuretics or water restriction [11].

Meanwhile, if not taken before, a history of events surrounding the drowning incident including rescue and resuscitation activities and any current or previous illness should be checked [21]. If the victim remains unresponsive without an obvious cause, a toxicology investigation and a computed tomography of head and neck should be considered [67].

Electrolytes, blood urea nitrogen, creatinine and hematocrit are not routinely recommended. Abnormalities are unusual [4,30] and correction of electrolyte imbalance is rarely needed [68].

Pneumonia is initially often misdiagnosed with the early radiographic appearance of water in the lungs. In a series of hospitalized cases, only 12% had pneumonia and needed antibiotics [69].

Prophylactic antibiotics tend to select out more resistant and aggressive organisms and are not routinely recommended [70].

In some cases, hypothermia is just a reflection of prolonged submersion time and a bad prognosis. In other victims, early hypothermia is an important reason why survival without neurological damage is possible [27,50,71]. Recent reports on drowning have documented good outcomes in post-resuscitation patients who were kept hypothermic or treated with therapeutic hypothermia, despite poor predicted outcomes [53,72]. The paradox in drowning resuscitation is that the hypothermic victim needs to be warmed initially in order to effectively resuscitate, but then may benefit from induced therapeutic hypothermia after successful resuscitation [3].

OUTCOME

With the progresses of intensive care therapy, prognostics are more and more based on neurologic outcome. Grades 1–5 drownings return home safely without sequelae in 95% of cases [4]; important medical complications of drowning other than neurological are rare and are almost all restricted to Grade 6. In hospital, permanent neurological damage is the most worrisome outcome of initial survival after CPR. Victims who remain comatose or deteriorate neurologically should undergo intensive assessment and care [73]. We need to answer questions such as: How can we know who we should make the effort to resuscitate? How long should we continue to resuscitate? How different should the treatment be? And what should we expect as life quality after successful resuscitation? Both at the rescue site and in the hospital, no one indicator for Grade 6 appears to be an absolutely reliable indicator of outcome [74]. Based on the largest submersion time registered in cold water (66 minutes) with complete recovery [11], resuscitation should be started without delay in each victim without a carotid palpable pulse who has been submerged for less than one hour, or who does not present obvious physical evidence of death (rigor mortis, putrefaction or dependent lividity). A long-time submersion with successful resuscitation is not only possible in cold or icy water: some anecdotal cases have been reported to survive in warm water without sequelae [4,75,76]. Multiple studies

have established that outcome is almost solely determined by a single fate factor – duration of submersion [3,4,11,28,57,75,77].

Basic and advanced life support enables victims to achieve the best outcome possible. After successful CPR, it is crucial to stratify neurological severity; this will allow comparison of different therapeutic approaches. Various prognostic scoring systems have been developed to predict which patients will do well with standard therapy and which are likely to have a significant cerebral anoxic encephalopathy and will require aggressive measures to protect the brain. One of the most powerful scoring systems is the evaluation of the consciousness level related to the Glasgow coma scale at the period immediately after resuscitation (first hour) (Conn & Modell Neurological Classification) [78]. Data suggest that patients who remain profoundly comatose (i.e. decorticate, decerebrate or flaccid) 2–6 hours after the drowning incident are brain-dead or have moderate to severe neurological impairment. Patients who are improving but remain unresponsive have a 50% likelihood of a good outcome. Most patients who are definitely improving and are alert or are stuporous or obtunded but respond to stimuli 2–6 hours after the incident have normal or near-normal neurological outcomes.

These prognostic variables are important in counselling family members of drowning victims in the early stages after the incident. They are helpful for deciding which patients are likely to have a good outcome with standard supportive therapy and which are candidates for intensive cerebral resuscitation therapies.

Drowning represents a tragedy that all too often is preventable. Perhaps the majority of cases are the end result of common sense violations, alcohol consumption or neglect of responsible childcare. This picture needs a radical preventive intervention.

REFERENCES

1. Word Health Orginisation *Global Report on Drowning: Preventing a Leading Killer.* 2014; Geneva: WHO.
2. Lu TH, Lunetta P, Walker S. Quality of cause-of-death reporting using ICD-10 drowning codes: A descriptive study of 69 countries. *BMC Med Res Methodol.* 2010; 10: 30.

3. Szpilman D, Bierens JJLM, Handley AJ, Orlowski JP. Drowning: Current concepts. *N Engl J Med.* 2012; 366: 2102–10.

4. Szpilman D. Near-drowning and drowning classification: A proposal to stratify mortality based on the analysis of 1,831 cases. *Chest.* 1997; 112: 660–5.

5. Venema AM, Groothoff JW, Bierens JJLM. The role of bystanders during rescue and resuscitation of drowning victims. *Resuscitation.* 2010; 81: 434–9.

6. Szpilman D, Elmann J, Cruz-Filho FES. Drowning classification: A revalidation study based on the analysis of 930 cases over 10 years. *World Congress on Drowning*, the Netherlands, Amsterdam, 26–28 June 2002.

7. Murray CJL. Quantifying the burden of disease: The technical basis for disability-adjusted life years. *Bull World Health Organ.* 1994; 72: 429–45.

8. Mitchell RJ, Williamson AM, Olivier J. Estimates of drowning morbidity and mortality adjusted for exposure to risk. *Inj Prev.* 2010; 16: 261–6.

9. Quan L, Bennett E, Branche CM. Interventions to prevent drowning. In Doll LS, Bonzo SE, Sleet DA, et al. (eds.). *Handbook of Injury and Violence Prevention.* New York: Springer; 2007, pp. 81–96.

10. Moran K, Quan L, Franklin R, Bennett E. Where the evidence and expert opinion meet: A review of open-water: Recreational safety messages. *Int J Aquat Res Educ.* 2011; 5: 251–70.

11. Orlowski JP, Szpilman D. Drowning. Rescue, resuscitation, and reanimation. Pediatric critical care: A new millennium. *Pediatr Clin North Am.* 2001; 48: 627–46.

12. Szpilman D, Webber J, Quan L, Bierens J, Morizot-Leite L, Langendorfer SJ, Beerman S, Løfgren B. Creating a drowning chain of survival. *Resuscitation.* 2014; 85(9): 1149–52. doi:10.1016/j.resuscitation.2014.05.034.

13. Nolan JP, Hazinski MF, Billi JE, et al. Part 1: Executive summary: 2010 International Consensus on Cardiopulmonary Resuscitation and Emergency Cardiovascular Care Science with Treatment Recommendations. *Resuscitation.* 2010; 81: e1–25.

14. Szpilman D, dos Santos Cruz Filho FE. One single variable for predicting the outcome after out-of-hospital-cardiac-arrest (OHCA): A reality or simply chasing El Dorado? *Resuscitation.* 2014; 85(4): P448–9.

15. Nolan JP, Nadkarni VM, Billi JE, et al. Part 2: International collaboration in resuscitation science: 2010 International Consensus on Cardiopulmonary Resuscitation and Emergency Cardiovascular Care Science with Treatment Recommendations. *Resuscitation.* 2010; 81: e26–31.

16. Young GB. Clinical practice. Neurologic prognosis after cardiac arrest. *N Engl J Med.* 2009; 361: 605–11.

17. Kuisma M, Alaspaa A. Out-of-hospital cardiac arrests of non-cardiac origin epidemiology and outcome. *Eur Heart J.* 1997; 18: 1122–8.

18. Idris AH, Berg RA, Bierens JJLM, et al. Recommended guidelines for uniform reporting of data from drowning: The "Utstein style." American Heart Association. *Circulation.* 2003; 108(20): 2565–74.

19. McCarney R, Warner J, Lliffe S, Van Haselen R, Griffin M, Fisher P. The Hawthorne effect: A randomised, controlled trial. *BMC Med Res Methodol.* 2007; 7: 30. doi:10.1186/1471-2288-7-30.

20. Van Beeck EF, Branche CM, Szpilman D, Modell JH, Bierens JJLM. A new definition of drowning: Towards documentation and prevention of a global public health problem. *Bull World Health Organ.* 2005; 83(11): 853–6.

21. Youn CS, Choi SP, Yim HW. Out-of-hospital cardiac arrest due to drowning: An Utstein Style report of 10 years of experience from St. Mary's Hospital. *Resuscitation.* 2009; 80: 778–83.

22. Sterba JA, Lundgren CE. Diving bradycardia and breath-holding time in man. *Undersea Biomed Res.* 1985; 12(2): 139–50.

23. Szpilman D, Elmann J, Cruz-Filho FES. Dry-drowning—Fact or myth? *World Congress on Drowning*, the Netherlands, Amsterdam, 26–28 June 2002, Poster Presentation, p. 176.

24. Lunetta P, Modell JH, Sajantila A. What is the incidence and significance of "dry-lungs" in bodies found in water? *Am J Forensic Med Pathol.* 2004; 25(4): 291–301.

25. Orlowski JP, Abulleil MM, Phillips JM. The hemodynamic and cardiovascular effects of near-drowning in hypotonic, isotonic, or hypertonic solutions. *Ann Emerg Med.* 1989; 18: 1044–9.

26. Grmec S, Strnad M, Podgorsek D. Comparison of the characteristics and outcome among patients suffering from out-of-hospital primary cardiac arrest and drowning victims in cardiac arrest. *Int J Emerg Med.* 2009; 2: 7–12.

27. Tipton MJ, Golden FS. A proposed decision-making guide for the search, rescue and resuscitation of submersion (head under) victims based on expert opinion. *Resuscitation.* 2011; 82: 819–24. doi:10.1016/j.resuscitation.2011.02.021.

28. Szpilman D, Soares M. In-water resuscitation—Is it worthwhile? *Resuscitation.* 2004; 63: 25–31.

29. Modell JH, Graves SA, Ketover A. Clinical course of 91 consecutive near-drowning victims. *Chest.* 1976; 70: 231–8.

30. Modell JH, Moya F, Newby EJ, Ruiz BC, Showers AV. The effects of fluid volume in seawater drowning. *Ann Intern Med.* 1967; 67: 68–80.

31. Polderman KH. Application of therapeutic hypothermia in the ICU: Opportunities and pitfalls of a promising treatment modality. Part 1: Indications and evidence. *Intens Care Med.* 2004; 30: 556–75.

32. Quan L, Pilkey D, Gomez A, Bennett E. Analysis of paediatric drowning deaths in Washington State using the child death review for surveillance: What the CDR tells us and doesn't tell us about lethal drowning injury. *Inj Prev.* 2011; 17(Suppl 1): 28–33.

33. Quan L, Kinder DR. Pediatric submersions: Prehospital predictors of outcome. *Pediatrics.* 1992; 90: 909–13.

34. López-Herce J, García C, Domínguez P, Rodríguez-Núñez A, Carrillo A, Calvo C, Delgado MA. Outcome of out-of-hospital cardiorespiratory arrest in children. *Pediatr Emerg Care.* 2005; 21: 807–15.

35. Claesson A, Svensson L, Silfverstolpe J, Herlitz J. Characteristics and outcome among patients suffering out-of-hospital cardiac arrest due to drowning. *Resuscitation.* 2008; 76: 381–7.

36. Pia F. Observations on the drowning of non-swimmers. *J Phys Educ.* 1974; 71(6): 164–7, 181.

37. Langendorfer S, Bruya L. *Aquatic Readiness. Developing Water Competence in Young Children.* Champaign, IL: Human Kinetics; 1995.

38. Langendorfer SJ. Applying a development perspective to aquatics and swimming. In Kjendlie PL, Stallman RK, Cabri J (eds.). *Biomechanics and Medicine in Swimming XI.* Oslo: Norwegian School of Sport Sciences; 2010, pp. 20–2.

39. Lanagan-Leitzel LK. Identification of critical events by lifeguards, instructors, and non-lifeguards. *Int J Aquat Res Educ.* 2012; 6(3): 203–14.

40. Lanagan-Leitzel LK, Moore CM. Do lifeguards monitor the events they should? *Int J Aquat Res Educ.* 2010; 4(3): 241–56.

41. Derks, E. (Producer). Piha Rescue [Television series]. New Zealand: South Pacific Video Productions; 2012.

42. Water Safety New Zealand. Drowning statistics 1980–2012 where the victim has been attempting to rescue others [Dataset]. 2013. Available at DrownBase™ database.

43. About.com Survival. How to make improvised floatation devices. 2013. Available at http://survival.about.com/od/3/a/How-To-Make-Improvised-Floatation-Devices.htm

44. Basic Water Rescue, The American National Red Cross—1998. Mosby Lifeline, Yardley Pennsylvania: Stay well, 1998.

45. Turgut A, Turgut B. A study on rescuer drowning and multiple drowning incidents. *J Saf Res.* 2012; 43: 129–32. doi:10.1016/j.jsr.2012.05.001.

46. Szpilman D, Brewster C, Cruz-Filho FES. Aquatic cervical spine injury—How often do we have to worry? *World Congress on Drowning,* the Netherlands, Amsterdam, 26–28 June 2002, Oral Presentation.

47. Watson RS, Cummings P, Quan L, Bratton S, Weiss NS. Cervical spine injuries among submersion victims. *J Trauma.* 2001; 51: 658–62.

48. Szpilman D. Aquatic cervical and head trauma: Nobody told me it could be a jump in the darkness! *World Conference on Drowning Prevention,* Danang, Vietnam, 17–21 May 2011, p. 153.

49. Wernicke P, Szpilman D. Immobilization and extraction of spinal injuries. In Bierens J (ed.). *Handbook on Drowning: Prevention, Rescue and Treatment*. Springer-Verlag, Heidelberg; 2015; 621–628.

50. Soar J, Perkins GD, Abbasc G, et al. European Resuscitation Council Guidelines for Resuscitation 2010. Section 8. Cardiac arrest in special circumstances: Electrolyte abnormalities, poisoning, drowning, accidental hypothermia, hyperthermia, asthma, anaphylaxis, cardiac surgery, trauma, pregnancy, electrocution. *Resuscitation*. 2010; 81: 1400–33.

51. Szpilman D, Handley A. Positioning the drowning victim. In Bierens JJLM (ed.). *Handbook on Drowning: Prevention, Rescue, and Treatment*. Berlin: Springer-Verlag; 2006, pp. 336–41.

52. Handley AJ, Becker LB, Allen M, van Drenth A, Kramer EB, Montgomery WH. Single-rescuer adult basic life support: An advisory statement from the Basic Life Support Working Group of the International Liaison Committee on Resuscitation. *Circulation*. 1997; 95(8): 2174–9.

53. Vanden HTL, Morrison LJ, Shuster M, et al. Part 12: Cardiac arrest in special situations: Drowning. 2010 American Heart Association Guidelines for Cardiopulmonary Resuscitation and Emergency Cardiovascular Care. *Circulation*. 2010; 122(3): S847–8.

54. International Life Saving Federation, Medical Committee. Clarification statement on cardiopulmonary resuscitation for drowning. Available at http://tinyurl.com/5u3mfdh

55. Kitamura T, Iwami T, Kawamura T, Nagao K, Tanaka H, Nadkarni VM, Berg RA, Hiraide A. Conventional and chest-compression-only cardiopulmonary resuscitation by bystanders for children who have out-of-hospital cardiac arrests: A prospective, nationwide, population-based cohort study. *Lancet*. 2010; 375: 1347–54.

56. Baker PA, Webber JB. Failure to ventilate with supraglottic airways after drowning. *Anaesth Intensive Care*. 2011; 39: 675–7.

57. Manolios N, Mackie I. Drowning and near-drowning on Australian beaches patrolled by life-savers: A 10-year study, 1973–1983. *Med J Aust*. 1988; 148: 165–71.

58. Beerman S, Lofgren B. Automated external defibrillator in the aquatic environment. In Bierens JJLM (ed.). *Handbook on Drowning: Prevention, Rescue, and Treatment*. Berlin: Springer- Verlag; 2006, pp. 331–6.

59. International Lifesaving Federation—Medical Position Statement (MPS 06). Who needs further medical help after rescue from the water. Available at http://www.ilsf.org/sites/ilsf.org/files/filefield/MPS-06%20Medical%20Help.doc

60. Gregorakos L, Markou N, Psalida V, et al. Near-drowning: Clinical course of lung injury in adults. *Lung*. 2009; 187: 93–7.

61. Diamond W, MacDonald RD. Submersion and early-onset acute respiratory distress syndrome: A case report. *Prehosp Emerg Care*. 2011; 15: 288–93.

62. Kochanek PM, Bayir H. Titrating oxygen during and after cardiopulmonary resuscitation. *JAMA*. 2010; 303: 2190–1.

63. Weiss SJ, Muniz A, Ernst AA, Lippton HL. The physiological response to norepinephrine during hypothermia and rewarming. *Resuscitation*. 2000; 45: 201–7.

64. Quan L, Cummings P. Characteristics of drowning by different age groups. *Inj Prev*. 2003; 9: 163–8.

65. Szpilman D, Elmann J, Cruz-Filho FES, Drowning Resuscitation Center. Ten-years of medical beach attendance in Rio De Janeiro-Brazil. *World Congress on Drowning*, the Netherlands, Amsterdam, 26–28 June 2002, Poster Presentation, p. 167.

66. Eggink WF, Bruining HA. Respiratory distress syndrome caused by near or secondary drowning and treatment by positive end-expiratory pressure ventilation. *Neth J Med*. 1977; 20(4–5): 162–7.

67. Rafaat KT, Spear RM, Kuelbs C, Parsapour K, Peterson B. Cranial computed tomographic findings in a large group of children with drowning: Diagnostic, prognostic, and forensic implications. *Pediatr Crit Care Med*. 2008; 9: 567–72.

68. Oehmichen M, Hennig R, Meissner C. Near-drowning and clinical laboratory changes. *Leg Med (Tokyo)*. 2008; 10: 1–5.

69. Berkel M, Bierens JJLM, Lierop C, et al. Pulmonary oedema, pneumonia and mortality in submersions victims: A retrospective study in 125 patients. *Intensive Care Med.* 1996; 22: 101–7.

70. Wood C. Towards evidence based emergency medicine: Best BETs from the Manchester Royal Infirmary. BET, 1: Prophylactic antibiotics in near-drowning. *Emerg Med J.* 2010; 27: 393–4.

71. Takano Y, Hirosako S, Yamaguchi T, et al. Nitric oxide inhalation as an effective therapy for acute respiratory distress syndrome due to near-drowning: A case report. *Nihon Kokyuki Gakkai Zasshi.* 1999; 37: 997–1002.

72. Guenther U, Varelmann D, Putensen C, Wrigge H. Extended therapeutic hypothermia for several days during extracorporeal membrane-oxygenation after drowning and cardiac arrest: Two cases of survival with no neurological sequelae. *Resuscitation.* 2009; 80: 379–81.

73. Warner D, Knape J. Recommendations and consensus brain resuscitation in the drowning victim. In Bierens JJLM (ed.). *Handbook on Drowning, Prevention, Rescue, Treatment.* Berlin: Springer Verlag; 2006, pp. 436–9.

74. Bierens JJ, van der Velde EA, van Berkel M, van Zanten JJ. Submersion in the Netherlands: Prognostic indicators and results of resuscitation. *Ann Emerg Med.* 1990; 19: 1390–5.

75. Szpilman D. A case report of 22 minutes submersion in warm water without sequelae. In Bierens J (ed.). *Handbook on Drowning: Prevention, Rescue and Treatment.* Springer-Verlag, Heidelberg; 2005, pp. 375–6.

76. Allman FD, Nelson WB, Gregory AP, et al. Outcome following cardiopulmonary resuscitation in severe near-drowning. *Am J Dis Child.* 1986; 140: 571–5.

77. Cummins RO, Szpilman D. Submersion. In Cummins RO, Field JM, Hazinski MF (eds.). *ACLS: The Reference Textbook: Vol II. ACLS for Experienced Providers.* Dallas, TX: American Heart Association; 2003, pp. 97–107.

78. Orlowski JP. Drowning, near-drowning, and ice water submersion. *Pediatr Clin North Am.* 1987; 34: 92.

10

Resuscitation techniques for lifeguards

JOOST BIERENS

INTRODUCTION

This chapter provides an overview on resuscitation techniques for lifeguards, with an emphasis on the typical aspects that are relevant for the resuscitation of asphyxic drowning victims and the practical and organizational consequences of performing resuscitations at or near a beach. This chapter does not describe resuscitation in situations of immersion hypothermia or the consequences of cervical spine injuries. Within the global effort to reduce drowning and the concept of the chain of survival in drowning, resuscitation is less important than prevention and rescue. However, beach lifeguards should possess the skills and knowledge to be able to achieve excellent resuscitation results. The 2015 Guidelines by the European Resuscitation Council (ERC) provide clear protocols for this [1–5].

BASIC LIFE SUPPORT AND AUTOMATED EXTERNAL DEFIBRILLATORS: GUIDELINES IN PRIMARY CARDIAC ARREST

More than 55 years ago, the first international guidelines for resuscitation were developed by Peter Safar, an Austrian anaesthesiologist working in Pittsburgh, PA, USA. The approach, which was revolutionary at the time, was that laypeople were put on the front line to reverse acute cardiac arrests by teaching them basic life support (BLS). Until then, only mouth-to-mouth ventilation had been taught to laypeople, which often proved to be successful in the resuscitation of drowning victims except for situations involving cardiac arrest. There had been a need for new guidelines because the number of cardiac arrests had increased dramatically. Studies had shown that 'hearts could be saved that are too good to die' [6,7]. Since then, resuscitation guidelines have been regularly updated to improve the quality and outcome of resuscitation. Each of these updates has been based on a compilation of evidence from a structured analysis of thousands of studies. In addition, the didactical aspects and efficacy of teaching BLS have been taken into account. This information is needed to increase the coverage of BLS-competent laypeople within different communities. This process is supervised by the International Liaison Commission of Resuscitation (ILCOR), in which all national resuscitation councils are congregated.

BLS guidelines are aimed at resuscitation by one layperson. If a layperson encounters someone who is unconscious or unresponsive and not breathing normally, the layperson calls for help and begins chest compressions. Occasional gasps, or agonal breaths, are ignored because this reflex can happen during the last phase of circulatory arrest. Medical dispatch or emergency services are called immediately. While starting cardiopulmonary resuscitation (CPR), other bystanders are requested to look for an automated external defibrillator (AED). After an initial series of 30 uninterrupted compressions, the patient is ventilated twice. Resuscitation is then continued with a compression–ventilation ratio of 30:2. As soon as possible during this sequence, the external defibrillator is attached; it then ascertains whether there is ventricular fibrillation (VF) or pulseless ventricular tachycardia (VT). If a shockable rhythm is confirmed, an electric shock is automatically delivered. If no shockable rhythm is detected, the voice prompt advises continued CPR. This cycle of events is repeated. While the AED is charging and analysing between shocks and immediately after each shock, the cycle of 30 uninterrupted chest compressions followed by two ventilations is resumed. This sequence continues for two minutes after which there is another AED analysis (Figure 10.1). The resuscitation is stopped at any moment when the victim coughs, moves, opens the eyes or speaks or until the pre-hospital system takes over [7].

In essence, the uniform BLS guidelines focus on a primary cardiac arrest situation, with an emphasis on the importance of immediate, uninterrupted, high-frequency chest compressions and the delivery of AED shocks as soon as possible. National resuscitation councils have limited freedom to adapt the ILCOR guidelines.

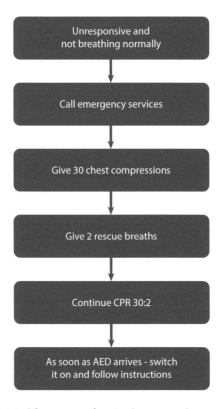

Figure 10.1 The algorithm of basic life support for single-person bystander CPR. (From Perkins GD, et al. Part 3: Adult basic life support and automated external defibrillation: 2015 International Consensus on Cardiopulmonary Resuscitation and Emergency Cardiovascular Care Science with Treatment Recommendations. *Resuscitation*. 2015; 95: e43–69. Copyright European Resuscitation Council - www.erc.edu - 2015_NGL_006. With permission.)

As a result, the BLS guidelines in some countries default in favour of chest compression–only resuscitation, in large part because of the educational efficacy [8]. Some other guidelines discourage mouth-to-mouth ventilation by pointing to the unpleasant sensations and the potential risks of infection. Most, but not all, guidelines have a short paragraph on paediatric resuscitation that deviates from the adult resuscitation guidelines with respect to palpation of the circulation [7].

In 2013, an estimated 16 million people around the world were trained in BLS [9–12]. In Europe, each year some 275,000 people are treated for cardiac arrest by ambulance crews. Most of these people also receive bystander resuscitation [13]. Lifeguards are expected to have the competency to perform BLS and use an AED [14,15].

WHY BLS AND AED PROTOCOLS IN DROWNING CASES SHOULD DIFFER FROM THESE GUIDELINES

The process of dying from primary cardiac arrest begins with a sudden and complete arrest of the circulation. In most situations, this is a ventricular fibrillation: uncoordinated contractions of heart muscles that disable the pump function of the heart. At the moment of circulatory arrest, there is an oxygen reserve in the lungs, arterial circulation and cells. During the arrest period, the oxygen content in the cells will decrease after the oxygen in the stagnant blood is used. However, when circulation is restarted quickly the oxygen reserve in the lungs will become available to the cells again.

In drowning, the physiological process is different: in general during at least the first one to two minutes underwater, the heart continues to beat and the circulation continues to transport available oxygen reservoirs to the cells. The oxygen reserve in the lungs and blood decreases as a result of the oxygen consumed by the cells and gradually all cells have to deal with hypoxia (lowered oxygen). To the brain, hypoxia initially means a decrease in consciousness. To the heart, it initially means a slower and reduced pumping function, which is reflected in a slower and weaker pulse. At a certain point, the oxygen

supply to the cells of the heart muscles becomes so low that the heart stops beating. At that point, the cells in the brain might already have started to suffer hypoxic damage, but this may temporarily be delayed when there has been a rapid decline in brain temperature [16,17]. However, in most cases the preceding and prolonged hypoxia will have caused gradual and severe neurological damage [18,19].

Therefore, when a drowning victim is taken out of the water, the situation is unlike that of a primary cardiac arrest. Even if the victim has been underwater for prolonged periods of time, there may still be a working, but severely hypoxic, heart. Circulation, often with very low heart rates, has been detected in drowning victims who have been underwater for prolonged periods [20–22]. Some of these drowning victims will show abnormal breathing patterns. This pattern is unlike the gasping in a primary cardiac arrest, which is a cerebral reflex and of no use for the reversal of the cardiac arrest. Breath-like movements in drowning is to compensate for and reverse hypoxia. If indeed cardiac arrest has occurred, in most instances it will be a full cardiac arrest preceded by a slow heart rate (bradycardia). A ventricular fibrillation is detected in 0%–10% of drowning victims (Table 10.1).

At the same time, the lungs of the drowning victims have often been heavily affected by the aspiration of water during the drowning process. This state can make ventilation very difficult. Moreover, because during submersion large quantities of water can be swallowed, there is a 20%–60% risk of vomiting [35,36]. Lifeguards should be trained in how to deal with all these typical aspects of resuscitation in a drowned person [14,37].

BEST PRACTICE IN DROWNING RESUSCITATION (PHYSIOLOGY-BASED)

Thus, there are major differences in what happens after a primary cardiac arrest and after an asphyxial cardiac arrest [16,17]. This may lead to a strong suggestion that these differences have important consequences for the optimal resuscitation of drowning victims. Unfortunately, formal research data are lacking. Drowning represents only a small minority of all resuscitations. No human or

Table 10.1 Frequency of ventricular fibrillation observed in resuscitation studies of drowning victims

Author	Year of publication	Drowning patients included	% of patients with ventricular fibrillation
Suominen et al. [23]	2002	48	6.2
Eich et al. [24]	2007	12	0
Grmec et al. [25]	2009	29	9.7
Youn et al. [26]	2009	130	2.3
Ballesteros et al. [27]	2009	20	5.0
Suominen et al. [28]	2010	9	0
Choi et al. [29]	2012	20	0
Nitta et al. [30]	2013	1737	1.7
Dyson et al. [31]	2013	336	6.0
Claesson et al. [32]	2014	499	8.0
Buick et al. [33]	2014	98	9.9
Kieboom et al. [34]	2015	160	2.0

animal studies have been performed to compare a standard resuscitation to one or more drowning-dedicated resuscitation techniques.

Based on an understanding of the different pathophysiological mechanisms, some of the best-practice advice in drowning has a solid basis in clear logic and common sense. This advice is also used in other domains of emergency medicine and resuscitation, such as in paediatric resuscitation and resuscitation after accidental hypothermia [6,38,39]. *Primum non nocere* ('first do no harm'): it makes no sense to immediately 'jump' on the chest of each victim that is taken from the water after a hectic rescue. Some will look dead at first sight, but may still have circulation. At the same time, it must be realized that up to 60% of patients who have been resuscitated have been diagnosed post-mortem with rib fractures, sternum fractures and other lethal consequences [40,41].

Instead: *treat first, what kills first*. The drowned victim is dying from lack of oxygen and oxygen has to be provided as soon as possible. Resuscitation after drowning therefore starts with ventilation. To have any effect, and because ventilation is often difficult in drowning victims, it is advised to start with five ventilations. A certain portion of drowning victims respond after ventilation-only CPR, probably because the presence of circulation was not detected or it was falsely assumed, based on the patient's appearance, that there was no circulation [20–22,36,42]. It should be noted that in a hypoxic

and hypercapnic situation, the oxygen-binding capacity of the erythrocytes is most effective [43].

Prioritizing chest compression to restore the circulation of deoxygenated blood or waiting for the analysis of an AED [44,45], which in over 90% of drowning resuscitation settings will say to start CPR because there is no VF (see Table 10.1), will contribute to enhanced hypoxic damage, notably in the brain cells. Instead, the focus should be on how to increase the oxygen content in lungs, arterial blood and cells by means of immediate and optimal ventilation and oxygenation.

In the education of resuscitation to the general public, these significant differences in resuscitation between primary cardiac arrest and drowning cardiac arrest are mentioned either marginally or not at all. Educational specialists fear that teaching about exceptions seriously disrupts an efficacy-driven educational programme for laypeople. There are good arguments for such a point of view when dealing with the general population, to maximize the coverage of BLS-trained people within communities. The quality of bystander CPR is already rather low and making extra categories and therapies may indeed confuse the students [46]. In addition, the very high incidence of primary cardiac arrest and the very low incidence of drowning-related cardiac arrest is very much in favour of one standard. In studies that included all causes of cardiac arrest, 0.4%–4.0% were drowning victims [25,30,32,33].

THE CONTENT OF A DROWNING RESUSCITATION COURSE

Lifeguard organizations may decide that their lifeguards should only be trained in the standard single-person CPR for cardiac arrest situations. There may be economic or political reasons to make such a suboptimal decision. Under no circumstances should lifeguard organizations teach or advise compression-only CPR for drowning situations. This type of CPR only repeats the process of hypoxic cardiac arrest in drowning and further interventions will become useless [8,47].

It should be realized that the standard resuscitation course prepares citizens for different situations than those lifeguards have to deal with. Bystanders most of all are interested in learning CPR to help people they know (parents, family, neighbourhood). In general, they arrive by chance at the scene of a cardiac arrest where they decide to perform CPR to the best of their knowledge. Most are cardiac arrest situations in a building, on the street or at another relatively convenient location with direct access to the patient and rapid arrival of ambulances.

Lifeguards are intentionally at the beach within a dedicated organizational structure; they have to respond frequently and with perfect quality performance. Resuscitation on a beach often occurs during unfavourable weather conditions, with unpredictable incoming waves and a lot of people. To prepare lifeguards for their formal duties, the inclusion of additional knowledge and skills in their resuscitation courses should be considered (Table 10.2).

Anecdotal data suggest that 50%–70% of all resuscitations by lifeguards are drowning victims and that 6%–9% of all lifeguards have resuscitation experience [51–53]. Most studies conclude that the success of resuscitation after drowning is at least as good as resuscitation after a primary cardiac arrest [22,54–57]. Importantly, most of the drowning resuscitation patients may have been healthy before the cardiac arrest and may return to a normal life. For lifeguards, it is therefore necessary and economic to learn the skills that allow them to master the optimal resuscitation techniques for drowning. These techniques are based on an understanding of the pathophysiology of drowning and practical experience. Lifeguards are intrinsically motivated to perform as well as possible and are willing to learn [58,59]. The most important elements of such techniques are summarized in Table 10.3. Figures 10.2 and 10.3 provide examples of how such resuscitation procedures may be performed.

When a team of lifeguards arrives at a drowning scene, they have to recognize first that it is a drowning situation. Most of the time, this will be immediately clear from the setting and the accounts of bystanders. If in doubt, treat a patient taken from the water as a drowning victim. A typical exception is the overweight tourist standing knee-deep in the water who suddenly collapses or the locally well-known older lady who goes for her daily swim and suddenly disappears underwater.

If a drowning victim makes atypical respiratory efforts, this means that there is a lack of oxygen.

Table 10.2 Important aspects for consideration in structuring resuscitation courses for lifeguards

- Lifeguards are generally recognized as the only formal body at the beach that is capable of providing medical care until an ambulance arrives [14]. It is expected by the public that they have a duty to act, behave and communicate in a professional manner. This expectation means that they need to have the competencies to deal with bystanders who have rescued a victim from the water and start CPR [22]; to deal with bystanders who want to interfere, either verbally or by action; to deal with family members and friends of the victim who observe the ongoing resuscitation; and to deal with initial after-care when the victim has been declared dead or transported by ambulance to a hospital [48].
- Lifeguards are often protected by special clothing that interferes with resuscitation performance. In addition, the conditions under which lifeguards have to operate are very different from classroom situations. As a result, they should train in realistic scenarios and settings [49].
- Lifeguards often act as teams where each member has a task. Team configuration changes and tasks often shift due to exhaustion, the need to solve technical problems, expansion of the team by more experienced lifeguards or involvement of trustworthy nurses or doctors who happen to be at the beach. Thus, there must be an understanding of the basics of crew resource management to apply an effective, coordinated and uninterrupted resuscitation [50].

The good news is that this is most likely a non-arrest situation. In most situations, it will be sufficient to provide oxygen with a non-rebreathing mask. Breathing and coughing are easier in an upright position if the patient can manage it [36,60]. If the respiratory efforts of the patients are inadequate, provide five effective mouth-to-mouth ventilations and supply the patient with oxygen as soon as possible. While watching to see whether the situation will improve, a second lifeguard can use the waiting time during the five inflations to check the carotid pulse. Although the palpation of the pulse has been removed from the resuscitation algorithm in cardiac arrest victims, a carotid

Table 10.3 Most important aspects of the resuscitation of drowning victims for lifeguards to know

- The first priority is ventilation. This should start as soon as possible, which often means mouth-to-mouth ventilation and oxygenation
- Compression-only CPR is useless in drowning cases
- Check circulation to avoid chest compression while the heart is beating
- Be prepared for ventilation to be difficult
- Apply AED only after ventilation and chest compression are orderly executed
- Work as a coordinated team
- Do not stop CPR at the beach before medical professionals have arrived

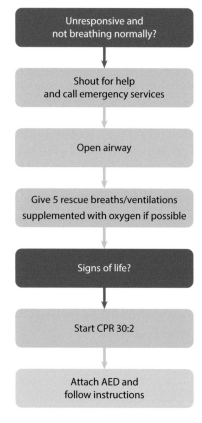

Figure 10.2 Example of the flow diagram for team resuscitation, as trained by the crews of the Royal Dutch Lifeboat Institution. A similar flow diagram may be used by lifeguards. The basic life support protocol for team CPR in drowning. (From Truhlář A, et al. European Resuscitation Council Guidelines for Resuscitation 2015: Section 4. Cardiac arrest in special circumstances. *Resuscitation*. 2015; 95: 148–201. Copyright European Resuscitation Council www.erc.edu 2015_NGL_006. With permission.)

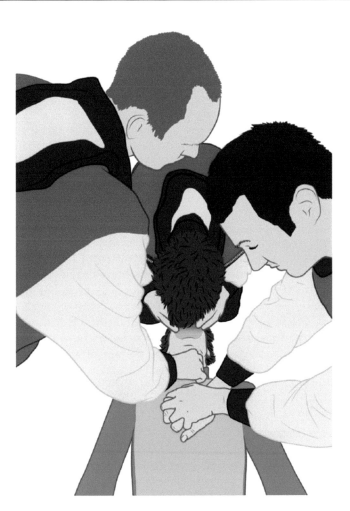

Figure 10.3 Position of persons in a resuscitation team setting, as trained by the crews of the Royal Dutch Lifeboat Institution. (1) The person at the head provides mouth-to-mask ventilation. (2) The person on the left side of the patient (on the right side of the picture) provides thoracic compressions. (3) The person on the right side of the patient (on the left side of the pictures) provides cricoid pressure when ventilation is ineffective (if the abdomen rises instead of the thorax during ventilation) and applies the automated external defibrillator as soon as basic life support functions well. (4) The fourth person (not pictured) is responsible for coordination and communication.

pulse can be detected by 90% of laypeople within one minute, and it provides valuable information in this situation. Many lifeguards do this intuitively [61–63].

If the victim does not make any respiratory efforts and has the characteristic bluish-white mottled skin, sometimes with foam or vomitus on the lips, the lifeguard should clean the lips and start five effective ventilations. Meanwhile, the carotid pulse should be checked by a second lifeguard. If pulsations are felt, the situation will generally improve after a few more ventilations, eventually with supplementary oxygen. If there are no pulsations, chest compressions should be started [1,36]. Depending on how the scenario-based training is organized locally, this could be a single-person or a two-person resuscitation.

If immediately available, oxygen should be provided through the oxygen inlet of a face mask [64]. There is some concern that excessively high concentrations of inspired oxygen may have a negative influence on the outcome of BLS in cardiac arrest [65–68]. In drowning resuscitation, these worries are considered irrelevant due to the need for oxygen; the drowning-induced damage at the alveolar-capillary level of the lung seriously decreases the diffusion of oxygen in the circulation, avoiding the risk of hyperoxygenation [69,70].

Only after ventilation, oxygenation and compressions are well established, should the AED be attached. The AED will only recognize a VF or VT and then initiate the shock procedure. In all other situations, such as bradycardia, sinus rhythm and other rhythm disorders, the AED is expected to advise continuing CPR [15,71]. It is therefore important to regularly check the carotid pulse in order to stop as soon as circulation can be detected.

The decision to start or stop resuscitation is always debatable. The current consensus is that in non-icy-cold water, which is the usual situation on a beach, resuscitation is useless after an observed submersion of more than 30 minutes [72,73]. For psychological, legal and professional reasons, it is often better to always start resuscitation when a victim is retrieved from the water, even after a long search period. It is never wise to stop resuscitation that has been started on the beach without further involvement by medical professionals. In addition, the local legal aspects need to be taken into account.

SPECIAL LIFEGUARDING SITUATIONS

Some studies have provided information related to special situations that should be introduced in the knowledge, skills and training of lifeguards.

The basis of good resuscitation is to be able to perform a well-organized, calm and focused resuscitation at the beach, on a boat or at the lifeguard station. Notably, when a lifeguard needs to continue resuscitation immediately following a rescue, it may seem impossible. After a rescue, a lifeguard may be exhausted and breathing heavily. This means that the lifeguard will be unable to control the frequency and depth of breathing. As a result, the victim may be over-inflated during mouth-to-mouth ventilation. In experimental settings, inflation volumes have been measured at up to 300% of the advised volume of 400 cc [74–76]. Such high inflation volumes lead to increased pressure in the thorax. This also increases the resistance against which the heart has to pump blood into circulation.

As a result, the output of the heart of some victims will decrease during chest compressions [77,78]. Moreover, the risk of stomach ventilation, regurgitation, vomiting and gastric perforation increases as a result of high inflation pressures [35,79–81]. At the same time, as a result of exhaustion from rescue efforts, the muscle function of the rescuer may be compromised. The rescuer may have difficulty performing chest compressions without leaning on the thorax and impacting on the correct depth of compressions. A lifeguard who is coming out of the water with a victim should therefore be assisted as soon as possible and, if possible, resuscitation should be conducted by other lifeguards [48,74–76,82].

There are also situations in which in-water ventilation or resuscitation in a rescue boat may be considered. One Brazilian study has shown that when a drowning victim is rescued on the ocean side of the surf, the lifeguard can better perform mouth ventilation while waiting for a rescue boat or helicopter, compared to dragging the victim immediately to shore and starting resuscitation on the beach [42,83,84]. Part of this better outcome was due to the fact that some of the victims ventilated behind the surf recovered while only receiving in-water ventilation. This finding generated several other studies that examined whether it is possible to improve the quality of ventilation during rescue swimming using respiratory aids. In an experimental setting, performed in the calm water of a lake, it has been shown that in-water ventilation with a supraglottic airway device (SGA) provides a fast rescue swim with only limited aspiration [85,86]. Until ventilation with a SGA is part of the BLS in drowning, however, such techniques are not advised for real-world situations.

Other studies have investigated the efficacy of BLS on board lifeboats and the application of an AED under moderate sea states [87–89] and showed that both are possible. More studies, especially in real situations, are needed to determine if it makes sense to train lifeguards on these resuscitation specialities.

Lifeguards can also be confronted with other unusual resuscitation situations, such as suffocation by collapsing sand tunnels [90,91] and suicidal drowning [92–94]. It should be considered that in such situations lifeguards can make use of telephone-assisted CPR from their dispatch

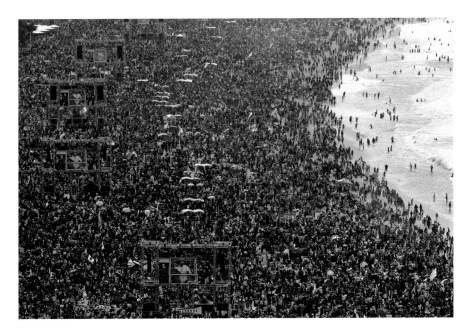

Figure 10.4 At some beaches, lifeguards must be prepared for resuscitation during mass events. This picture is from the visit of Pope Francis to Copacabana Beach in Rio de Janeiro, Brazil, in 2013. Over three million people attended the event. There were 142 rescues and no fatal.

centres where protocols for such situations should be available [95]. Another element that should be anticipated on some beaches is how to deal with several drownings during mass events at beaches (Figure 10.4) [96].

CURRENT DEVELOPMENTS THAT ARE NOT YET ACCEPTED

Within the various lifeguard systems, techniques have been accepted or are under consideration that may further improve the quality of resuscitation on beaches.

Cricoid pressure

A common experience of lifeguards who have ventilated a drowning victim is that ventilation can be difficult and sometimes even impossible. The most relevant cause is the loss of surfactant activity in the alveoli due to the aspirated water in the lungs and the narrowing of the airways, which increases resistance. Surfactant is a lipoprotein located at the air–water interface of the alveoli that reduces surface tension and increases the compliance of the lungs. When washed away, the alveoli collapse

and behave according to the law of LaPlace, which states that the smaller the balloon, the more pressure is needed to inflate it [97,98]. The aspirated water results in a local type of acute respiratory arrest (acute respiratory distress syndrome) that may occur over minutes [89,99]. The other reasons for the high inflation pressure are bronchospasm and abdominal counter-pressure due to a stomach full of swallowed water. In such a situation with high inflation pressure, the inflated air will move in the direction with the lowest resistance: the stomach. Thus, instead of the anticipated rise and fall of the chest during conventional ventilation, the lifeguard only observes a further expansion of the abdomen during unusually forceful ventilations. The inflated air in the stomach further adds to the counter-pressure that has to be overcome to inflate the lungs.

This is a common situation in drowning. If this situation occurs, a prolonged time is needed for ventilation, which increases the period of interruption of chest compressions. This is not considered harmful [100].

Sometimes, this treatment still does not allow ventilation. No air can be inflated at all. In such a hopeless situation, consideration can be given to the use of cricoid pressure (Figure 10.5); by means of a gentle (3–4 kg) pressure on the cricoid ring during ventilation, the oesophagus is closed and high pressure can be applied, which will inflate the lungs. Typically, the pulmonary resistance decreases after a few inflations and the use of cricoid pressure should be stopped. The technique of applying cricoid pressure has been used for centuries in drowning resuscitation (since 1774) [101]; it is safe and easy to learn [102–107]. The technique was introduced as part of the BLS training of Dutch lifeboat crews with good training results [108].

The lifeboat crew of the Royal Dutch Lifeboat Institution has learned to apply cricoid pressure as a last-resort measure in case high resistance of the lungs make the initial ventilation of the lungs impossible. This situation only occurs if the abdomen rises with each well-performed ventilation and there is no active rise and passive fall of the thorax.

During the cricoid pressure, the entrance of the oesophagus is closed, while the trachea remains open. The cricoid pressure is only applied during the ventilation and is stopped as soon as ventilation becomes effective.

Airway devices

Airway devices range from simple mouth covers to avoid mouth-to-mouth contact to devices that, even in the hands of well-trained and experienced medical professionals such as anaesthesiologists, are sometimes difficult to handle. Based on limited research data, it seems that only mouth-to-mouth ventilation with a protective shield, mouth-to-mask ventilation using both hands and bag-mask ventilation (where one rescuer uses both hands to position the mask and the second rescuer squeezes the balloon) can be taught to lifeguards. There are no studies that have investigated the quality of ventilation with these devices in real practice.

Some lifeguard organizations use bag-mask devices without proper training or without regular retraining, allow the lifeguards to fumble with the bag-mask devices, sometimes single-handed, and accept that this allows a longer hypoxic period. Teaching such techniques without a proper system that regularly controls the competencies of the trainees violates basic medical regulations. Such a control system needs to be an integrated part of the training program. Other lifeguard organizations insist on using barrier devices to protect lifeguards from infections in all circumstances. However, the risk of acquiring infections is extremely low. There has been no report of HIV transmission by mouth-to-mouth ventilation [80,109]. A barrier device will not always be immediately available and strict adherence to this rule delays the immediate delivery of oxygen. Moreover, most lifeguards do not routinely train in the provision of ventilation with a barrier device and retention of the technique is low [110,111]. In most situations, straightforward mouth-to-mouth ventilation is the most effective and immediately available method to ventilate a drowning victim [112,113].

The supraglottic airway device (SGA) seems to be a potentially promising replacement for each of these techniques. It has been demonstrated with manikins that even untrained persons are able to insert an SGA [114]. Several studies have also shown excellent results with lifeguards inserting the device into a manikin [85,86,115]. A case series is needed to evaluate the efficiency, efficacy and problems of using SGAs on the beach to further guide any introduction of these devices into training programs for lifeguards. Notably the required high inflation pressure in many drowning victims may be a problem in real-life situations [116].

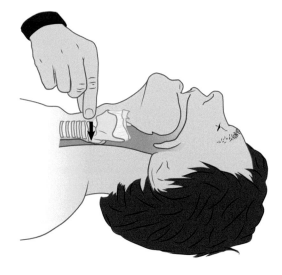

Figure 10.5 The cricoid pressure.

Pulse oximetry

Pulse oximetry may be considered to non-invasively measure the oxygen saturation in the arterial blood of a drowning victim during or while recovering from drowning. Their value in cold, peripherally vasoconstricted individuals is, however, questionable. One pilot study concludes that the current generation of pulse oxymeters is not yet reliable for people taken from the water [117]. Infrared spectrometry may become a more useful alternative [118].

Thoracic thumpers

Thoracic thumpers have been developed to increase the efficacy of chest compression and to reduce the fatigue and increase the comfort and safety of ambulance crews. In pre-hospital studies, the device has not been shown to improve outcome [119,120]. When this device can be purchased at a reasonable price, it may be of interest to further consider the role of thoracic thumpers, notably when resuscitation has to be performed over long distances on land or at sea [121–123]. The price is currently a barrier to including this device on the priority list [124].

Suction devices

Most drowning victims vomit or have water and foam in the oral cavity. Suction devices have been introduced to remove these substances. There is no evidence that suctioning of the airways improves the outcome. On the other hand, suctioning delays more important measures such as starting ventilation, thoracic compressions and oxygen provision.

To avoid aspiration, it is advised that a breathing victim should be placed in a stable lateral position, if possible with the head downwards on a slope to allow free drainage of fluids. If debris or vomitus are blocking effective ventilation, they should be

removed manually [99]. In some situations, there is already a lot of foam coming out of the mouth of the victim. It makes no sense to remove the foam: it keeps coming. The treatment here is intubation by medical professionals (which can be extremely difficult because there is no view of the vocal cords) and ventilation with positive end expiratory pressure [37].

QUALITY OF RESUSCITATION

The outcome of resuscitation is defined by local implementation, educational efficacy and medical science (Figure 10.6) [125].

Local implementation

In general, it should not take too much effort to implement the resuscitation tasks and responsibilities of beach lifeguards within the local health structure. Most of all this requires good organization with the local ambulance services. When resuscitation occurs at a beach, the local ambulance services will take over at a certain point. Matching of telecommunication, good communication about the names of locations (frequent beachgoers often use slang names unfamiliar to others), best and worst locations for rendezvous, exchange of uniform equipment and the understanding and acceptance of mutual protocols are helpful to facilitate a smooth interface between the two organizations. The same organization should be implemented with helicopter services in case they need to land on the beach to assist and transport drowning victims. Other activities relevant for local implementation are joint training and exercises, including other relevant parties such as lifeboat crews, police, firefighters, general practitioners and emergency departments. At some beaches, it may be useful to include beach cleaners or beach restaurant personnel in the chain of survival [2].

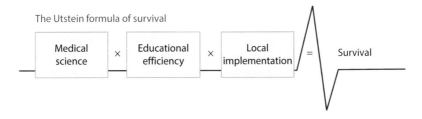

Figure 10.6 The Utstein formula of survival.

Something to consider is a backup medical advice structure with the local general practitioners, hospital or dispatch centre. Several of the aspects to be considered for a good local implementation are included in the ILS position statement 'Medical priorities in lifesaving' [124].

Training

The quality of resuscitation depends very much on the training and retraining provided. After resuscitation skills have been learned, the retention of these skills is a problem. Within six months, the performance of resuscitation decreases by almost 40%, depending on age and experience [126,127]. Skills decay faster than knowledge [128]. Retraining of BLS can be formally organized but self-learning, using computers and posters, is also effective in BLS skill retention [87,126]. For optimal training in drowning situations, interactive scenario-based training on the beach and at sea are important. Instructors responsible for such training should, most of all, be able to organize good feedback and debriefing to all participants [44,129,130]. The local or national lifesaving organization should consider regular evaluation of training programs. This evaluation should include the quality of the training programme as well as the level of knowledge and skills of the lifeguards [131,132].

Research

As discussed, there is a good understanding of what is best for a drowning patient at a beach from pathophysiological, practical and anecdotal points of view. However, much more research is needed to establish the evidence [133]. It would be beneficial if beach lifeguards collected data on each resuscitation in an "Utstein for drowning" based registry [134,135] or initiated studies related to understanding and performance of drowning resuscitation, the efficacy of training and the feasibility and cost–benefit of equipment [100]. Because the number of drownings at life-guarded beaches is extremely low, registration-based studies will need the collaboration of many beaches around the world, covering several hundred of million beach visitors each year. Such a global effort however is needed to collect more evidence on important issues such as, for example, the role of SGA, other airway management devices and cricoid pressure during ventilation, pulse-oximetry and other on-site monitoring, in-water resuscitation, spinal immobilisation and thoracic thumpers [136].

CONCLUSION

This chapter has provided an overview on the resuscitation techniques for lifeguards. Based on the view that the BLS courses given to the lay public are inappropriate for the optimal resuscitation of a drowning victim, the adaptation of drowning-focused resuscitation techniques was described. In addition, some common scenarios were described related to the environment where drowning resuscitation may be needed. Some potentially useful technical equipment was introduced with the clear reservation that each item needs further investigation in local settings before they can be applied. Finally, it was emphasized that the success of resuscitation never depends on the moment of resuscitation alone, but largely on its implementation within the local health system, training and retraining of lifeguards, and current and future research data [125,133].

REFERENCES

1. Szpilman D, Bierens JJ, Handley AJ, Orlowski JP. Drowning. *N Engl J Med.* 2012; 366(22): 2102–10.
2. Szpilman D, Webber J, Quan L, Bierens J, Morizot-Leite L, Langendorfer SJ, Beerman S, Løfgren B. Creating a drowning chain of survival. *Resuscitation.* 2014; 85(9): 1149–52.
3. Szpilman D, Morizot-Leite L, de Vries W, Beerman S, Neves F, Martinho R, Smoris L, Løfgren B, Webber J. First aid courses for the aquatic environment. In Bierens J (ed.). *Drowning: Prevention, Rescue, Treatment.* 2nd ed. Heidelberg: Springer; 2014, pp. 659–66.
4. Perkins GD, Travers AH, Berg RA, Castren M, Considine J, Escalante R, Gazmuri RJ, Koster RW, Lim SH, Nation KJ, Olasveengen TM, Sakamoto T, Sayre MR, Sierra A, Smyth MA, Stanton D, Vaillancourt C. Basic Life Support Chapter Collaborators. Part 3: Adult basic life support and automated external defibrillation: 2015 International Consensus on Cardiopulmonary Resuscitation and

Emergency Cardiovascular Care Science with Treatment Recommendations. *Resuscitation*. 2015; 95: e43–69.

5. Truhlář A, Deakin CD, Soar J, Khalifa GE, Alfonzo A, Bierens JJ, Brattebø G, Brugger H, Dunning J, Hunyadi-Antičević S, Koster RW, Lockey DJ, Lott C, Paal P, Perkins GD, Sandroni C, Thies KC, Zideman DA, Nolan JP. Cardiac arrest in special circumstances section Collaborators. European Resuscitation Council Guidelines for Resuscitation 2015: Section 4. Cardiac arrest in special circumstances. *Resuscitation*. 2015; 95: 148–201.

6. Safar P. *Cardiopulmonary Cerebral Resuscitation*. A manual for physicians and paramedical instructors, prepared for the World Federation of Societies of Anaesthesiologists. Stavanger: Asmund S. Laerdal; 1981.

7. Safar P, Bircher NG. *Cardiopulmonary Cerebral Resuscitation*. 3rd ed. London: WB Saunders; 1988.

8. Perkins GD, Handley AJ. Chest-compression-only versus standard CPR. *Lancet*. 2011; 377(9767): 716.

9. Berdowski J, Berg R, Tijssen JGP, Koster RW. Global incidences of out-of-hospital cardiac arrest and survival rates: Systematic review of 67 prospective studies. *Resuscitation*. 2010; 81(11): 1479–87.

10. Anderson ML, Cox M, Al-Khatib SM, Nichol G, Thomas KL, Chan PS, Saha-Chaudhuri P, et al. Rates of cardiopulmonary resuscitation training in the United States. *JAMA Intern Med*. 2014; 174(2): 194–201.

11. American Heart Association Year report 2012–2013. Available at http://www.heart.org/idc/groups/heart-public/@wcm/@adt/documents/downloadable/ucm_449081.pdf

12. American Heart Association Year report 2013–2014. Available at http://www.heart.org/idc/groups/heart-public/@wcm/@cmc/documents/downloadable/ucm_469976.pdf

13. Atwood C, Eisenberg MS, Herlitz J, Rea TD. Incidence of EMS-treated out-of-hospital cardiac arrest in Europe. *Resuscitation*. 2005; 67: 75–80.

14. ILS Medical Position Statement—MPS 11: Critical skills for lifesavers. Available at http://www.ilsf.org/about/position-statements

15. ILS Medical Position Statement—MPS 04: Automated External Defibrilation used lifesavers and lifeguards. Available at http://www.ilsf.org/about/position-statements

16. Bierens J, Lunetta P, Tipton M. Pathophysiology of drowning. In Bierens J (ed.). *Drowning: Prevention, Rescue, Treatment*. 2nd ed. Heidelberg: Springer; 2014, pp. 545–60.

17. Bierens JJ, Warner DS. Drowning resuscitation requires another state of mind. *Resuscitation*. 2013; 84(11): 1467–9.

18. Vaagenes P, Safar P, Moossy J, Rao G, Diven W, Ravi C, Arfors K. Asphyxiation versus ventricular fibrillation cardiac arrest in dogs. Differences in cerebral resuscitation effects—A preliminary study. *Resuscitation*. 1997; 35: 41–52.

19. Topjian AA, Berg RA, Bierens JJ, Branche CM, Clark RS, Friberg H, Hoedemaekers CW, et al. Brain resuscitation in the drowning victim. *Neurocrit Care*. 2012; 17(3): 441–6.

20. Quan L, Wentz KR, Gore EJ, Copass MK. Outcome and predictors of outcome in pediatric submersion victims receiving Prehospital care in King County, Washington. *Pediatrics*. 1990; 86: 586–93.

21. Kyriacou DN, Arcinue EL, Peek C, Kraus JF. Effect of immediate resuscitation on children with submersion injury. *Pediatrics*. 1994; 94(2 Pt 1): 137–42.

22. Venema AM, Groothoff JW, Bierens JJ. The role of bystanders during rescue and resuscitation of drowning victims. *Resuscitation*. 2010; 81(4): 434–9.

23. Suominen P, Baillie C, Korpela R, Rautanen S, Ranta S, Olkkola KT. Impact of age, submersion time and water temperature on outcome in near-drowning. *Resuscitation*. 2002; 52(3): 247–54.

24. Eich C, Bräuer A, Timmermann A, Schwarz SK, Russo SG, Neubert K, Graf BM, Aleksic I. Outcome of 12 drowned children with attempted resuscitation on cardiopulmonary bypass: An analysis of variables based on the "Utstein Style for Drowning." *Resuscitation*. 2007; 75(1): 42–52.

25. Grmec S, Strnad M, Podgorsek D. Comparison of the characteristics and outcome among patients suffering from out-of-hospital primary cardiac arrest and drowning victims in cardiac arrest. *Int J Emerg Med.* 2009; 2(1): 7–12.

26. Youn CS, Choi SP, Yim HW, Park KN. Out-of-hospital cardiac arrest due to drowning: An Utstein Style report of 10 years of experience from St. Mary's Hospital. *Resuscitation.* 2009; 80(7): 778–83.

27. Ballesteros MA, Gutiérrez-Cuadra M, Muñoz P, Miñambres E. Prognostic factors and outcome after drowning in an adult population. Acta Anaesthesiol Scand. 2009; 53(7): 935–40.

28. Suominen PK, Vallila NH, Hartikainen LM, Sairanen HI, Korpela RE. Outcome of drowned hypothermic children with cardiac arrest treated with cardiopulmonary bypass. *Acta Anaesthesiol Scand.* 2010; 54(10): 1276–81.

29. Choi SP, Youn CS, Park KN, Wee JH, Park JH, Oh SH, Kim SH, Kim JY. Therapeutic hypothermia in adult cardiac arrest because of drowning. *Acta Anaesthesiol Scand.* 2012; 56(1): 116–23.

30. Nitta M, Kitamura T, Iwami T, Nadkarni VM, Berg RA, Topjian AA, Okamoto Y, et al. Out-of-hospital cardiac arrest due to drowning among children and adults from the Utstein Osaka Project. *Resuscitation.* 2013; 84(11): 1568–73.

31. Dyson K, Morgans A, Bray J, Matthews B, Smith K. Drowning related out-of-hospital cardiac arrests: Characteristics and outcomes. *Resuscitation.* 2013; 84(8): 1114–18.

32. Claesson A, Lindqvist J, Herlitz J. Cardiac arrest due to drowning—Changes over time and factors of importance for survival. *Resuscitation.* 2014; 85(5): 644–8.

33. Buick JE, Lin S, Rac VE, Brooks SC, Kierzek G, Morrison LJ. Drowning: An overlooked cause of out-of-hospital cardiac arrest in Canada. *CJEM.* 2014; 16(4): 314–21.

34. Kieboom JK, Verkade HJ, Burgerhof JG, Bierens JJ, Rheenen PF, Kneyber MC, Albers MJ. Outcome after resuscitation beyond 30 minutes in drowned children with cardiac arrest and hypothermia: Dutch nationwide retrospective cohort study. *BMJ.* 2015; 350: h418. doi: 10.1136/bmj.h418.

35. Manolios N, Mackie I. Drowning and near-drowning on Australian beaches patrolled by life-savers: A 10-year study, 1973–1983. *Med J Aust.* 1988; 148(4): 165–7, 170–1.

36. Szpilman D. Near-drowning and drowning classification: A proposal to stratify mortality based on the analysis of 1,831 cases. *Chest.* 1997; 112: 660–5.

37. US Lifeguard standards. Available at http://www.lifeguardstandards.org/pdf/USLSC_FINAL_APPROVAL_1-31-11.pdf

38. Biarenta D, Bingham R, Eich C, López-Herce J, Maconochie I, Rodríguez-Núez A, Rajkag T, Zideman D. European Resuscitation Council guidelines for resuscitation 2010 section 6. Paediatric life support. *Resuscitation.* 2010; 81: 1364–88.

39. Brugger H, Durrer B, Elsensohn F, Paal P, Strapazzon G, Winterberger E, Zafren K, Boyd J, ICAR MEDCOM. Resuscitation of avalanche victims: Evidence-based guidelines of the international commission for mountain emergency medicine (ICAR MEDCOM): Intended for physicians and other advanced life support personnel. *Resuscitation.* 2013; 84(5): 539–46.

40. Kralj E, Podbregar M, Kejžar N, Balažic J. Frequency and number of resuscitation related rib and sternum fractures are higher than generally considered. *Resuscitation.* 2015; 93: 136–41. doi: 10.1016/j.resuscitation.2015.02.034.

41. Kashiwagi Y, Sasakawa T, Tampo A, Kawata D, Nishiura T, Kokita N, Iwasaki H, Fujita S. Computed tomography findings of complications resulting from cardiopulmonary resuscitation. *Resuscitation.* 2015; 88: 86–91.

42. Szpilman D, Soares M. In-water resuscitation—Is it worthwhile? *Resuscitation.* 2004; 63(1): 25–31.

43. Oxygen-hemoglobin dissociation curve. Available at http://en.wikipedia.org/wiki/Oxygen–hemoglobin_dissociation_curve

44. Bobrow BJ, Vadeboncoeur TF, Stolz U, Silver AE, Tobin JM, Crawford SA, Mason TK, Schirmer J, Smith GA, Spaite DW. The influence of scenario-based

training and real-time audiovisual feedback on out-of-hospital cardiopulmonary resuscitation quality and survival from out-of-hospital cardiac arrest. *Ann Emerg Med.* 2013; 62(1): 47–56.

45. Cheskes S, Schmicker RH, Christenson J, Salcido DD, Rea T, Powell J, Edelson DP, et al. Perishock pause: An independent predictor of survival from out-of-hospital shockable cardiac arrest. *Circulation.* 2011; 124(1): 58–66.

46. Soar J, Monsieurs KG, Balance JHW, Barelli A, Biarent D, Greif R, Handley AJ, et al. European Resuscitation Council guidelines for resuscitation 2010. Section 9. Principles of education in resuscitation. *Resuscitation.* 2010; 81: 1434–44.

47. ILS Medical Position Statement—MPS 15: Compression-only CPR. Available at http://www.ilsf.org/about/position-statements

48. Moen S, Berg vd JP, Bongers M, Hoogeveen RM, Puts MWJ, Bierens JJLM Resuscitation experience identified by Focus Group Studies. Conference abstracts WCDP2015, Potsdam. Available at http://www.wcdp2013.org/fileadmin/Documentation/Presentations/wcdp_abstracts_web.pdf

49. Abelsson A, Rystedt I, Suserud BO, Lindwall L. Mapping the use of simulation in prehospital care—A literature review. *Scand J Trauma Resusc Emerg Med.* 2014; 22: 22. doi: 10.1186/1757-7241-22-22.

50. Edwards S, Siassakos D. Training teams and leaders to reduce resuscitation errors and improve patient outcome. *Resuscitation.* 2012; 83(1): 13–15.

51. Fenner PJ, Harrison SL, Williamson JA, Williamson BD. Success of surf lifesaving resuscitations in Queensland, 1973–1992. *Med J Aust.* 1995; 163(11–12): 580–3.

52. De Vries W, Bierens JJLM. Frequency of resuscitations by lifeguards. Occurrence of cardiac arrest on beaches (AP-019). *Resuscitation.* 2008; 77: S44. doi: 10.1016/j.resuscitation.2008.03.138.

53. Moran K, Webber J. Surf lifeguard perceptions and practice of cardiopulmonary resuscitation (CPR). *Int J Aquat Res Educ.* 2012; 6: 24–34.

54. Bierens JJLM, van der Velde EA, van Berkel M, van Zanten JJ. Submersion in the Netherlands: Prognostic indicators and results of resuscitation. *Ann Emerg Med.* 1990; 19: 1390–5.

55. Brüning C, Siekmeyer W, Siekmeyer M, Merkenschlager A, Kiess W. Retrospective analysis of 44 childhood drowning accidents. *Wien Klin Wochenschr.* 2010; 122(13–14): 405–12.

56. Claesson A, Lindqvist J, Ortenwall P, Herlitz J. Characteristics of lifesaving from drowning as reported by the Swedish Fire and Rescue Services 1996–2010. *Resuscitation.* 2012; 83(9): 1072–7.

57. Vähätalo R, Lunetta P, Olkkola KT, Suominen PK. Drowning in children: Utstein style reporting and outcome. *Acta Anaesthesiol Scand.* 2014; 58(5): 604–10.

58. de Vries W, Turner NM, Monsieurs KG, Bierens JJ, Koster RW. Comparison of instructor-led automated external defibrillation training and three alternative DVD-based training methods. *Resuscitation.* 2010; 81(8): 1004–9.

59. Kovačič U, Kosec L. Effectiveness and limitations of learning cardiopulmonary resuscitation with an automated external defibrillator in the curriculum of First Aid courses among lay people. *Critical Care.* 2012; 16(Suppl 1): P268.

60. Szpilman D, Handley A. Positioning of the drowning victim. In Bierens J (ed.). *Drowning: Prevention, Rescue, Treatment.* 2nd ed. Heidelberg: Springer; 2014, pp. 629–34.

61. Bahr J, Klingler H, Panzer W, Rode H, Kettler D. Skills of lay people in checking the carotid pulse. *Resuscitation.* 1997; 35: 23–6.

62. Lapostolle F, Le Toumelin P, Agostinucci JM, Catineau J, Adnet F. Basic cardiac life support providers checking the carotid pulse: Performance, degree of conviction, and influencing factors. *Acad Emerg Med.* 2004; 11: 878–80.

63. Breckwoldt J, Schloesser S, Arntz HR. Perceptions of collapse and assessment of cardiac arrest by bystanders of out-of-hospital cardiac arrest (OOHCA). *Resuscitation.* 2009; 80: 1108–13.

64. ILS Medical Position Statement—MPS 09: The use of oxygenation by lifesavers. Available at http://www.ilsf.org/about/position-statements

65. Yeh ST, Cawley RJ, Aune SE, Angelos MG. Oxygen requirement during cardiopulmonary resuscitation (CPR) to effect return of spontaneous circulation. *Resuscitation.* 2009; 80(8): 951–5.

66. Neumar RW. Optimal oxygenation during and after cardiopulmonary resuscitation. *Curr Opin Crit Care.* 2011; 17(3): 236–40.

67. Bosson N, Gausche-Hill M, Koenig W. Implementation of a titrated oxygen protocol in the out-of-hospital setting. *Prehosp Disaster Med.* 2014; 29(4): 403–8.

68. Angelos MG, Yeh ST, Aune SE. Post-cardiac arrest hyperoxia and mitochondrial function. *Resuscitation.* 2011; 82(Suppl 2): S48–51.

69. Kochanek PM, Bayir H. Titrating oxygen during and after cardiopulmonary resuscitation. *JAMA.* 2010; 303(21): 2190–1.

70. Kochanek P, Bayir H. Oxygen monitoring and the use in the drowning victim. In Bierens JJLM (ed.). *Drowning.* Heidelberg: Springer; 2015.

71. Løfgren B, Beerman S. Automated external defibrillators in the aquatic environment. In World congress on Drowning. Handbook on Drowning: prevention, rescue, treatment. *Drowning.* Heidelberg-Berlin: Springer; 2006; 331–35.

72. Tipton MJ, Golden FS. A proposed decision-making guide for the search, rescue and resuscitation of submersion (head under) victims based on expert opinion. *Resuscitation.* 2011; 82(7): 819–24.

73. Tipton MJ, Golden F. Comments on editorial "rescue and resuscitation or body retrieval—The dilemmas of search and rescue efforts in drowning incidents." *Resuscitation.* 2011; 82(12): e1; author reply e5. doi: 10.1016/j.resuscitation.2011.07.007.

74. Claesson A, Karlsson T, Thorén AB, Herlitz J. Delay and performance of cardiopulmonary resuscitation in surf lifeguards after simulated cardiac arrest due to drowning. *Am J Emerg Med.* 2011; 29(9): 1044–50.

75. Moran K, Webber J. Too much puff, not enough push. Surf lifeguard simulated CPR performance. *Int J Aquat Res Educ.* 2012; 6: 13–23.

76. Barcala-Furelos R, Abelairas-Gomez C, Romo-Perez V, Palacios-Aguilar J. Effect of physical fatigue on the quality CPR: A water rescue study of lifeguards: Physical fatigue and quality CPR in a water rescue. *Am J Emerg Med.* 2013; 31(3): 473–7.

77. Pepe PE, Roppolo LP, Fowler RL. The detrimental effects of ventilation during low-blood-flow states. *Curr Opin Crit Care.* 2005; 11(3): 212–18.

78. Grasso S, Mascia L, Del Turco M, Malacarne P, Giunta F, Brochard L, Slutsky AS, Marco Ranieri V. Effects of recruiting maneuvers in patients with acute respiratory distress syndrome ventilated with protective ventilatory strategy. *Anesthesiology.* 2002; 96(4): 795–802.

79. Becker LB, Berg RA, Pepe PE, Idris AH, Aufderheide TP, Barnes TA, Stratton SJ, Chandra NC. A reappraisal of mouth-to-mouth ventilation during bystander-initiated cardiopulmonary resuscitation. A statement for healthcare professionals from the Ventilation Working Group of the Basic Life Support and Pediatric Life Support Subcommittees, American Heart Association. *Resuscitation.* 1997; 35(3): 189–201.

80. Safar P, Bircher N, Pretto E Jr, Berkebile P, Tisherman SA, Marion D, Klain M, Kochanek PM. Reappraisal of mouth-to-mouth ventilation during bystander-initiated CPR. *Circulation.* 1998; 98(6): 608–10.

81. Spoormans I, Van Hoorenbeeck K, Balliu L, Jorens PG. Gastric perforation after cardiopulmonary resuscitation: Review of the literature. *Resuscitation.* 2010; 81(3): 272–80.

82. Abelairas-Gómez C, Romo-Pérez V, Barcala-Furelos R, Palacios-Aguilar J. Efecto de la fatiga física del socorrista en los primeros cuatro minutos de la reanimación cardiopulmonary posrescate acuático. *Emergencias.* 2013; 25: 184–90.

83. Perkins GD. In-water resuscitation: A pilot evaluation. *Resuscitation.* 2005; 65(3): 321–4.

84. ILS Medical Position Statement—MPS 08: In-water resuscitation. Available at http://www.ilsf.org/about/position-statements

85. Winkler BE, Eff AM, Eff S, Ehrmann U, Koch A, Kähler W, Muth CM. Efficacy of ventilation and ventilation adjuncts during in-water-resuscitation. A randomized cross-over trial. Resuscitation. 2013; 84(8): 1137–42.

86. Winkler BE, Eff AM, Ehrmann U, Eff S, Koch A, Kaehler W, Georgieff M, Muth CM. Effectiveness and safety of in-water resuscitation performed by lifeguards and laypersons: A crossover manikin study. Prehosp Emerg Care. 2013; 17: 409–15.

87. de Vries W, Bierens JJ. Instructor retraining and poster retraining are equally effective for the retention of BLS and AED skills of lifeguards. Eur J Emerg Med. 2010; 17(3): 150–7.

88. Tipton M, David G, Eglin C, Golden F. Basic life support on small boats at sea. Resuscitation. 2007; 75(2): 332–7.

89. Barcala-Furelos R, Arca-Bustelo Á, Palacios-Aguilar J, Rodríguez-Núñez A. Quality of cardiopulmonary resuscitation by lifeguards on a small inflatable boat. Resuscitation. 2015; 90: e1–2. doi: 10.1016/j.resuscitation.2015.02.007.

90. Zarroug AE, Stavlo PL, Kays GA, Rodeberg DA, Moir CR. Accidental burials in sand: A potentially fatal summertime hazard. Mayo Clin Proc. 2004; 79(6): 774–6.

91. Heggie TW. Sand hazards on tourist beaches. Travel Med Infect Dis. 2013; 11(2): 123–5.

92. Avis SP. Suicidal drowning. J Forensic Sci. 1993; 38: 1422–6.

93. Stemberga V, Bralic M, Coklo M, Cuculic D, Bosnar A. Suicidal drowning in Southwestern Croatia: A 25-year review. Am J Forensic Med Pathol. 2010; 31(1): 52–4.

94. Byard RW, Houldsworth G, Ross AJ. Characteristic features of suicidal drownings. A 20-year study. Am J Forensic Med Pathol. 2001; 22(2): 134–8.

95. Clawson J. Drowning: A dispatch perspective. In Bierens J (ed.). Drowning: Prevention, Rescue, Treatment. 2nd ed. Heidelberg: Springer; 2014, pp. 595–600.

96. Zlotnik H. Population: Crowd control. Nature. 2013; 501: 30–1.

97. West JB. Respiratory Physiology. The Essentials. 9th ed. Baltimore: Wolters Kluwers; 2012.

98. van Berkel M, Bierens JJ, Lie RL, de Rooy TP, Kool LJ, van de Velde EA, Meinders AE. Pulmonary oedema, pneumonia and mortality in submersion victims; a retrospective study in 125 patients. Intensive Care Med. 1996; 22: 101–7.

99. Modell J. Aspiration. In Bierens J (ed.). Drowning: Prevention, Rescue, Treatment. 2nd ed. Heidelberg: Springer; 2014, pp. 561–4.

100. Beesems SG, Wijmans L, Tijssen JG, Koster RW. Duration of ventilations during cardiopulmonary resuscitation by lay rescuers and first responders: Relationship between delivering chest compressions and outcomes. Circulation. 2013; 127(15): 1585–90.

101. Salem MR, Sellick BA, Elam JO. The historical background of cricoid pressure in anesthesia and resuscitation. Anesth Analg. 1974; 53(2): 230–2.

102. Petito SP, Russell WJ. The prevention of gastric inflation—A neglected benefit of cricoid pressure. Anaesth Intensive Care. 1988; 16(2): 139–43.

103. Moynihan RJ, Brock-Utne JG, Archer JH, Feld LH, Kreitzman TR. The effect of cricoid pressure on preventing gastric insufflation in infants and children. Anesthesiology. 1993; 78(4): 652–6.

104. Parry A. Teaching anaesthetic nurses optimal force for effective cricoid pressure: A literature review. Nurs Crit Care. 2009; 14(3): 139–44.

105. Rice MJ, Mancuso AA, Gibbs C, Morey TE, Gravenstein N, Deitte LA. Cricoid pressure results in compression of the postcricoid hypopharynx: The esophageal position is irrelevant. Anesth Analg. 2009; 109(5): 1546–52.

106. Johnson RL, Cannon EK, Mantilla CB, Cook DA. Cricoid pressure training using simulation: A systematic review and meta-analysis. Br J Anaesth. 2013; 111(3): 338–46.

107. Bhatia N, Bhagat H, Sen I. Cricoid pressure: Where do we stand? J Anaesthesiol Clin Pharmacol. 2014; 30(1): 3–6.

108. Herman NL, Carter B, Van Decar TK. Cricoid pressure: Teaching the recommended level. *Anesth Analg*. 1996; 83(4): 859–63.

109. Bierens JJ, Berden HJ. Basic-CPR and AIDS: Are volunteer life-savers prepared for a storm? *Resuscitation*. 1996; 32(3): 185–91.

110. Paal P, Falk M, Gruber E, Beikircher W, Sumann G, Demetz F, Ellerton J, Wenzel V, Brugger H. Retention of mouth-to-mouth, mouth-to-mask and mouth-to-face shield ventilation. *Emerg Med J*. 2008; 25(1): 42–5.

111. Queiroga AC, Barcala-Furelos R, Abelairas-Gómez C, Farto-Ramírez O, Prieto-Saborit JA, Rodríguez-Núñez A. Cardiopulmonary resuscitation quality among lifeguards: Self-perception, knowledge, and performance. *Am J Emerg Med*. 2014; 32(11): 1429–30.

112. Adelborg K, Dalgas C, Grove EL, Jørgensen C, Al-Mashhadi RH, Løfgren B. Mouth-to-mouth ventilation is superior to mouth-to-pocket mask and bag-valve-mask ventilation during lifeguard CPR: A randomized study. *Resuscitation*. 2011; 82: 618–22.

113. Umesh G, Krishna R, Chaudhuri S, Tim TJ, Shwethapriya R. E-O technique is superior to E-C technique in manikins during single person bag mask ventilation performed by novices. *J Clin Monit Comput*. 2014; 28(3): 269–73.

114. Bickenbach J, Schälte G, Beckers S, Fries M, Derwall M, Rossaint R. The intuitive use of laryngeal airway tools by first year medical students. *BMC Emerg Med*. 2009; 9: 18. doi: 10.1186/1471-227X-9-18.

115. Adelborg K, Al-Mashhadi RH, Nielsen LH, Dalgas C, Mortensen MB, Løfgren B. A randomised crossover comparison of manikin ventilation through Soft Seal®, i-gel™ and AuraOnce™ supraglottic airway devices by surf lifeguards. *Anaesthesia*. 2014; 69(4): 343–7.

116. Baker PA, Webber JB. Failure to ventilate with supraglottic airways after drowning. *Anaesth Intensive Care*. 2011; 39: 675–7.

117. Montenij LJ, de Vries W, Schwarte L, Bierens JJ. Feasibility of pulse oximetry in the initial prehospital management of victims of drowning: A preliminary study. *Resuscitation*. 2011; 82(9): 1235–8.

118. Eichhorn L, Erdfelder F, Kessler F, Doerner J, Thudium MO, Meyer R, Ellerkmann RK. Evaluation of near-infrared spectroscopy under apnea-dependent hypoxia in humans. *J Clin Monit Comput*. 2015; 1–9.

119. Axelsson C, Karlsson T, Axelsson Å, Herlitz J. Mechanical active compression-decompression cardiopulmonary resuscitation (ACD-CPR) versus manual CPR according to pressure of end tidal carbon dioxide (PETCO2) during CPR in out-of-hospital cardiac arrest (OHCA). *Resuscitation*. 2009; 80(10): 1099–103.

120. Smekal D, Johansson J, Huzevka T, Rubertsson S. A pilot study of mechanical chest compressions with the LUCAS device in cardiopulmonary resuscitation. *Resuscitation*. 2011; 82: 702–6.

121. Kyrval HS. Automatic mechanical chest compression during helicopter transportation. *Ugeskr Laeger*. 2010; 172(46): 3190–1.

122. Putzer G, Braun P, Zimmermann A, Pedross F, Strapazzon G, Brugger H, Paal P. LUCAS compared to manual cardiopulmonary resuscitation is more effective during helicopter rescue-a prospective, randomized, cross-over manikin study. *Am J Emerg Med*. 2013; 31(2): 384–9.

123. Barcala-Furelos R, Abelairas-Gomez C, Romo-Perez V, Palacios-Aguilar J. Influence of automatic compression device and water rescue equipment in quality lifesaving and cardiopulmonary resuscitation. *Hong Kong J Emerg Med*. 2014; 21(5): 291.

124. ILS Medical. ILS Medical Position Statement—MPS Position Statement—MPS 07: Medical priorities. Available at http://www.ilsf.org/about/position-statements

125. Søreide E, Morrison L, Hillman K, Monsieurs K, Sunde K, Zideman D, Eisenberg M, et al. Utstein formula for survival collaborators. The formula for survival in resuscitation. *Resuscitation*. 2013; 84(11): 1487–93.

126. de Vries W, Turner NM, Monsieurs KG, Bierens JJ, Koster RW. Comparison of instructor-led automated external defibrillation training and three alternative DVD-based training methods. *Resuscitation*. 2010; 81(8): 1004–9.

127. Iserbyt P, Schouppe G, Charlier N. A multiple linear regression analysis of factors affecting the simulated Basic Life Support (BLS) performance with Automated External Defibrillator (AED) in Flemish lifeguards. *Resuscitation.* 2015; 89: 70–4.

128. Yang CW, Yen ZS, McGowan JE, Chen HC, Chiang WC, Mancini ME, Soar J, Lai MS, Ma MH. A systematic review of retention of adult advanced life support knowledge and skills in healthcare providers. *Resuscitation.* 2012; 83(9): 1055–60.

129. Andersen PO, Jensen MK, Lippert A, Østergaard D, Klausen TW. Development of a formative assessment tool for measurement of performance in multi-professional resuscitation teams. *Resuscitation.* 2010; 81(6): 703–11.

130. Walker ST, Sevdalis N, McKay A, Lambden S, Gautama S, Aggarwal R, Vincent C. Unannounced in situ simulations: Integrating training and clinical practice. *BMJ Qual Saf.* 2013; 22(6): 453–8.

131. van Heukelom JN, Begaz T, Treat R. Comparison of postsimulation debriefing versus in-simulation debriefing in medical simulation. *Simul Healthc.* 2010; 5(2): 91–7.

132. Cook DA. Twelve tips for evaluating educational programs. *Med Teach.* 2010; 32(4): 296–301.

133. Warner DS, Bierens JJLM, Beerman S, Katz LM. Drowning—A cry for help. *Anesthesiology.* 2009; 110: 1399–401.

134. Idris AH, Berg RA, Bierens J, Bossaert L, Branche CM, Gabrielli A, Graves SA, et al. Recommended guidelines for uniform reporting of data from drowning: The "Utstein style." *Circulation.* 2003; 108(20): 2565–74.

135. Idris AH, Berg RA, Bierens J, Bossaert L, Branche CM, Gabrielli A, Graves SA, et al. Recommended guidelines for uniform reporting of data from drowning: The "Utstein style." *Resuscitation.* 2003; 59(1): 45–57.

136. Wernicki P, Espino M. Evidence-based standards in lifesaving: The conclusions of the United States Lifeguard Standards Coalition. In: Bierens J, ed. *Drowning, Prevention, Rescue, Treatment.* Berlin Heidelberg: Springer-Verlag: 2015. pp. 331–6.

PART 4

Performance

11

Recognition, vigilance and surveillance techniques

JENNY SMITH (NEE PAGE)

INTRODUCTION

Surprisingly, given the long history associated with looking out to sea and keeping watch, there has been little research examining the best method of surveying a prescribed area of open water [1]. *Visual scanning* refers to the use of the visual system to pass information about the outside world to the brain. For lifeguards, it is defined as 'observing, encoding and making an assessment of the water area that is being surveyed' [2]. Visual search is a challenging behavioural task [3,4] especially when the target behaviour is rare, as in drowning [5].

Consider the demands of beach lifeguarding: lifeguards have to observe and extract relevant cues and then make decisions about very complex environments [6]. Furthermore, lifeguards can be required to perform these tasks for long periods of time. For example, in the United Kingdom a beach lifeguard could observe continually for up to six hours, although most professional bodies will encourage regular breaks. However, early lab-based non-lifeguard-related research suggested that vigilance capacity cannot be maintained at an optimal level for more than 30 minutes [7]. The performance of lifeguards can also be affected by monotony, stress and fatigue (for a review, see Ref. [8]). Indeed, a survey

that was carried out with 839 lifeguards found that lifeguards reported a number of distracting thoughts (e.g. about relationships and weekend plans) and felt bored and nervous when lifeguarding [9]. It was also found that the scanning (measured by head movements) of pool lifeguards declined later in the day and suggested that this may be caused by fatigue or boredom [10]. However, there is little scientific evidence to support these claims. The particular environment (temperature, lighting levels, solar radiation and noise) in which beach lifeguards work can negatively impact on their performance. For example, both heat and noise can affect vigilance in non-lifeguard-related tasks [11–13]. When the beach is busy, stress and fatigue high and the weather hot, it would appear to be nearly impossible for anyone to see everything that is happening at the beach. In such conditions, a lifeguard's ability to process visual information, remain attentive and make sound judgments may be compromised [14].

To help inform the performance of beach lifeguards several reports have been produced. The International Life Saving Federation produced a report [8] which stated four key guidelines for scanning. First, several basic and key observation techniques must be employed to enable the lifeguard to adequately observe all the people in their area of responsibility. Second, visual scanning requires the guard to sweep their area of responsibility continually, looking from side to side, checking each person or group of persons briefly to ascertain any of the previously defined indications of difficulty or distress. Third, watch swimmers close to shore as well as those offshore and, finally, watch all classifications of bathers, waders and swimmers with equal intensity to locate trouble.

USLSC RECOMMENDATIONS

To further inform lifeguards' performance, the United States Lifeguard Standards Coalition (USLSC) published a thorough review with recommendations that aimed to have a positive influence on the training of lifeguards [15]. Topics covered included scanning techniques, vigilance, inattentional blindness, visual and behavioural cues, breaks (interruptions of duty), age, hearing, vision etc. Of interest to this chapter are scanning techniques, vigilance and visual and behavioural cues, and the aim of this chapter is to update the reader with the innovative research that has been conducted since the publication of the USLSC report in these three key areas. Before the most recent research is reviewed, the aim, method and key findings from the USLSC report in these three areas will be briefly outlined.

The USLSC report [15] aimed to give evidence-based statements across a variety of key areas. The literature used as evidence was assessed and the implications were presented using the following groupings:

- **Standard**
  - The anticipated benefits of the recommended intervention clearly exceed the harm, and the quality of the supporting evidence is excellent. In some clearly identified circumstances, strong recommendations may be made when high-quality evidence is impossible to obtain but the anticipated benefits strongly outweigh the harms.
- **Guideline**
  - The anticipated benefits exceed the harm, but the quality of evidence is not as strong. In some clearly identified circumstances, recommendations may be made when high-quality evidence is impossible to obtain but the anticipated benefits outweigh the harms.

- **Option**
  - Courses that may be taken when either the quality of evidence is suspect, or the level or volume of evidence is small, or carefully performed studies have shown little clear advantage to one approach over another.
- **No recommendation**
  - A lack of pertinent evidence; the anticipated balance of benefits and harm is unclear.

The key findings from the USLSC report outlined listed below.

Scanning techniques

What evidence is there to support the effectiveness of scanning techniques in identifying patrons in need of assistance?

- **Standards**
  - None
- **Guidelines**
  - Lifeguard-certifying agencies and supervisors should provide training programs and in-service protocols that cover the following:
    - Emphasize scanning all fields within a scanning zone using maximal head movements.
    - Require new lifeguards to practise scanning with supervision and feedback.
    - Emphasize that, when individuals within a population are similar in appearance, it takes longer to identify potential drowning incidents.
    - Inform lifeguards that distractions greatly affect the scanning process.
    - When training aquatic supervisors, include information regarding the benefits of supervision and frequent encouragement.
- **Options**
  - A plan should be in place to provide backup support when rule-enforcement duties or incidents affect the ability of a lifeguard to effectively scan.
  - Because scanners tend to observe what is in front of the total viewing area and spend less time searching areas to the right and left of the visual field, lifeguard employers

should consider reducing the field of view assigned to lifeguards. This could be done by placing lifeguards closer together along a linear beach or at the corners of a pool versus along the sides.

- Since the probability of finding a target decreases as the number of patrons increases, consider increasing the lifeguard staff and dividing scanning responsibilities among them when the number of patrons rises.
- **No recommendation**
  - None

Vigilance

What evidence is there that has identified external factors that positively influence vigilance among lifeguards?

- **Standards**
  - Supervision and regular encouragement during each 30 minutes of watch improve vigilance; therefore, supervision of lifeguards should include regular contact and encouragement.
- **Guidelines**
  - Because sleep deprivation decreases vigilance even after a recovery night of sleep, training and in-service protocols should emphasize the need for lifeguards to obtain a full night's sleep before assuming lifeguard duties.
  - Lifeguard employers should screen candidates for untreated sleep apnea because these individuals have a decreased ability to maintain vigilance. This could be ascertained on application for employment.
  - Reasonable steps should be taken to protect lifeguards from high ambient temperatures. Steps might include providing sun protection for outdoor activities (e.g. sun shades, protective clothing), using air conditioning and adjusting indoor temperatures and/or decreasing the length of shifts.
  - Training relating to the use of different intervention options should be incorporated.
- **Options**
  - Consumption of caffeinated, non-sugared drinks has been demonstrated to benefit vigilance. (**Note:** Negative health impacts of caffeine, if any, were not reviewed.)

- Use of recreational drugs among lifeguards should be prohibited because chronic use decreases vigilance, even when the user is not under the influence.
- Aerobic exercise can positively impact a subsequent vigilance task. Lifeguards should consider including exercise periods during their breaks as a way to subsequently improve vigilance.
- Aquatic facilities should incorporate into their operational plans the foregoing evidence-based interventions that positively influence vigilance (standards, guidelines and options above).
- **No recommendation**
  - None

Visual and behavioural cues

What visual and behavioural cues are useful for identifying high-risk patrons?

- **Standards**
  - Consumption of alcohol is a visual and behavioural cue that an individual may be at greater risk of drowning. Lifeguard-certifying agencies should emphasize this fact in lifeguard training.
- **Guidelines**
  - Individuals who are under the influence of alcohol should be discouraged or excluded from participating in aquatic activities.
- **Options**
  - None
- **No recommendation**
  - None

UNIVERSITY OF PORTSMOUTH AND RNLI RESEARCH PROGRAMME

Given the lack of published experimental evidence to inform these reports and the fact that the Royal National Lifeboat Institution (RNLI) were interested in enhancing their own standard operating procedures for beach lifeguards, the University of Portsmouth and the RNLI embarked on a programme of research to provide a stronger evidence base. For the remainder of this chapter this programme of work is summarized and the recommendations it led to are presented. Other experimental research in this area is also reviewed in order to provide a comprehensive and exhaustive overview of work in this field.

Four key questions will be addressed here:

1. Do experienced and less experienced lifeguards employ similar search strategies?
2. How does attention change based upon the visual display?
3. How does communication influence attention?
4. Do scanning techniques help?

Before the first question is addressed it is important to understand the methods that were adopted in these studies. Specifically, all simulated studies (i.e. those that did not use real beach footage) involved at least one swimmer who submerged. It should be highlighted that there were no other contextual behaviours such as those identified in the instinctive drowning response (see Ref. [16] for a review of these behaviours) present to help the lifeguards detect the person submerging. Additionally, all the studies reviewed utilized an eye tracker to understand where the participants were looking when viewing the pool or beach scenes. Generally the eye trackers used in these studies operate by illuminating the eye with the beam from a near infrared source, while the optical system focuses an image of the eye onto a solid-state video sensor (eye camera). A second solid camera is focused on the scene being viewed by the participants. The illuminator, optics and both cameras are mounted on a pair of glasses or headband. Each participant was required to look at a sequence of markers (for example, see Figure 11.1) to calibrate their eye positioning (pupil and corneal reflection) with a specific point on the screen. This calibration was recorded by the system, which enabled all other gaze points to be accurately determined.

For most studies, the raw data film was loaded onto a computer and a frame-by-frame analysis was conducted using Windows Media Player, where the location of the cross hair was recorded (Figure 11.2) using a grid square format (Figure 11.3). Once these analyses had been completed the number of fixations (for the purpose of these studies a fixation was defined as the eye remaining within a specific grid square for >100 or 120 milliseconds [depending on the capture rate of the specific eye tracker used]), fixation duration (how long each fixation was) and fixation location (where the fixations were) were calculated.

Figure 11.1 Calibration screen.

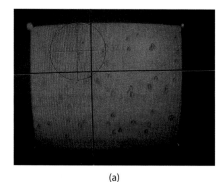

(a)

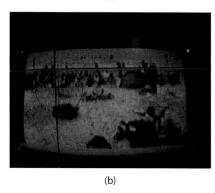

(b)

Figure 11.2 Cross hair examples (a and b).

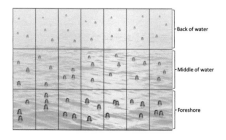

Figure 11.3 Grid system (grid unseen by participants, used only for analysis purposes).

Question 1: Do experienced and less experienced lifeguards employ similar search strategies?

A study was conducted to investigate whether experienced lifeguards employed similar visual search strategies as less experienced lifeguards. Within this study 69 lifeguards wearing an eye tracker watched a uniform display of 63 identical swimmers in the water for 12 minutes in two conditions [1,17]. In the non-biased condition, lifeguards were given instructions to watch the display as if they were looking out into the sea. On every occasion, unknown to the lifeguard, a person disappeared after 10 minutes in the middle on the left hand side of the screen (grid square 8, Figure 11.3). In the biased condition, lifeguards were given instructions to 'watch the display as if they are looking out into the sea and that there is a rip in the right hand side of the water'. In this condition, and again unknown to the lifeguard, a person disappeared after 10 minutes in the middle on the right hand side of the screen (grid square 14, Figure 11.3).

The tests were conducted using a counterbalanced (crossover) design in which half of the lifeguards saw the non-biased condition first and half saw the biased condition first. The results showed that experienced lifeguards were 4.9 times more likely to detect the person disappearing. The eye tracking data showed that there were no significant interaction effects between the experienced and less experienced lifeguards, surf and non-surf lifeguards and male and female lifeguards in terms of the number of fixations or fixation duration (data analysed from 2 to 10 minutes). These data also showed changes to the visual search pattern when the lifeguards were told about the rip (biased condition);

the instruction influenced the search patterns causing the lifeguards to search more on the right of the water. Between 40% and 42% of the lifeguards did not detect the person disappearing even though they fixated in the correct grid square in the 3.5 seconds before the person submerged in both conditions. This data suggests that, although the search pattern may be directed towards a relevant area within a display, almost half of the lifeguards did not detect the person disappearing and therefore their attention may not have been focused. This supports the notion that lifeguards may look at areas, but not be effective at extracting cues from them. Twenty-five percent of the lifeguards in the biased condition and 36% of the lifeguards in the non-biased conditions did not fixate in the direct location of the person disappearing, but were able to identify that person. This provides evidence to suggest that peripheral vision is being utilized by some lifeguards.

A more recent study used beach footage rather than a simulated beach scene to investigate what knowledge and visual search patterns were used by experienced and less experienced beach lifeguards in the lead-up to the successful and unsuccessful detection of hazards. The study attempted to determine whether experience and success are characterized by a specific knowledge base and trainable search patterns [18]. These authors used the study design in Figure 11.4:

It was hypothesized that

1. Less experienced lifeguards would identify a similar number of hazards but would require a greater amount of time to detect them than the experienced lifeguards in the video and video control groups.

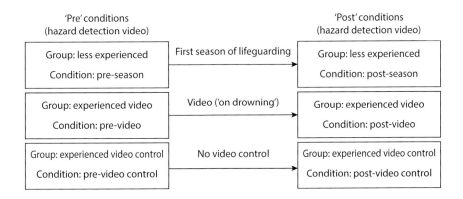

Figure 11.4 Study groups.

2. Less experienced lifeguards would detect more hazards at the end of the season compared to the beginning of the season.
3. Experienced lifeguards who watched the Pia video *On Drowning* (1970) (video group) would detect an increased number of hazards from pre- to post-video conditions compared to the video control group.
4. All lifeguards would respond in similar ways to each hazard.
5. Experienced lifeguards would have longer mean fixation durations, have a greater percentage time fixating and have shorter time spent fixating on hazards than less experienced lifeguards in the pre- and post-video conditions.

For the video stimuli, footage of complex beach scenes that represented real life, demanding decision-making scenarios was captured. Prior to the video capture, a focus group of experienced lifeguards and the head of lifeguards from the RNLI determined the behaviours that needed to be included in the video. Following on from this, lifeguards (not in uniform) were asked to partake in the hazardous behaviours, among natural busy beach scenes. Once the videos were captured the focus group met again to decide the most realistic clips to be used for the study.

The less experienced group data were collected at the beginning (pre-season) and end (post-season) of their first season working for the RNLI. The experienced video group data were collected before (pre-video) and immediately after (post-video) watching the Pia video *On Drowning* (1970). The experienced video control group data were collected before a 15-minute rest (the approximate duration of the Pia video) (pre-video control) and then immediately after the rest period data (post-video control). Each testing session in the pre- and post-conditions followed a similar procedure (Figure 11.4).

A mobile eye tracker was worn by each lifeguard during testing. The lifeguards were trained, using a video to (1) press a button when they saw a hazard, (2) verbally indicate what the hazard was, (3) show where the hazard was using a laser pen and (4) say how they would intervene. They then had two 30-second practice attempts. After that they watched 20 minutes of real beach footage projected onto a large screen under the two conditions outlined above.

The key findings from this study were that experienced lifeguards perceived more hazards than less experienced lifeguards when watching identical displays; the time taken to detect the hazards were similar for experienced and less experienced lifeguards (reject H1). The experience gained during the lifeguards' first season did not implicitly improve their hazard detection rates (reject H2). Furthermore, watching the 1970 Pia video *On Drowning* did not improve the experienced lifeguards' hazard detection rates (reject H3). Less experienced lifeguards used more active responses when intervening with hazards than the experienced lifeguards (reject H4). Experienced compared to less experienced lifeguards, had similar eye-tracking patterns in the lead-up to hazards (reject H5).

Lanagan-Leitzel and colleagues have also been conducting research into attention, but the focus of this work has been pool rather than beach lifeguard performance. However, the findings may be applicable given the similar study designs. In a study that used sixty 30-second clips of aquatic scenes to investigate how lifeguards monitor critical events, it was found that lifeguards fixate more than naïve participants (31.32 vs 26.64 fixations, respectively), but not more than briefly trained participants (29.80 fixations). It was also found that there were no significant differences in fixation duration. Lifeguards detected a greater percentage of the critical events than naïve participants (54% vs 41.4%, respectively), but not briefly trained participants (49.2%) [19]. Furthermore, subsequent analyses were conducted based on clips where the target 'objects' moved more than $1°$ of visual angle (and therefore multiple fixations would be needed to monitor the object). Similar to the overall analyses, lifeguards monitored more critical events (20.9/29) and had more fixations (74.7) than naïve participants (16.4/29 and 51.4), but were not significantly different compared to briefly trained participants (20.2/29 and 82.8). With regard to fixation location, lifeguards had fewer fixations off the water (10.7%) than naïve participants (19.5%), but were not significantly different to the briefly trained participants (13%). Interestingly, for submersion behaviour, the percentage of fixations was similar between the three groups.

In a later study using two-minute clips of aquatic scenes, it was found that experienced instructors identified significantly more critical events (average 52.9, SD 8.70) out of the 323 total than certified lifeguards (average 25.2, SD 3.99) [20]. Students who were involved in lifeguard training identified an average (SD) of 16.3 (3.39) critical events at the beginning of the semester and 18.7 (6.17) events at the end of the semester. The non-lifeguards reported an average (SD) of 29.6 (4.97) events, which did not differ significantly from the certified lifeguards. Specific events were examined to determine if they were frequently reported by any participant group. The highest rate of agreement was among the lifeguard instructors, but there were no events identified by every lifeguard instructor. Fourteen events were identified by at least 70% of the lifeguard instructors. The lifeguards did not agree with each other in relation to the frequency of the detection of the events, any better than the non-lifeguards or the students on the lifeguarding course. Each event was scrutinized to determine what features were present that could attract a lifeguard's attention. The categories that emerged from the explanations focused on instinctive drowning response behaviours (submersion, splashing), patron weakness indicators (young child, water depth, weakness), physical danger warnings (bad water conditions, horseplay, vehicle presence), problems with unattended children, an obstructed view, a new person entering the scene or a general comment such as 'mask hinders breathing' or 'people swimming in [to shore]' [20].

PRACTICAL IMPLICATIONS AND RECOMMENDATIONS

1. The surveillance pattern used by lifeguards can be altered by instruction and detection rates improve as a consequence.
2. Putting a new lifeguard on the beach for one season may not significantly change their surveillance-related knowledge; therefore, bespoke surveillance training should be introduced.
3. Watching a narrow-focused drowning video will not enhance the range of hazards detected by experienced lifeguards. However, if continued professional development is required to understand drowning in more detail then the Pia video *On Drowning* (1970) may be appropriate.
4. Less experienced lifeguards should be trained to adopt less active intervention strategies; this could facilitate their detection of more hazards.
5. Training should be surveillance knowledge-based rather than eye-movement focused, but a combination of the two may be most appropriate.

Question 2: How does attention change based upon the visual display?

To investigate whether lifeguards' attention changes based upon the visual display, we [21] manipulated a simulation in two ways. First, we manipulated the number of swimmers in three scenarios (43, 53 and 63 swimmers unevenly distributed [95% of swimmers in the foreshore, 3% in the middle of the water, 2% at the back of the water]). We also manipulated the distribution of the swimmers within the simulation (63 swimmers in uniform distribution vs 63 swimmers in the unevenly distributed condition). Thirty-one lifeguards watched a five-minute video in the four conditions while wearing an eye tracker. The lifeguards were informed that at any point in the five minutes a person or people might or might not submerge. The lifeguards were required to highlight with a laser pen if, and where, a person submerged. The lifeguards were unaware that a predefined swimmer submerged after 4.5 minutes in each of the conditions. The person submerged in different areas between conditions but in the same areas within conditions across participants. The swimmer took five seconds to submerge.

We found that the detection rates were not significantly different across the four conditions, suggesting that lifeguards were equally as effective at detecting people in trouble in the evenly distributed conditions as they were in the unevenly distributed conditions. There was a significant difference between the total numbers of fixations across the four conditions, with lifeguards fixating significantly more in the evenly distributed condition compared to all other conditions. There was no significant difference in the total number of fixations between any of the unevenly distributed conditions. There was a significant difference between the average fixation duration across the four conditions with lifeguards fixating for significantly shorter durations in the evenly distributed condition compared to all other conditions. There was no significant difference in the average fixation duration between any of the unevenly distributed conditions.

PRACTICAL IMPLICATIONS AND RECOMMENDATIONS

1. Lifeguards are equally efficient at detecting swimmers in trouble in the water regardless of distribution and number in the water up to at least 63 in the present scenario.
2. Lifeguards change their surveillance patterns based on the *distribution* of swimmers in the water.
3. Lifeguards do not change their surveillance patterns based on subtle changes in the *number* of swimmers in the water. This suggests that training programmes for surveillance should take distributions of swimmers into account. Such a programme should include instruction on cue utilization, use of peripheral vision and optimization of scanning patterns.
4. Further research should focus on providing more content for such training.

Question 3: How do communication and *a priori* instructions influence attention?

To investigate how communication and *a priori* instructions influence attention we [22] conducted a study with five conditions where lifeguards performed the following:

1. Natural scan of a simulated beach scene alone; each lifeguard tested separately.
2. Natural scan of the same scene when two lifeguards work together; no communication.
3. Self-determined scan when two lifeguards work together; communication allowed prior to testing (lifeguards come to their own agreement) and during testing.
4. Prescribed scan when two lifeguards work together; *a priori* instruction to cover 50% of the screen each (left vs right).
5. Natural scan alone (repeat condition 1 to determine learning effects).

In all conditions lifeguards wore an eye tracker. They watched five minutes of animated beach footage projected onto a large screen in the five conditions listed above, in an evenly distributed 63 swimmer condition. The lifeguards were informed that at any point in the five-minute video a person or people might or might not submerge. They were required to highlight with a laser pen if, and where, a person submerged. The lifeguards were unaware that a predefined swimmer submerged after 1.5, 2.5, 3.5 and 4.5 minutes in each of the conditions. The people submerged in different areas between conditions. The swimmers took five seconds to submerge. The conditions were presented in a standardized order.

We found that there was no association between the number of detections and the five conditions. However, there was a significant difference between Conditions 1 and 5, suggesting that a learning effect had taken place due to the training received in the three paired conditions. There were also no significant differences in the number of fixations between the five conditions. The fixation duration in Condition 1 was significantly longer than Conditions 3, 4 and 5. There were no significant differences in fixation duration between Conditions 2 and 3, 2 and 4, 3 and 4, or 3 and 5. The fixation duration in Condition 4 was significantly longer than Condition 5 and the fixation duration in Condition 2 was significantly longer than Condition 5. There were no significant differences in the total duration of joint fixations between the three paired conditions. There were also no significant differences in the Euclidian distances between gaze points between the three paired conditions. Lifeguards spent the majority of their time fixating on the right side of the water unless they were specifically instructed (either by the researcher or by mutual agreement with each other) to look at other places (Conditions 3 and 4). When asked to develop their own search strategy (Condition 3), the lifeguards opted for a number of differing strategies including the following: looking left versus right; top versus bottom; horizontal versus vertical scanning; both scanning the whole screen randomly.

PRACTICAL IMPLICATIONS AND RECOMMENDATIONS

1. Video-based surveillance training is likely to improve detection rates of beach lifeguards watching a virtual scene. Consideration should be given to this training.

2. Higher detection rates (of simulated drowning individuals) are not statistically associated with any of the specific conditions. However, the median value increases from two detections (working alone) to three detections (working in pairs), and the detection percentage also increases suggesting that there is practical value in working together.

3. Some eye movement variables (e.g. mean fixation duration) change when working together, but the change is so small that there would be no value in training eye movements in isolation.

4. There is very little overlap in the area of the scene being looked at by the lifeguards at the same time when working together in silence and when able to communicate when viewing uniform displays (i.e. the scene used in this study). This suggests that even when fixating on the same side of the water (Condition 2) lifeguards still looked at different regions within that side. It is important to determine if this conclusion also applies to a more natural and complex beach scene.

5. When lifeguards work together, the division of their field of view horizontally may be more effective than dividing the beach vertically. The most frequent technique used was to divide the beach vertically. Future research should investigate whether dividing the display horizontally is the most effective strategy when working in pairs and viewing more natural and complex beach scenes.

Question 4: Do scanning techniques help?

Some lifeguard training agencies advocate the use of specific scan techniques and patterns [15]. However, no specific research has been conducted to support these recommendations. One study examined the physiology of the eye and the field of vision while scanning in order to assess which scanning techniques cover 100% of the required zone with the middle 40° of the visual field [23]. The assumption was that if a signal is detected in the middle field, the lifeguards can then bring it into the inner field (1°), which enables them to determine whether a person is in trouble. This study identified three techniques that were theoretically considered to be 100% effective if followed by the lifeguard, but given the physiological nature

of the paper the authors did not provide specific evidence that these scanning patterns were indeed effective.

To understand whether scanning techniques helped lifeguard performance, we [24] examined the effects of prescribed and free scanning on coverage of the primary zone and the detection rates of beach lifeguards. A secondary aim was to examine the impact of an auditory prompt on the detection rates of beach lifeguards when free scanning. More specifically, we aimed to determine the percentage of time spent covering the primary zone and the rates of detection of a submerging individual by beach lifeguards when using the following techniques: (a) free scan technique; (b) parallel scan technique; (c) spoke scan technique and (d) free scan technique with an auditory prompt. In addition to this, the study used subjective analyses to determine whether lifeguards were able to adopt specific scan strategies and the degree to which they felt confident that the techniques were effective.

It was hypothesized that (i) lifeguards would have the ability to adopt the prescribed scan patterns after the training interventions; (ii) lifeguards would have no significant differences in their perceptions of the effectiveness of the two prescribed scan patterns; (iii) lifeguards would have significantly higher detection rates in the free scan conditions compared to the prescribed scan conditions; (iv) lifeguards would produce significantly more fixations of shorter duration in the prescribed scan conditions than the free scan conditions; (v) lifeguards would cover significantly more of the primary zone in the free scan conditions compared to the prescribed scan conditions; (vi) there would be no significant difference in detection rates or how much time is spent covering the primary zone between the parallel and spoke scan conditions; and (vii) lifeguards would have significantly higher detection rates in the auditory prompt condition compared to the non-cued free scan condition.

A mobile eye tracker was worn by each lifeguard during testing. They watched five minutes of animated beach footage projected onto a large screen in four conditions presented above in an unevenly distributed 43 swimmer condition with 95% of swimmers in the foreshore, 3% in the middle third of the water and 2% at the back of the water.

The lifeguards were informed that at any point in the five minutes a person or people might or might not submerge. The lifeguards were required to highlight with a laser pen if and where a person submerged. The lifeguards were unaware that a predefined swimmer submerged after 4.5 minutes in each of the conditions. The person submerged in different areas between conditions. The conditions were presented in a counterbalanced order. For analysis purposes the *primary zone* was defined as the zone that covered where 100% of the swimmers were.

It was found that most lifeguards had the ability to adopt the prescribed scanning patterns after the training intervention. Lifeguards had no significant differences in their perceptions of the effectiveness of the two prescribed scan techniques. Detection rates were not significantly greater in the free scan conditions compared to the prescribed scan conditions. The prescribed scan conditions resulted in more fixations of shorter duration than the free scan conditions. Lifeguards spent significantly more time in the primary zone in the two free scan conditions than they did in the prescribed scan conditions. There were no significant differences in either the detection rates (free scan, 14%; parallel scan, 11%; spoke scan, 18%; free scan with auditory prompt, 20%) or how much time was spent covering the primary zone between the parallel and spoke scan conditions.

PRACTICAL IMPLICATIONS AND RECOMMENDATIONS

1. Most lifeguards can adopt prescribed scanning patterns if they are trained using a short video.
2. Lifeguards only appear to be approximately 52%–57% confident that parallel and spoke scan patterns are effective.
3. Lifeguards are equally efficient at detecting swimmers in trouble in the water regardless of the type of scanning pattern adopted.
4. Lifeguards cover the primary zone for a greater amount of time when using free scan patterns. This suggests that, at present, training programmes for surveillance should not be specifically focused on training lifeguards to use prescribed scan techniques.

CONCLUSIONS

Our understanding of how beach lifeguards scan a beach scene has improved in recent years. As a consequence of recent research we know that experienced lifeguards with more than one season of experience perform better than inexperienced lifeguards, that lifeguards change their surveillance patterns based on the *distribution* of swimmers in the water but not based on subtle changes in the *number* of swimmers in the water, working together aids effectiveness, and that pre-prescribed scanning techniques are not more effective than natural scanning techniques. We suggest that lifeguards would benefit from a training programme aimed at making naïve lifeguards experienced as soon as possible.

REFERENCES

1. Page J, Bates V, Long G, Dawes P, Tipton M. Beach lifeguards: Visual search patterns, detection rates and the influence of experience. *Ophthal Physl Opt.* 2011; 31: 216–24.
2. Fenner P, Leahy S, Buhk A, Dawes P. Prevention of drowning: Visual scanning and attention span in lifeguards. *J Occup Health Safety Aust.* 1999; 15: 61–6.
3. Duncan J, Humphreys GW. Visual search and stimulus similarity. *Psychol Rev.* 1989; 96: 433–58.
4. Wolfe JM. Visual search. In Pashler H (ed.). *Attention.* Sussex, UK: Psychology Press; 1998, pp. 13–74.
5. Schwebel DC, Lindsay S, Simpson J. Brief report: A brief intervention to improve lifeguard surveillance at a public swimming pool. *J Pediatr Psychol.* 2007; 32: 862–8.
6. Harrell WA, Boisvert JA. An information theory analysis of lifeguards scanning. *Percept Mot Skills.* 2003; 97: 129–34.
7. Mackworth NH. *Researches on the Measurement of Human Performance.* Medical Research Council Special Report Series 268. London: Her Majesty's Stationary Office; 1950.
8. Richardson WJ. *Recognition and Observation of Potential Rescue Victims in an Open Water Environment.* Report from International Life Saving Federation International Medical Rescue Conference, San Diego, US Lifesaving Association Manual of Open Water Lifesaving. 1997.

9. Griffiths RC, Griffiths TJ. Internal noise distractions in lifeguarding. *Int J Acad Res Educ.* 2012; 6: 56–71.

10. Harrell WA. Lifeguards' vigilance: Effects of child-adult ratio and lifeguard positioning on scanning by lifeguards. *Psychol Rep.* 1999; 84: 193–7.

11. Epstein Y, Keren G, Moisseiev J, Gasko O, Yachin S. Psychomotor deterioration during exposure to heat. *Aviat Space Environ Med.* 1980; 51: 607–10.

12. Griffiths T, Steel D, Vogelsong H. Operation Baywatch: Results of the national lifeguard survey. *Parks Recreat.* 1997; 32: 62–8.

13. Wyon DP, Wyon I, Norin F. Effects of moderate heat stress on driver vigilance in a moving vehicle. *Ergonomics.* 1996; 39: 61–75.

14. Brener J, Oostman M. Lifeguards watch but they don't always see. *World Water Park Magazine*, 5 September 2002, pp. 14–16.

15. United States Lifeguards Standards Coalition. *An Evidence Based Review and Report.* United States Lifeguards Standards Coalition, San Deigo; 2011.

16. Pia F. Reflections on lifeguard surveillance programs. In Fletemeyer JR, Freas SJ (eds.). *Drowning: New Perspectives in Intervention and Prevention.* London, UK: CRC Press; 1999, pp. 231–43.

17. Page J, Bates V, Long G, Dawes P, Tipton M. *Surveillance and Detection Rates of Beach Lifeguards.* Royal National Lifeboat Institution, Poole, UK; 2010.

18. Page J, Long G, Dawes P, Tipton M. *Towards an Understanding of the Differences in Hazard Detection and Associated Responses of Experienced and Less Experienced Beach Lifeguards.* Royal National Lifeboat Institution, Poole, UK; 2014.

19. Lanagan-Leitzel LK, Moore CM. Do lifeguards monitor the events they should? *Int J Acad Res Educ.* 2010; 4: 241–56.

20. Lanagan-Leitzel LK. Identification of critical events by lifeguards, instructors, and non-lifeguards. *Int J Acad Res Educ.* 2012; 6: 203–14.

21. Page J, Long G, Dawes P, Tipton M. *The Impact of the Number and Distribution of Swimmers in the Water on Beach Lifeguard Surveillance and Detection.* Royal National Lifeboat Institution, Poole, UK; 2011.

22. Page J, Long G, Lunt H, Dawes P, Tipton M. *The Impact of a Priori Instructions and Communication on Surveillance and Detection Rates of Beach Lifeguards that Are Working Together.* Royal National Lifeboat Institution, Poole, UK; 2014.

23. Hunsucker J, Davison S. How lifeguards overlooks victims: Vision and signal detection. *Int J Aquat Res Educ.* 2008; 1: 59–74.

24. Page J, Long G, Dawes P, Tipton M. *Enhancing Detection Rates of Beach Lifeguards: Determining the Best Scanning Technique.* Royal National Lifeboat Institution, Poole, UK; 2012.

12

Lifeguard swimming performance in surf

MIKE TIPTON AND ANDREW BYATT

INTRODUCTION

This chapter considers the topic of swimming in the surf. It covers the limited amount of science that has looked specifically at this issue as well as the skills involved in swimming efficiently in the surf and ways of developing those skills.

THE SCIENCE

As part of the research to support the development of their fitness standard for beach lifeguards (BLG), Reilly et al. [1,2] reported that the time taken to cover 200 m out to sea (variable surf conditions) and in a pool did not differ. However, in the sea this distance was covered by a combination of running and swimming, with running being significantly faster; in the pool only swimming was undertaken. It follows that swimming in the sea must have been slower than swimming in the pool, because the same overall time was taken despite the initial advantage of running when in the sea.

This information led to questions about the differences in performance when swimming in different types of water and the impact of experience on the ability to swim in surf. Anecdotally, those from surf beaches report a skill factor when swimming in the surf, but this area has received little or no peer-reviewed published research. The literature associated with surf beach lifeguards reveals more about their physical capabilities and characteristics than their surf swimming skill [3–5]; where swimming skill is defined as the non-fitness-related component of performance. Even in pool swimming, there is clearly a skill factor that is independent of fitness [4]; however, this skill component had never been quantified for surf swimming. To address this, Tipton et al. [6] examined the swim performance of a group of beach lifeguards with (SE) and without (NSE) experience of swimming in the surf.

Sixty-five BLG had their surf swimming experience assessed by a series of questions designed specifically to examine the frequency and severity of surf swimming experience to produce a score for each lifeguard on a scale from 0 to 310. On the basis of this score, the BLG were divided into two distinct groups: 30 BLG had little or no surf swimming experience (NSE, score of 0–85), and 35 had a high level of surf swimming experience (SE, score of 110–310). The BLG with NSE had an average score of 25 on the surf experience questions; the corresponding score for the BLG with SE was 267. Each BLG undertook the following tests:

1. An initial maximum effort 200-m pool swim (25-m pool).
2. A maximum effort 200-m calm sea swim (Gyllingvase, Falmouth, UK).
3. A maximum effort 200-m surf sea swim (Perranporth, Cornwall, UK).
4. A final maximum effort 200-m pool swim (25-m pool).
5. A 50-m maximum effort swim, 25-m underwater/25-m over water pool swim.
6. Maximum effort swim bench ergometer test. A 30-second swim bench test. Measures: strokes/min; stroke length; distance/min; force/stroke; force peak; force average; time to force peak; length to force peak; power per stroke; power average; work/stroke; work average.
7. Static anthropometric measures. The following measurements were taken: height, weight, age, arm length, shoulder circumference, skinfold thickness at four sites (biceps, triceps, subscapular, suprailiac crest).

The tests listed in f and g were undertaken because authors have attempted to develop simple, indirect tests and indices that predict swimming aerobic power and performance. These tests include simulated swimming [7], the measurement of upper body anaerobic power [8], anthropometry (lean body weight has been found to predict VO_{2max} in trained swimmers [9]), an arm stroke index (number of strokes divided by swimming velocity [10]) and swim bench tests [11]. Upper body anaerobic power (peak sustained workload) has been reported to predict swimming performance in events up to 400 m [8]; this relationship underpins the use of arm ergometry (cranking) to simulate swimming and predict performance. The correlations reported by Tipton et al. [12] between in-water casualty-towing VO_{2max} and both upper body anthropometric measures and push-ups support the conclusion that upper body strength is an important characteristic for rescue swimming. Swim bench tests of upper body strength and power have been reported to provide higher correlations with swimming performance than isometric upper body strength measures because of their greater specificity [9].

The environmental conditions at Gyllingvase were zero metres wave height, 16°C water temperature and 18°C air temperature. The environmental conditions at Perranporth were 1.0–1.5 m wave height, 19°C water temperature and 18°C air temperature. All 200-m swims were undertaken wearing BLG-issue swimming costumes only. On the basis of the initial 200-m pool swim times, an attempt was made to match a BLG with NSE to a BLG with SE. The matched subjects then undertook tests b–d together; this ensured that the two groups were competitive and experienced the same sea states. Tests b–g were conducted on the same day; at least 2.5 hours elapsed between successive swims.

The BLG started their pool swims in the water. For the sea swims, they waded into the water until they were immersed to the waist; the timed swims started from this position. This prevented the ability to run into the sea from influencing the results and increased the likelihood of isolating the skill factor in surf swimming.

The NSE was an average of 9.3 seconds slower on the 200-m pool swim when compared to the BLG with SE. In order to compare the sea swims directly, 9.3 seconds were subtracted from the individual sea swim times of the NSE group to normalize their data. The swim time results of the study are presented in Figure 12.1.

In both groups, the time taken to swim 200 m was greater in a calm sea than in the pool and greater in a surf sea than in the calm sea. The calm sea swim times of the two groups did not differ significantly. The NSE group was significantly slower swimming 200 m in the surf, by a mean swim time of 58.3 seconds (before normalization) when compared to the experienced group.

The average time to swim 25 m underwater followed by 25 m over water was 38.3 seconds for the SE group and was significantly longer at 40.4 seconds for the NSE. However, when comparing only the underwater 25-m swims, the two groups (NSE = 22.2 seconds and SE = 21.3 seconds) did not differ.

In terms of predicting surf swim time, regression analysis identified surf experience as the only statistically significant predictor. That none of the swim bench or anthropometric variables and tests of power and strength predicted surf swim time was perhaps to be expected. Tanaka et al. [11] identified that dry-land resistance training did not improve swimming performance despite the

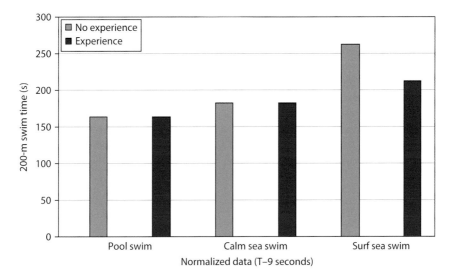

Figure 12.1 Normalized pool swim times of NSE (swim times minus 9 seconds) and SE swimmers in the swimming tests (n = 65).

fact that there were significant power gains on the biokinetic swim bench and during a tethered swim over a 14-week period. One reason given for this was that some of the tests did not evaluate swimming skill in the specific scenario under examination. In addition, the bench test was much shorter (30 seconds) than the swim times required. One conclusion from these findings is that training for surf swimming should directly and specifically address the skills and capacities associated with the task (see 'The skill of surf swimming' section).

It is clear that there is a significant and quantifiable skill component associated with swimming in the surf. Comparing the surf swim times when pool swimming performance is matched, the presence of surf experience reduced the 200-m surf swim time from an average of 262–213 seconds. This reduction represents an improvement of 18%. This percentage is an indication of the skill component of surf swimming, which is not attributed to pool swimming ability. Instead, it is likely to be experience-based and due to attributes such as navigational skills, surf awareness and confidence. However, the change in an individual's surf swim time relative to an increase in their surf experience is dependent on a wide range of influences. Therefore, it is likely to be highly variable at an individual level and not particularly predictive at this level.

The finding that two BLG with similar 200-m pool times may perform very differently in surf

has some important implications. While pool times predict the time to reach 200 m out to sea by running/wading and swimming in calm sea and surf, clearly pool swimming time is not an indicator of an individual's ability to swim in surf. Care should therefore be taken when allocating BLG to surf beaches on the basis of pool swim times. When trying to swim 200 m out to sea in surf, a large proportion of the subjects without surf swimming experience were unable to cover the distance in less than the required 3.5 minutes [1,2]. Indeed, just fewer than 50% of those with surf swimming experience achieved this time but, as noted, during an actual emergency the BLG should be able to wade/run for a significant proportion of the 200 m on a surf beach, thereby reducing the time taken to reach a casualty.

As experience of swimming in the surf can significantly improve surf swimming times, consideration should be given to providing BLG operating on surf beaches with formal training in the skills associated with swimming in the surf. These skills and the training associated with them are outlined and discussed in the sections that follow.

THE SKILL OF SURF SWIMMING

Note: The guidance presented here is based on practical application and observation by experienced surf swim coaches rather than comprehensive academic research.

The skill of surf swimming can be broken down into a number of components. A programme for improving surf swimming should focus on the components that are likely to be most frequently used in the environmental conditions by the individual(s) concerned. Surf swimming performance should be assessed by an experienced and qualified surf swim coach. The coach should be able to effectively analyze surf swimming performance by providing appropriate feedback and practices for improvement specific to the individual needs of each participant.

It is good practice to assess individuals against each surf swimming component using a measurement tool, both pre- and post-intervention, to ensure the programme is effective for the individuals involved and allow evaluation of the intervention. The effectiveness may be measured using an appropriate grading scale or time-based activities, for example. Although timing can be used as a performance measure over set distances, the ocean is an environment with consistently changing variables, which often makes accurate comparison of times from day to day unreliable.

Swimming from shore to patient

The primary skill components considered when swimming from shore to patient in surf conditions are listed below:

COMPONENT 1: WADING

Wading is a form of modified running through water used by surf swimmers. It is considered important in surf swim performance, as running is approximately five times faster than swimming. The surf swimmer is aiming to utilize this advantage by adapting the running technique through water.

Effective wading is based on the following assessment points and observations:

Assessment form: Wading

Assessment point	Observations
Appropriate initial running speed	The greater the initial running speed prior to reaching the water's edge, the greater the momentum that is carried into wading.
	Appropriate initial running speed is considered to be a balance between the maximum speed the individual can achieve, the expected increase in water depth and the individual's wading ability/fitness. Running too fast into a depth of water where the individual cannot adequately wade results in tripping/stumbling or stopping. Running too fast also contributes to fatigue throughout the swim.
Progressive knee/ ankle clearance, as water depth increases	As water depth increases, the hip gradually increases into a greater angle of abduction and internal rotation (during hip flexion) with a flexed knee position. This motion allows the knee and ankle to clear the depth of the water being encountered.
	Without adequate hip abduction, internal rotation and knee flexion, the knee and ankle drag/catch the water. This drag prematurely slows wading momentum and increases the energy required to continue wading. If the individual is unable to continue to wade, the slower alternatives of dolphin dives, swimming or walking through water will be required.
Progressive arm swing height as water depth increases	Arm swing height increases progressively with the increase in water depth, in order to counterbalance the altered leg movements described above. Arm height typically increases until both wrist and elbow reach just above shoulder height.
	As depth increases, inexperienced surf swimmers are often unable to maintain contralateral arm–leg timing when wading. This limits the momentum that can be maintained by the surf swimmer and increases the energy required to continue.

Continued

Assessment point	Observations
Appropriate posture	The individual's posture is upright and slightly angled forwards to allow momentum to be maintained forwards through increasing depth of water. The torso should not be bent forward/flexed at the hips as this is associated with reduced ability for hip flexion and water clearance for the legs. Being too upright or leaning backwards decreases the momentum, slows wading down and requires greater energy for legs to drive through the water.
Momentum maintained as water depth increases	Rhythm is key to maintaining momentum from running to wading to dolphin dives. The speed at which the arms and legs move through the water progressively decreases with increasing water depth; this reduces stumbling or stopping. When encountering small waves while wading, the surf swimmer often performs an extra high wading step to clear the oncoming wave and then maintain wading momentum, rather than stopping or slowing down. Stopping wading and hop–skip actions slow the surf swimmer down and require the surf swimmer to expend increased amounts of energy to return to optimal speed.
Wading until correct water depth	When wading on a beach with a shallow gradient or gradual increase in water depth, wading is typically continued until mid-thigh depth or until dolphin dives become the quicker option for the individual's fitness level. Very experienced individuals with appropriate fitness and flexibility may be able to wade until groin depth. Some beaches may have a gradual gradient for a given distance and then have a sudden increase in gradient, meaning that dolphin dives or swimming become the preferred option sooner than mid-thigh depth. This point is discussed below in the 'Component 2: Dolphin diving' section.

COMPONENT 2: DOLPHIN DIVING

Dolphin diving is the term used for the action of performing multiple dives through the water when pushing off with the feet from the seabed. Dolphin dives are often used as a transition between wading and swimming.

Assessment form: Dolphin diving

Assessment point	Observations
Appropriate starting depth	Dolphin dives start when the water depth is too deep for effective wading to continue and when dolphin dives would be considered faster than the individual's swimming speed. On a beach with a gradual gradient, this would typically be water around mid-thigh depth. On a beach where there is a sudden increase in water depth, it can be appropriate to start when the legs are in much shallower water. Swimmers should always ensure there is adequate water depth for dolphin dives for safety reasons.
Momentum carried from wading to dolphin dives	Experienced surf swimmers will continue momentum from wading directly into the first dolphin dive. To enable this, the surf swimmer accurately judges when the final wading step will be taken and transfers their weight forward into the dive position in one fluid motion. They use appropriate head positioning looking to the direction of travel and subsequently the entrance point in the water.

Continued

Assessment point	Observations
	Typically, the first dolphin dive involves the whole body exiting the water and re-entering in a streamlined position with the following order of entry: hands, elbows, head, shoulders, hips, knees, feet. The streamlined position is maintained through the water.
Preparation and push-off for subsequent dolphin dive	When momentum of the dive slows, the swimmer will typically touch/grab the sand with the hands. The feet are quickly placed into a track start 'set' type position in the sand behind the hands for an immediate push-off forward and upwards into the next dolphin dive.
	Typically, there is no delay, standing or upright positioning of the body between dolphin dives. This may occur on occasion to assist with timing of dives between waves or for fatigued swimmers.
	A judgement is taken whether to dive under or over oncoming waves when performing dolphin dives. Typically, the quicker option of diving over a wave is used to avoid the opposing drag associated with a wave. When the height of a wave is too great to clear by dolphin diving over the wave, diving under the wave is undertaken as the most appropriate option.
Subsequent dolphin dive execution	Subsequent dolphin dives should aim to maintain a streamlined entry and maximum forward momentum with each dive, with the following order of entry: hands, elbows, head, shoulders, hips, knees, feet.
	However, depending upon water depth, the level of fatigue and pacing required, the entire body may not completely clear the water with each dive. The hands re-enter the water almost immediately after push-off. The head may have re-entered the water before the hips and knees exit. This positioning gives a more dolphin type appearance to the action, whereby this component gains its name.
Appropriate finishing depth	On a beach with a gradual gradient and increase in depth, the finishing depth of the dives would be at approximately belly button depth or when dolphin diving becomes slower than swimming.
	Momentum from the final dolphin dive should then be carried directly into the first swimming stroke.

COMPONENT 3: NEGOTIATING SURF AND SWIMMING TO PATIENT

After wading and dolphin diving, the swimmer begins to swim to the patient and negotiates waves with head-down surface dives when applicable.

Assessment form: Negotiating surf and swimming to patient

Assessment point	Observations
Continuing swimming to patient	The swimmer maintains head-down freestyle swimming stroke through small choppy conditions, rather than swimming head-up or aiming to swim over each 'bump' in the ocean.

Continued

Assessment point	Observations
	The swimmer periodically checks that their direction remains towards the patient. This check is done approximately every four to eight strokes or at appropriate opportunities, e.g. when on top of a swell rather than in the trough of a swell. The check is performed within the cycle of the normal swimming stroke, so torso rotation is maintained and stroke rhythm is affected minimally. Typically, visual checks do not involve the head looking forward for more than a single stroke.
Diving at appropriate time	When approaching waves, the swimmer aims to be fully submersed to the appropriate depth, typically 0.5–1.0 m prior to the wave reaching the swimmer by performing a head-down surface dive.
	Inexperienced or fatigued swimmers often swim straight into the wave, perform the dive too late, too shallow or a pencil (feet-down) type dive, rather than maintaining momentum from their swimming position.
Appropriate depth of dive	The depth of the dive remains as shallow as possible while aiming to clear the turbulence and drag created by the wave. This optimal depth is often reported to be around one-third of the depth of the wave's height. Often swimmers report noting the bubbles under the water and aiming to clear the significantly aerated patches throughout their dive.
	When negotiating very powerful waves where white water cannot be avoided, experienced surf swimmers may dive to the bottom and grab onto the sand to avoid being pulled backwards and may even attempt to take some steps forward on the seabed while underwater.
Approach to the surface	After diving to negotiate a wave, the swimmer will aim to return to the surface at the optimal angle considering conditions, often 15–45 degrees. Experienced swimmers will use dolphin kicks while underwater and aim to surface at an area of minimal aeration.
	Momentum should then be maintained directly into the first stroke of swimming.

COMPONENT 4: USING THE PREVAILING CONDITIONS

There are a number of prevailing conditions that should be considered and utilized. The following table considers waves, rip currents and sand banks. The swimmer should also maintain an awareness of other conditions, e.g. wind, tide, inshore holes, natural, man-made structures and other water users.

Assessment form: Use of the prevailing conditions

Assessment point	Observations
Use of sand banks for wading, where appropriate	Where the surf swim entry point is close to a sand bank, the experienced surf swimmer will make an informed judgement about whether it is more time efficient to run and wade across the nearby sand bank rather than swimming. Where the water is shallower, it should be quicker wading than swimming.
Use of rip currents when swimming, where appropriate	Where the surf swim entry point is close to a current for the swimmer to utilize, the experienced surf swimmer will make an informed judgement about whether it is more time efficient to swim slightly off course to utilize the assisting current and avoid oncoming waves rather than maintaining a direct line to the patient.
	Inexperienced surf swimmers often battle into waves when a close-by channel and associated rip current are available to speed the path out to the patient.

CONCLUSION

Surf swimming is a skill that has specific components that can be improved by coaching. Agencies responsible for recruiting beach lifeguards and allocating them to specific beaches should be cautious of making assignments simply based on pool or calm open water swim times. The provision of surf swim training for those lifeguarding on surf beaches should be considered and an appropriate assessment and improvement scheme used.

REFERENCES

1. Reilly TJ, Wooler A, Tipton MJ. Occupational fitness standards for beach lifeguards phase 1: The physiological demands of beach lifeguarding. *Occup Med.* 2006; 56: 6–11.
2. Reilly TJ, Iggleden C, Gennser M, Tipton MJ. Occupational fitness standards for beach lifeguards phase 2: The development of an easily administered fitness test. *Occup Med.* 2006; 56: 12–17.
3. Gayton PH. The physique of New Zealand surf life savers. *N Z J Health Phys Educ Recreat.* 1975; 8: 114–20.
4. Gulbin JP, Fell JW, Gaffney PT. A physiological profile of elite surf ironmen, full time lifeguards and patrolling surf life savers. *Aust J Sci Med Sport.* 1996; 28: 86–90.
5. VanHeest JH, Mahoney CE, Herr L. Characteristics of elite open-water swimmers. *J Strength Cond Res.* 2004; 18: 302–5.
6. Tipton MJ, Reilly TJ, Rees A, Spray G, Golden F. Swimming performance in the surf: The influence of experience. *Int J Sports Med.* 2008; 29(11): 895–8.
7. Kimura Y, Yeater RA, Martin RB. Simulated swimming: A useful tool for evaluation the VO_2max of swimmers in the laboratory. *Br J Sp Med.* 1990; 24: 201–6.
8. Hawley JA, Williams MM. Relationship between upper body anaerobic power and freestyle swimming performance. *Int J Sports Med.* 1991; 12: 1–5.
9. Costill DL, Kovaleski J, Porter DA, Kirwan J, Fielding R, King DS. Energy expenditure during front crawl swimming: Predicting success in middle-distance events. *Int J Sports Med.* 1985; 6: 266–70.
10. Lavoie JM, Leone M, Bongbele J. Functional maximal aerobic power and prediction of swimming performances. *J Swim Res.* 1988; 4: 17–19.
11. Tanaka H, Costill DL, Thonas R, Fink WJ, Widrick JJ. Dry-land resistance training for competitive swimming. *Med Sci Sports Exerc.* 1993; 25: 952–9.
12. Tipton MJ, Reilly TR, Iggleden C, Rees A. *Fitness and Medical Standards for Beach Lifeguards.* Report to the RNLI. Portsmouth, UK: University of Portsmouth; 2002.

PART 5

Standards

13

Medical standards for beach lifeguards

DAVID ANTON

INTRODUCTION

The key to understanding medical standards for beach lifeguards is risk management. Risk management drives whether a beach is guarded in the first place and then drives how many lifeguards, and with what skills, are deployed on a beach. Continuation of this process reveals that lifeguarding is a 'safety critical task' and dictates that the risk that lifeguards themselves pose to the safe operation of the lifeguarding system must be assessed. Questions about adequate fitness and visual acuity are dealt with in other chapters. This chapter deals with what medical standards are appropriate. Readers wanting detailed information about what standards will be applied to a particular condition are referred to (in) the references at the end of this chapter; these standards are regularly reviewed and updated by the appropriate authorities. Issues of physical disability are dealt with objectively through the application of standards of physical fitness.

STANDARDS FOR BEACH LIFEGUARDS

Beach lifeguards are an interesting occupational group; they are disproportionately young, in comparison with most occupational groups, are physically fit and are highly motivated. They work in an environment that is potentially lethal to them as well as the group that they exist to protect. The environment itself can be one of extremes, with sudden wide variation in exercise levels and temperature on transition between beach and water. Physical fitness standards alone do not guarantee fitness for the job, as a number of medical causes exist such as insulin-dependent diabetes, epilepsy and certain cardiac rhythm disorders that can suddenly incapacitate physically fit individuals. Sudden incapacitation is not the only concern. Beach lifeguards have to be capable of maintaining alertness and vigilance over prolonged periods of time, and the effects of psychological and psychiatric conditions on these abilities have to be considered. Finally, it has to be remembered that if a lifeguard is 'taken ill', it is his/her own colleague(s) that will be responsible for attending to them; illness in the lifeguard inevitably reduces cover for the beach by more than the one afflicted lifeguard.

By taking the risk management approach it becomes clear that it is, primarily, the effect of the beach lifeguard's health on public safety that is the driver for the medical standards. The application of medical standards provides a secondary benefit in terms of individual safety to the lifeguards themselves.

WHAT STANDARDS ARE APPROPRIATE?

Considerations of public safety apply to many professional occupational groups. When the UK Royal National Lifeboat Institution (RNLI) started providing a beach lifeguarding service in the early 2000s, medical standards for other, broadly comparable groups were examined, as well as standards in other countries. No national medical standards for beach lifeguards from other countries were available for review. Three occupational groups were looked at in detail: seafarers [1], commercial vehicle drivers [2] and commercial aircrew [3]. Although standards for these three groups are written around different aspects of the transport industry they have, in common with lifeguarding, the need to minimize the effects of sudden and subtle incapacitation on task performance. All three groups attempt to limit medical risk to a level of a 1%–2% risk of an incapacitating event per year. The advantage of using such comparator groups is that the medical standards are well documented, particularly so in the case of civil aviation, subject to regular peer review and nationally and/or internationally accepted. It also means that, since these comparable standards are regularly reviewed by the appropriate national and/or international bodies, by monitoring these changes and their relevance to lifeguarding, lifeguarding standards can be kept up to date without the need for the lifeguard organization to have its own specialist review panels. This system also avoids the need to write a new set of standards from scratch, as well as avoiding the need to set up an internal process to review the continuing relevance of certain standards. Clearly, where the needs of lifeguarding are demonstrably different, different standards may be applied, but guidance from comparable occupational groups can still be used. Two major differences between lifeguards and such comparator groups exist however. First, the comparator groups usually have a much larger 'older' population, and the standard setting for these groups has to take into account the effects of ageing on organ systems and how

that increases risk. Second is the availability of first aid and medical care; this is relatively rapidly available for lifeguards, albeit at the price of significantly degrading safety on the beach.

LEGAL POSITION

Other very important differences exist. Unlike many comparator groups, the medical standards for lifeguarding are not enshrined in law. Indeed, the operation within the United Kingdom of the Equality Act 2010 [4] (slightly different legislation applies in Northern Ireland and other places) means that employment decisions taken in the United Kingdom on the basis of an individual's medical state can be automatically discriminatory. It is important therefore in order to be legally defensible, in the United Kingdom at least, that decisions taken by a lifeguard 'employer' be both 'legitimate' in objective and 'proportionate' in operation. Similar legislation applies in many other jurisdictions.

PHYSICAL FITNESS, MEDICAL FITNESS AND RISK MANAGEMENT

Matters are complicated by the fact that an applicant lifeguard may be physically fit to do the job, in the sense of being able to meet the physical goals, but still be rejected medically because of an underlying medical condition. The concept of individual rights not infrequently leads to the claim that the applicant has the right to decide whether or not to shoulder the burden of risk himself. This claim, of course, ignores the concept of public safety, and the right of an individual to incur their own risk should not be allowed to override the right of the public to expect that those who are there to safeguard them are as free of avoidable risk as can reasonably be achieved. This way of thinking needs to be clearly communicated to lifeguards. A secondary benefit of using standards derived from groups with a comparable need to minimize risk is that they are freely available for all to view, and applicants can see that they are not being treated in an arbitrary way. Furthermore, where problems arise after individuals have been accepted, the comparable standards indicate mechanisms whereby the individuals can be assessed to establish continuing fitness.

Matters are further complicated when applicants are supported by their own doctors, who will normally be unaware of the complexities of the working environment, against the decision of the employer's doctor. This is a common problem in occupational medicine. Part of the difficulty lies in the fact that the evidence for some medical conditions is not that robust, and different specialists will have different views of the risk. This tends to be particularly true when a condition is episodic and unpredictable. Clearly, the fact that other 'safety critical' occupational groups use similar standards helps to remove the charge of arbitrariness from beach lifeguard medical decisions. Provided that the medical evidence has been carefully assessed and, where necessary, appealed through an appropriate mechanism, the advice of the beach lifeguard employer's doctor (who should be an accredited specialist in occupational medicine) should stand.

The adoption of a risk-based system of assessment both simplifies and complicates medical assessment. It simplifies it in the sense that the need for standards becomes obvious; it complicates it in the sense that different circumstances will result in different decisions. This possibility can give rise to perceptions of unfairness. For example, it may be that a very well controlled insulin-dependent diabetic is accommodated within a small team of lifeguards on a particular beach. A risk assessment and management plan allows for a 'safe system of work' with a small increase in managed, controlled and known risk. It will almost inevitably not be possible to accommodate a second similarly affected individual, because managing the further increase in risk impacts too much on the primary task of guarding the public. What is achievable in terms of accommodation of increased risk is also a function of budget. Budgets for beach lifeguarding are always constrained and managers have to take difficult decisions on the allocation of resources.

Further consideration of risk management makes clear that setting medical standards is only part of managing the risk. Not only must standards be set, but they must be applied and maintained. This task requires a medical system that is robust and thorough. Difficulty is encountered because of the frequently seasonal nature of lifeguarding, which leads to a surge of applicants for part-time employment just prior to the opening of the season. Management naturally wants these applications processed expeditiously and efficiently. In most cases where there are no relevant medical conditions this is not a problem, but where queries about health

exist, these need to be properly and carefully evaluated. Seasonal appointment results in some form of screen being conducted annually. For full-time lifeguard employees, routine medical review can take place at greater intervals, particularly where an occupational health department is available for sickness absence and other management referral.

A useful concept to be held in mind is that of the efficiency/thoroughness trade-off. It is very hard, and requires careful thought, not to compromise safety in the pursuit of efficiency. It should be remembered that the medical process is part of overall beach safety and, in behavioural safety terms, is just as subject to errors and violations as operations on the beach. These errors and violations must be avoided.

PARTICULAR PROBLEMS

Four areas commonly give rise to problems with new applicant and current beach lifeguards.

1. Insulin-dependent diabetes mellitus
   Insulin-dependent diabetes mellitus (IDDM) is a frequent chronic disease of childhood. La Porte et al. [5] quote a 50-fold geographic variation in the incidence of the disease ranging from 0.7 per 100,000 in Shanghai to 35.3 per 100,000 in Finland. In the United States, there is considerable racial and ethnic variation ranging from 3.3 per 100,000 in African Americans in San Diego, CA, to 20.6 per 100,000 in whites in Rochester, MN. The incidence of IDDM continues to increase worldwide.

   The particular risk is one of insulin-induced hypoglycaemia, although certain drugs used in the management of type 2 diabetes can also induce 'hypos'. The concern is not just of loss of consciousness due to hypoglycaemia, but also of the effects on cognition of the descent into hypoglycaemia. Carter et al. [6] refer to the UK Driver Vehicle Licensing Agency receiving around 300 police notifications per annum of presumed driver impairment due to this cause. IDDM is an absolute bar to flying as a commercial pilot, and the general rule for lifeguards is the same. However, there is considerable variation in how individuals exist with their illness, and there is a small group of highly motivated, extremely well controlled, physically very fit individuals who engage in water sports and

who wish to be lifeguards. The assessment of these individuals is not easy and should be conducted by an experienced occupational physician in conjunction with a consultant diabetologist. For a very thorough treatment of the issues of IDDM and safety critical employment, the reader is referred to the chapter on diabetes in the UK Maritime and Coastguard Agency *Approved Doctor's Manual: Seafarer Medical Examinations* [1]. The applicant individual will need to present thorough records of treatment and monitoring and have good hypoglycaemic awareness and understanding of their condition. Depending on the assessment, the applicant should either be assessed as unfit or issued with a waiver 'fit with restrictions' and, in the latter case, will have to enter into a dialogue with management about whether these restrictions can be safely accommodated. As previously noted, the issuing of a waiver for one individual does not indicate that this is a general position for all applicants with the same condition. There are two steps in the process. First, medically, it must be established whether this individual is potentially fit enough to work on a beach and safe enough with appropriate accommodation. Second, managerially, it must be ascertained whether the individual's requirements can be met safely within a particular beach lifeguard team.

2. Epilepsy

   Epilepsy is a disease with onset generally at the extremes of life. Neligan and Sander [7] state that the overall incidence of the disease in developed countries is around 50 per 100,000 and is higher in resource-poor countries, in the range of 100–190 cases per 100,000. Epilepsy is defined as a tendency towards recurrent, unprovoked seizures, and an individual must experience at least two seizures to qualify for the diagnosis. A history of seizure requires very careful evaluation as the diagnosis is not uncommonly inaccurate, although loss of consciousness for whatever reason will make an individual unfit to be a beach lifeguard without further investigation. Once made, the diagnosis disqualifies the individual from all classes of medical certification as a commercial pilot. For both seafarers and heavy goods and public service vehicle drivers, licensing is only

considered if the applicant has been fit-free, off anticonvulsant medication, for a period of 10 years. Similar standards are applied to beach lifeguards.

The single seizure is treated slightly differently. A history of a single seizure makes an applicant or current beach lifeguard unfit pending further investigation. In the absence of an identified cause, where any period of disqualification will depend on the cause identified, the lifeguard will remain unfit for a period of four years. If after this period they have been seizure- and medication-free, they can be reconsidered for work as a beach lifeguard as their risk of a seizure approximates that of the population at large.

3. Mental disorders, alcohol and substance abuse

   Mental disorders, alcohol and substance abuse all have adverse effects on personal performance through changes to perception, cognition, mood, risk-taking and thought processes. Fitness determinations are made difficult by the fact that these conditions exist over a wide spectrum of severity, which can vary with time, and sufferers commonly have a different view of the potential impact of their condition to the examining doctor. These difficulties are compounded by the lack of simple objective tools to assess impairment.

   Certain principles can be applied. Evidence of 'cure' is only achievable by observation of normal function over time when the applicant is off both medication and out of therapy. Periods of time for demonstration of normal function will typically vary between one year for relatively mild cases of mood disorder through to a minimum of five years for psychotic illness. Substance abusers will typically need to demonstrate that they have been 'clean' or 'dry' for a period of time within these bounds.

4. Post-traumatic stress and post-traumatic stress disorder

   This is something of a special case, as these are conditions that arise in healthy individuals. Lifeguards can be witness to, and indeed participants in, very traumatic events. Normally, individuals will cope well with these events and will require no intervention.

In the United Kingdom, the National Institute for Health and Care Excellence Guidelines [8,9] specifically note that 'the systematic provision to an individual alone of brief, single session interventions (often referred to as debriefing) that focus on the traumatic event, should *not* be routine practice'. Where individuals have mild symptoms, a period of watchful waiting for four weeks after the event is appropriate and these individuals can be allowed to remain at work. A follow-up contact by a professional with experience in trauma illness should occur around the four-week point. Individuals with more persistent or severe symptoms will usually need to be removed from work and referred either for trauma-focused cognitive behavioural therapy or eye movement desensitisation and reprocessing. Individuals will need careful assessment and regular monitoring after such therapy before they can return to the beach.

CONCLUSION

Medical standards for beach lifeguards ultimately derive from a process of risk assessment. A range of standards exist for broadly comparable occupational groups, particularly in the transport industry. Such standards have the further benefit of being internationally comparable or, in some cases, internationally agreed.

REFERENCES

1. *Approved Doctor's Manual, Seafarer Medical Examinations*. Maritime and Coastguard Agency, UK Government. Available at www.gov.uk/government/uploads/system/uploads/attachment_data/file/285747/mca_doctors_manual_links.pdf
2. Driver & Vehicle Licensing Agency. *"At a Glance Guide to the Current Medical Standards of Fitness to Drive" for Medical Practitioners*. Swansea, United Kingdom: Drivers Medical Group, DVLA.
3. Manual of Civil Aviation Medicine, International Civil Aviation Organisation, Doc 8984. ISBN 978-92-9231-959-5. 3rd ed., 2012. Available at www.icao.int/publications/Documents/8984_cons_en.pdf
4. Equality Act 2010, UK HMSO.
5. La Porte, R.E., Matsushima, M., and Chang, Y.-F. *Diabetes in America*, 2nd ed. National Diabetes Data Group, National Institute of Diabetes and Digestive and Kidney Diseases, National Institute of Health, NIH Publication No. 95-1468, 1995. Available at www.diabetes/niddk.nih.gov/dm/pubs/America/pdf/chapter3.pdf
6. Carter, T., Major, H.G., Evans, S.A., and Colvin, A.P. Chapter 28. In Palmer, K.T., Brown, I., and Hobson, J. (eds.). *Fitness for Work*. Health and transport safety: fitness to drive. 5th ed. Oxford University Press; 2013, pp. 564–571.
7. Neligan, A., and Sander, J.W. In Rugg-Gunn, F.J., and Smalls, J.E. (eds.). *Epilepsy 2013 from Membranes to Mankind: A Practical Guide to Epilepsy*. The Incidence and prevalence of Epilepsy. The Epilepsy Society; Chalfont St. Peter, UK; 2013, pp. 331–42.
8. National Institute of Health and Care Excellence. *Post-Traumatic Stress Disorder (PTSD): The Management of PTSD in Adults and Children in Primary and Secondary Care*. NICE Guidelines [CG26]. London: NIHCE; 2005.
9. National Institute of Health and Care Excellence. *Post-Traumatic Stress Disorder (PTSD)*. Evidence Update 49. NIHCE. Manchester, UK; 2013.

14

Eyesight standards for beach lifeguards

POLONA JAKI AND MIKE TIPTON

INTRODUCTION

This chapter reviews the requirements for beach lifeguards' eyesight. This includes not only visual acuity but also many often hotly debated issues such as colour blindness and the use of sunglasses, swimming goggles and contact lenses. Where advice can be based on scientific evidence, this evidence is presented; where this cannot be done, a recommendation is based on clinical experience.

VISUAL ACUITY

There is no universally accepted standard for beach lifeguard eyesight; different agencies have adopted alternative requirements and tests. In 2011, the US Lifeguard Standards Coalition published an evidence-based review and report on US lifeguard standards: 22 relevant literature sources were identified. The studies with the highest level of evidence included one that looked specifically at developing visual acuity standards in lifeguarding [1], and another that examined the same but pertaining specifically to beach lifeguards [2]. The coalition concluded that further research was needed to determine if corrective devices (contact lenses and glasses) are acceptable for use in a lifeguarding setting. There was enough evidence to recommend that there should be validated minimum visual

acuity standards for lifeguarding, but not enough evidence to propose such a standard. Each facility was encouraged to require testing of corrected and uncorrected vision and then to develop appropriate standards for their venues.

As the above information suggests, the international picture is mixed. For example, the vision requirements for bay and ocean lifeguards in the city of San Diego, California, include uncorrected vision no worse than 20/40 (see text below for explanation of these figures) in both eyes together with 'acceptable' colour vision. Vision between 20/20 and 20/40 in both eyes together must be corrected to 20/20 both eyes together with glasses or contact lenses. Monocular vision is not acceptable. Those who have undergone any type of refractive vision surgery such as laser-assisted *in situ* keratomileusis (LASIK), radial keratotomy or photo refractive keratectomy a year or longer prior to being medically considered for a lifeguard position must be substantially free of vision problems such as impaired vision at night or under dim lighting conditions; sensitivity to glare; starbursts experienced around light sources such as street lights or headlights, hazing or blurring of vision, eye irritation and pain, progressive regression of visual acuity and daily changes in visual acuity (http://agency.governmentjobs.com/sandiego/job_bulletin.cfm?JobID=334906, 2013). In the United Kingdom, the Royal National Lifeboat

Institution (RNLI) allows beach lifeguards to wear glasses on the beach, provided lifeguards meet the RNLI's eyesight standard of 6/24, 6/36 (correcting to 6/6, 6/12). A new applicant who wears glasses or contact lenses or who has had eye surgery is asked to see an optician for a sight test and is not passed medically fit until this is confirmed.

It has been recommended that there should be a corrected and uncorrected visual acuity (distance and near) for each eye at least every two years. Other considerations for a vision standard have been recommended to include peripheral vision, colour vision, depth prescription, contrast sensitivity, LASIK surgery, the influence of brightness, visual perception, visual memory and contact lenses. It is further recommended that lifeguard agencies, the US Lifeguard Association and International Life Saving Federation require all lifeguards to wear polarized sunglasses with ultraviolet protection and institute a well-researched vision policy (Art Clarke, OD, NJ State Park Service, Water Safety Supervisor, http://www.slideshare.net/ILS/03-25-ppt-arthur-clarke-vision-standards). We consider these issues and present relevant research in the remainder of this chapter.

It is accepted that the majority of the surveillance demands of beach lifeguards are within 100 m of the shore and that those bathers going further out to sea can usually be tracked as they go. Nevertheless, it is possible that individuals could find themselves further out to sea without having been tracked from the shore (e.g. a man overboard from a passing boat, fast rip or when lifeguards are distracted by another incident). It therefore seems reasonable that if beach lifeguards have accepted responsibility for supervising up to, for example, 300 m out to sea, that they should have sufficient visual acuity to function up to these distances.

It can be calculated that to see a 25 cm diameter head at 300 m should require a visual acuity of 6/17. To discriminate the features of a head at this distance is likely to require 6/3, beyond the capability of most individuals. However, it is important to consider the use of binoculars: a beach lifeguard must be able to locate/detect something in the water with the naked eye as a cue to instigating further investigation with binoculars (beach lifeguards do not normally scan using binoculars). Some organizations have an eyesight standard for beach lifeguards that require acuity to be, at worst, 6/12 in one eye,

uncorrected. The use of correction in the form of spectacles is usually not recommended due to the consequent restriction of the visual field and the ease with which they could be lost or damaged when removed during an emergency.

The standard measure for determining the quality of central vision is to measure visual acuity.* This property is measured as angular resolution, where two closely spaced dots can still be recognized separately (also known as 'minimum separable') until the angle between them, measured from the eye, becomes too small to detect. However, in tasks such as seeing people in need of rescue in the water, it is not only this visual property that is critical for success. Some other functions of central vision also come into play, for example 'minimum cognizable' – the ability to recognize the object – which primarily depends on experience in given circumstances, and 'looming detectors' – the ability to judge if some object is approaching or drifting away slowly, when this occurs beyond the stereoscopic vision domain.

The most commonly used, rapid, simple and economical test of visual acuity is the optotype or chart test. One such test is the Snellen chart (rows of letters of decreasing font size [3]); other optotype alternatives include the Landolt C, Sloan, BSI (British Standard Institution) and E charts. The standard definition of visual acuity is the ability of the eye to resolve a spatial pattern separated by a visual angle of one minute of arc. With the Snellen chart, normal visual acuity is recorded as 20/20 (feet) or 6/6 (metres) using a diffusely illuminated chart without glare. This means that at 6 m the test subject should be able to see the same as a 'normal' person with good eyesight. A score of 6/12 means

---

* *Myopia* is short-sightedness: Light from a distant object forms an image before it reaches the retina (the eye is too long, or the cornea or crystalline lens is too strong). This condition results in clear vision when looking at close objects but distant objects appear blurred. A concave lens (minus-powered) is placed in front of the eye to move the image back to the retina. *Hypermetropia* is long-sightedness: The image of a nearby object is formed behind the retina (the eye is too short, or the cornea or crystalline lens does not refract the light enough). This condition results in blurred vision when looking at close objects and clearer vision when looking at distant objects. A convex (plus-powered) lens is placed in front of the eye, moving the image forward to focus on the retina.

that a test subject can see the same at 6 m as a 'normal' person with good eyesight can see at 12 m. The maximum acuity of the human eye without visual aids is generally thought to be about 6/4. The Snellen fraction may also be expressed as a decimal, where 6/6 =1; 6/12 = 0.5.

An alternative method for assessing visual acuity is to record the minimum angle of resolution (MAR). The MAR relates to the resolution required to resolve the elements of a letter. Thus, 6/6 equates to a MAR of one minute of arc, 6/12 equates to two minutes of arc and so on. LogMAR is the $\log_{10}$ of the MAR.

The Snellen chart has one letter on the first row, two on the second and so on down to eight, after which the number remains the same but the size diminishes (Table 14.1). Problems with the number and spacing of letters on this chart have led to various attempts to improve it and one chart, designed by Bailey and Lovie [4], has emerged

as the test of choice in vision research. This chart overcomes many of the shortcomings of the Snellen chart by having five letters on each line, with the spacing between each letter and each row related to the width and height of the letters, respectively. Each row is thus a scaled-down version of the row above, so the task remains the same as the test subject reads down the chart. The progression of the letter sizes is uniform, increasing in a constant ratio of 1.26 (0.1 log unit steps) from the bottom to the top of the chart. The result is usually recorded as a logMAR score. As letter size changes in units of 0.1 logMAR units per row, each letter can be assigned a score of 0.02 (five letters per row); thus 0.02 is added for each letter incorrectly read and, as such, the final logMAR score takes account of every letter read correctly. Visual acuity obtained with standard adult logMAR acuity tests is greater at low acuity levels than for acuity scores within the normal range.

Both the Snellen and logMAR [Bailey–Lovie or Early Treatment Diabetic Retinopathy Study (ETDRS)] charts measure just one aspect of visual capability: the ability to resolve small high-contrast letters (Figure 14.1). While this relates well to the ability to read text, it may correlate less well to the ability to see a person in difficulty in the water; this task involves the ability to locate/detect dynamic objects of various sizes in a range of contrasts. Additionally, a person with 6/6 (logMAR 0) vision does not necessarily have 'perfect' vision; again, these scores simply indicate the ability to resolve static images from distance.

Table 14.1 The relationship between the different acuity scales

Snellen	Decimal	MAR	LogMAR
6/60	0.10	10	1.000
6/24	0.25	4	0.602
6/12	0.50	2	0.301
6/6	1.00	1	0.000
6/4	1.50	0.667	–0.176

Note: To convert logMAR to Snellen: Inverse log × 6. MAR, minimum angle of resolution.

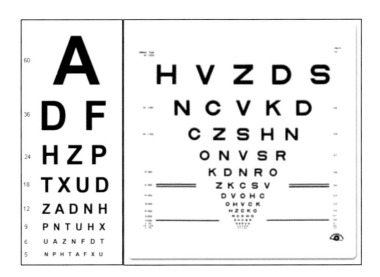

Figure 14.1 Optotypes for detecting visual acuity: Snellen (left) and ETDRS (right) charts.

Tipton et al. [2] attempted to determine, in an operational scenario, the visual acuity required by beach lifeguards in order to identify a human head at 300 m. The authors hypothesized that this would be better than that calculated (6/17) due to factors associated with location/detection, colour, contrast, lighting and movement in the operational scenario.

Prior to the experiment, 21 (16 males, 5 females, all under 35 years) volunteer beach lifeguards underwent a range of tests to ensure normal vision (mean [range] visual acuity 6/4.8 [6/3.8–6/5]). They then undertook a series of tests on two beaches in the United Kingdom, during which their vision was blurred (using spherical lenses placed within a trial frame; Figure 14.2) to a visual acuity at which they could not identify the targets presented to them (approximately 6/70). These targets were human heads or equivalent sized buoys. The participants looked out to calm seas or across a wet beach, and their visual acuity was improved every minute by reducing the refractive blur in 0.25 dioptre increments until they could identify the target to the point at which they would investigate it further using binoculars. The tests were performed on the same day, in good weather, with uniform lighting conditions and a sea state of 0–1 (calm). The results are presented in Table 14.2.

The variability between participants was probably due to the differing ability of individuals to adjust to the lenses and the central processing

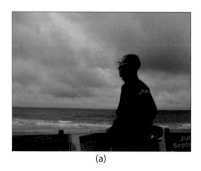
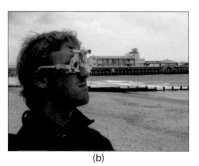

(a)   (b)

Figure 14.2 (a) Participant looking for a head-out immersed human at 300 m. (b) Ophthalmic trial frames for altering visual acuity.

Table 14.2 Results of tests to determine the visual acuity necessary to identify different objects in beach scenes at two beaches

Condition	LogMAR mean (SD)	Snellen
(i) B: locate and identify a human head within a 300 m radius out to sea (volunteer immersed to neck)	0.11 (0.06)	6/8
(i) W: locate and identify a human head within a 300 m radius out to sea (volunteer immersed to neck)	0.06 (0.17)	6/7
(ii) B: identify an arm waving at 300 m in the sea (volunteer immersed to neck)	0.33 (0.16)	6/13
(iii) B: identify a human immersed to the waist at 300 m in the sea	0.74 (0.15)	6/33
(iv) B: locate and identify a human head within a 100 m radius out to sea (volunteer immersed to neck)	0.86 (0.23)	6/43
(ii) W: identify a buoy at 200 m out to sea (n = 8)	0.28 (0.18)	6/11
(iii) W: identify a buoy at 100 m out to sea (n = 8)	0.78 (0.25)	6/36
(iv) W: identify a buoy on the wet beach at 300 m	0.23 (0.19)	6/10
(v) W: identify a buoy on the wet beach at 200 m	0.48 (0.13)	6/18
(vi) W: identify a buoy on the wet beach at 100 m	0.87 (0.15)	6/44

Note: n = 21 unless stated otherwise; B = Bournemouth Beach, UK (dry sand); W = Weston Beach, UK (wet sand).

required to search, see and identify a head in the sea. This also explains why the measured visual acuity required to see a human head at 300 m in the sea was 6/7, rather than the theoretical figure of 6/17.

As a consequence of these tests, it was recommended that a beach lifeguard should have binocular visual acuity of 6/7 or better. As this would exclude some individuals, the authors suggested that consideration could be given to allowing beach lifeguards to wear glasses. It seemed logical to base the requirement for uncorrected eyesight on what the beach lifeguard must see when they have removed their glasses and are moving towards a casualty; by this time the beach lifeguard will have detected the casualty. As the visual acuity required to maintain sight of a casualty is less than that required to locate/detect them in the first place, it was suggested that it would be reasonable to require a beach lifeguard to have uncorrected vision, in their worst eye, that is at least equivalent to that required to see a head from a 200–300 m distance, or an arm waving from 300 m. The average for these activities is 6/14.

In terms of the Snellen chart, the process is simplified if the levels of visual acuity, determined in the study of Tipton et al. [2], are translated into values that can be easily and accurately assessed by an optometrist. Thus, it was recommended that the corrected vision for beach lifeguards should be 6/7 tested to 6/9 in the best eye, and 6/14 tested to 6/18 in the worst eye. The unaided acuity should be no worse than 6/18 in either eye.

Those with 6/6 vision may suffer from other visual problems such as colour blindness, reduced contrast or difficulty tracking moving objects. Additional eyesight tests and other factors associated with the vision of beach lifeguards are considered below. A separate chapter deals with surveillance. The information presented below was obtained from questionnaire studies, reviews of the literature and discussions with those suitably qualified or experienced in ophthalmology, physiology, medicine, vigilance and signal detection.

USE OF SWIMMING GOGGLES DURING RESCUES

No studies examining the use of swimming goggles during beach rescues could be found in the literature. The following benefits and possible disadvantages were identified.

Benefits

- Reduce the chance of seawater contacting, and thus irritating, the surface of the eye (cornea and conjunctiva).
- If they function correctly, goggles will improve vision underwater.

Disadvantages

- May erroneously be considered to improve surface vision during swimming.
- Reduce visual acuity at the surface of the sea. Swimming goggles are normally made of polycarbonate, which does not have very good optical properties, and thus visual acuity is impaired as a result.
- Reduced visual field. Swimming goggles normally have small viewing lenses and are encapsulated in rubber or other material. As a consequence peripheral vision is reduced.
- Distortion of depth perception. The viewing lenses of swimming goggles are not normally aligned, which might lead to impaired stereopsis, and thus distort stereopsis.
- Swimming goggles do not always prevent water entry and thus cannot be considered a method of preventing the risk of losing contact lenses. Flooded goggles are worse than no goggles as vision is then impaired above the water.
- An immersion victim who is struggling may disturb the goggles, causing them to flood.
- In the event that the rescuer must dive underwater to reach the victim, the air compartment within the swimming goggles cannot be equalized; this may cause rupture of the small blood vessels in the eye surface depending on depth.
- There are logistic and ergonomic difficulties associated with the use of swimming goggles. They would have to be put on at the time of an emergency. They can only be adjusted when actually in the water, as this is when it will become apparent that they are leaking; this adjustment will take time.

RECOMMENDATION

Beach lifeguards should not use swimming goggles during rescues. This being the case, it would be wise for them to train and be assessed without goggles.

TESTS OF OBSERVATIONAL CAPABILITY OF LIFEGUARDS

The following tests were considered; they may be repeated annually:

Visual acuity: Distant (and near vision)

See above 'Visual acuity' section.

'Near vision' is the vision for objects 2 feet or closer to the viewer (within an arm's distance from the body). The purpose in testing near vision is to determine how people can cope with near tasks, such as reading the first aid kit instructions.

TEST

The test chart is held at the distance preferred by a person. The test is performed with spectacles on if they are normally used. The smallest size able to be read correctly is recorded.

The use of glasses could be considered while on duty surveying the sea. However their use with sunglasses can be problematic; they restrict the visual field and they are easily lost or damaged during an emergency when they would have to be removed. Prescription sunglasses could be allowed, but the lifeguard would normally be required to provide these, and they should make sure that they have a spare pair. Prescription sunglasses should meet all of the criteria described in the section 'Use of sunglasses' below.

Contact lenses could be allowed, as they are less likely to demonstrate any of the above disadvantages. It is probable that the advantages (recruitment, visual acuity, observational ability) of allowing lifeguards to use contact lenses outweigh the potential disadvantages associated with their use (may get displaced during an emergency). Disposable contact lenses are recommended for reasons of hygiene, resistance to infection and cost if lost. Orthokeratology (ortho-K) lens wear modality (aka corneal refractive therapy) can also be considered as an option for beach lifeguards, as these lenses are worn overnight and preserve the corrective effect during the following day, when not in place. However, they are only suitable for correcting moderate amounts of myopia and astigmatism.

RECOMMENDATION

Consideration could be given to allowing beach lifeguards to wear glasses while surveying the sea.

Contact lenses (preferably disposable) or ortho-K–wearing modality could be permitted.

Contrast sensitivity

Contrast sensitivity function (CSF) is a property of a healthy retina, which is able to enhance contrast areas in the visual field by 'lateral inhibition' – a *within-retina* process of horizontal signal coding. It is considered an important property of visual function, as objects in real life do not usually appear in full contrast, but in subtle shades of different tints. In poor lighting conditions, CSF is believed to play a more important role for visual acuity in most real-life visual tasks.

Good contrast sensitivity is maintained as long as the optical media stay regular and clear. In subjects with healthy eyes and near to normal visual acuity, the CSF is expected to be normal. However, lifeguards who have the start of cataracts or opacities in their corneas, who have undergone any refractive surgery procedure (especially LASIK or LASEK laser surgery or implantation of implantable contact lens) or who have had their cataracts removed may have poor contrast vision despite good visual acuity. This happens due to irregular or, sometimes, hazed optical media.

TEST

Contrast sensitivity tests incorporate a variety of targets presented in different shades of grey. These targets can either be letters or stripes of varying width. Contrast sensitivity determines the lowest contrast level which can be detected by a person for a given size target. Examples of such tests are Regan charts, Ginsburg's sine wave grating patterns and the Pelli–Robson letter sensitivity chart (Figure 14.3).

Contrast sensitivity is presented as a curve, which plots the lowest contrast level a patient can detect for a specific size target. The *x*-axis of the curve is for spatial frequency, while the *y*-axis is for contrast sensitivity. Low spatial frequencies are thick gratings and high spatial frequencies are thin gratings. Contrast sensitivity is the inverse of contrast level. The higher the contrast sensitivity, the lower the contrast level at which a person can detect a target.

RECOMMENDATION

A test for contrast sensitivity is not necessary if lifeguards have 6/12 acuity as a minimum, but it

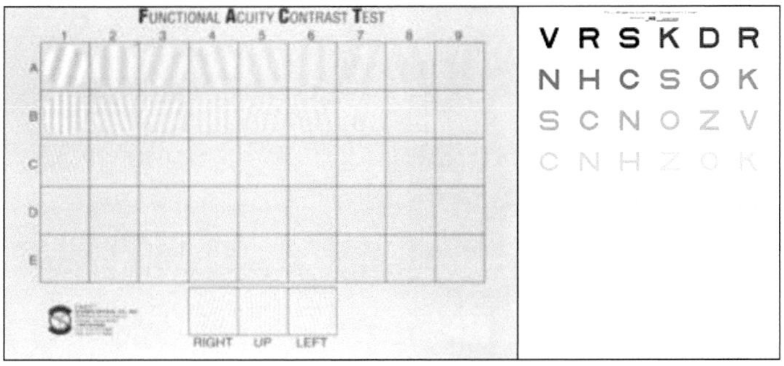

Figure 14.3 Ginsburg's functional acuity contrast test (left) and Pelli–Robson letter sensitivity chart (right) for measurement of visual contrast sensitivity.

should be performed if an individual has undergone any refractive surgery procedure, including cataract removal.

Visual field (peripheral and central)

Visual field is the entire area that can be seen when the eye is directed forward, including that which is seen within the peripheral vision.

TEST

The monocular confrontation field test (mainly for outer limits and larger scotomas) is used in combination with either the Amsler grid test (for the central 10 degrees) or perimetry.

The monocular confrontation field test is a test evaluating mainly the outer limits of the visual field and the presence of larger scotomas. It is performed by having the subject sit facing the investigator at a distance of 60 cm. When the test is performed for the left eye, the subject should cover his right eye with his right hand and look at the investigator's left eye. When performing the test on the right eye, the left eye is covered with the left hand, and the subject looks at the investigator's right eye. The investigator extends his hand and moves his index finger from the outer limits of the subject's visual field inwards, maintaining a distance of 30 cm between his hand and the subject. The subject is requested to inform the investigator as soon as he sees the investigator's finger in his visual field. Throughout the examination the subject should keep his gaze on the investigator's eye (and not on the moving finger). The investigator continues moving his fingers across the visual field until the subject no longer sees them. This procedure is repeated in the horizontal, vertical and diagonal planes. In this manner,

the temporal, nasal, upper and lower limits of the visual field are defined. The subject should also be requested to note if, at any stage, he ceases to see the fingers (i.e. they suddenly disappear for a brief moment during the passage through the visual field); this reflects the presence of larger scotomas.

The Amsler grid test for the central 10 degrees of visual field uses the Amsler recording chart. This chart consists of a grid of black lines on a white background. The chart is 10 cm × 10 cm, with the grid comprising 0.5 cm squares. The subject is requested to look at a black dot drawn in the centre of the grid at a distance of 30 cm. While conducting the test, the subject wears near correction, and one eye is occluded. The subject is requested to indicate whether any parts of the grid are blurred or distorted in any way. In addition, the subject is requested to mark with a pen the position of these abnormalities on the chart. In this manner, the test detects any abnormalities in the central 10 degrees of field of vision.

Perimetry: For accurate assessment of the visual field an apparatus called a perimeter is used (Figure 14.4). The subject is seated at the device with one eye covered and the chin resting on a chin rest. The subject is requested to keep his gaze on a central target of the perimeter. Current automated perimeters continuously assess the subject's gaze with a video monitor. The subject is requested to signal immediately each time he sees the target. In this manner, the entire field of vision is mapped out. The normal monocular visual field extends approximately 100 degrees to the temporal (outer) side, 60 degrees to the nasal and inferior sides and 50 degrees to the superior side from the central point (cross of the horizontal and vertical meridian). It has no scotoma (depressed vision) except that caused by a blind spot.

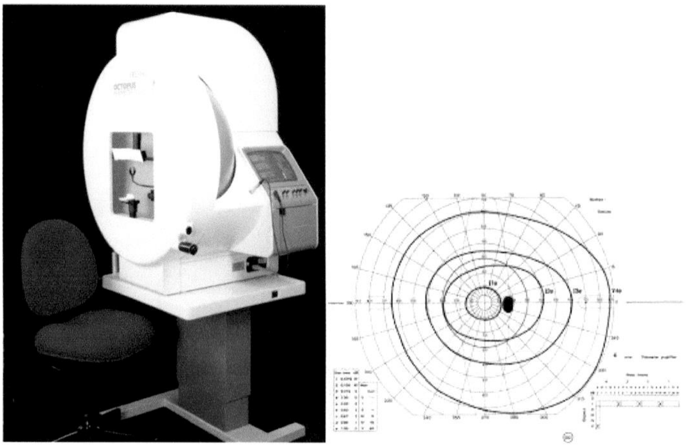

Figure 14.4 Perimeter test equipment and visual field of the right eye.

RECOMMENDATION

The visual field should be tested; this test identifies scotomas in the visual field as well as the early signs of chorioretinal or optic nerve disease.

Depth perception test

Depth perception can be tested simply by having the patient place the end of one finger to the tip of the examiner's finger coming in horizontally end to end. More refined testing is done using the Titmus test (viewing a large fly, four-circle sets and animal figures with 3D glasses). Good quality of stereopsis is a hallmark of good binocular visual function.

RECOMMENDATION

The test is desirable but not necessary.

Colour vision [5] test

Polychromatic Ishihara plates are used to detect red–green deficiencies and Hardy-Rand–Rittler plates are used to identify blue–yellow colour deficiencies.

RECOMMENDATION

Colour vision, and testing for it, is desirable but not necessary.

The tests recommended above, if adopted, should be undertaken every year before the start of the season.

USE OF SUNGLASSES

It is widely accepted that solar radiation, particularly UV radiation, can damage the eyes and sunglasses are recommended to provide protection against ocular tissue damage.

Sunglasses are essentially optical filters; they should be capable of filtering ultraviolet radiation, as well as visible blue light (glare). The former is necessary to reduce the detrimental effect on the intraocular lens and retina, and the latter to reduce the detrimental effect of blue light on the retina. The displacement of the cut-off margin towards the red end of the colour spectrum results in both enhanced contrast sensitivity and attenuated colour vision.

There are three forms of sun glare:

- Disability glare: This arises from light in the eye not forming part of the retinal image. It is caused by scattering of light in the media of the eye or other extraocular media (e.g. sunglasses). It can also be caused by fluorescence of the crystalline lens, which dilutes the contrast of the focused image and makes objects less visible. Tinted lenses cannot control disability glare because a lens that attenuates the scattered light will attenuate the image in the same proportion. Disability glare due to fluorescence of the crystalline lens can be reduced by UV-absorbing spectacles, sunglasses or contact lenses, especially those that absorb wavelengths in the range 340–360 nm.

- Reflected glare: This is caused by specular reflection from a reflective surface such as water. Reflected glare most frequently arises from horizontal surfaces (e.g. the surface of the sea) and polarized lenses in sunglasses are orientated to take account of this.
- Discomfort glare: This is the sensation of pain or discomfort from bright light sources in the visual field. Sunglasses can reduce discomfort glare, even if they cannot reduce disability glare, other than that caused by lens fluorescence.

Thus, sunglasses should accomplish the following:

- Reduce visible light sufficiently to diminish discomfort glare
- Have polarizing lenses when reflected glare from horizontal surfaces (e.g. the sea) must be attenuated
- Substantially reduce the UV dose to the cornea and lens

Sunglasses should not introduce secondary hazards by impeding vision or by being constructed from easily broken materials. Small lenses, no matter how good, will allow UV light to reach the eye. Lenses should be optically regular and a focal to maintain visual acuity and comfort. Lens transparency should be as good as prescription lenses and should not be hazy or fluorescing as this will impair vision, reduce contrast and increase disability glare. Coloured lenses can have a dramatic effect on the detection and recognition of colours. The ability to see a colour depends on the sunglass lens transmitting sufficient light in the bandpass of wavelengths emitted by the coloured signal, for the visual threshold to be exceeded. Grey tint ('neutral density filter') allows colours to appear more realistic; brown tint distorts colour perception but increases contrast, acuity and depth perception [6–12]. For best colour perception, Prevent Blindness America recommend lenses that are neutral grey, amber or brown. This organization also recommends that people who wear contact lenses that offer UV protection should still wear sunglasses.

There are no definitive studies on the ideal cut-off wavelengths for humans without some sort of eye pathology. Thus, it is difficult to make a firm recommendation about the ideal cut-off wavelength and allow a choice of sunglasses based on optimal contrast sensitivity and colour vision. Most studies suggest a cut-off wavelength of 450 nm. To minimize glare (an advantage for lifeguards looking out to sea) the cut-off wavelength could be raised to 480 nm.

Another important characteristic of sunglasses which needs to be considered is their ability to transmit light. Their transmittance should be such that only frequencies that are not detrimental to the eyes and vision are allowed to penetrate. Thus, in addition to filtering unwanted frequencies, sunglasses should also reduce the percentage of the light they allow to penetrate. Transmittance is defined in terms of percentage of the total light available after filtration. Again, there are no extensive or specific studies on this topic relevant to beach lifeguarding. From one study conducted on US Army sunglasses, it would appear that a sunglass transmittance of 23% results in a minimal decrease in visual performance relative to normal clinical test conditions.

RECOMMENDATION

The sunglasses used by beach lifeguards should have a cut-off wavelength of 480 nm, transmittance should be about 23% and the glasses should reduce the visual field as little as possible.

USE OF BINOCULARS

There is only one main disadvantage of binoculars: they reduce the visual field.

Compensation of vision:

- Visual anomalies are either spherical or astigmatic by nature. Spherical anomalies refer to situations where light entering the eye is refracted equally at all angles. However, this refraction is either too large or too small and results in impaired vision. Astigmatic anomalies refer to situations where the light entering the eye is not refracted equally at all angles. In this case, the eye has different refractive powers in two meridians, which are normally perpendicular to each other [13].
- Spherical anomalies are corrected with spherical lenses and astigmatism anomalies with

cylindrical lenses. Since binoculars incorporate spherical lenses, they can compensate for spherical but not astigmatic anomalies. Thus, astigmatism, which is a cylindrical anomaly, cannot be compensated for with binoculars.

- If visual acuity of 6/18 in the worst eye is acceptable, it is redundant to discuss the ability of binoculars to compensate for reductions in visual acuity because of possible astigmatic underlying causes. If the criterion were much more conservative (6/6), then compensation with binoculars would be more meaningful.

REFERENCES

1. Seiller B. Sunglasses: Lifeguard vision project; Behind the ongoing programme to test the vision of lifeguard candidates. *Parks and Recreation*, 1997. Available at http://findarticles.com/p/articles/mi_m1145/is_n2_v32/ai_19203762/?tag=content;col1

2. Tipton MJ, Reilly T, Scarpello E, McGill J. Visual acuity standards for beach lifeguards. *Br J Ophthalmol.* 2007; 91(11): 1570–1.

3. Currie Z, Bhan A, Pepper I. Reliability of Snellen charts for testing visual acuity for driving: Prospective study and postal questionnaire. *Br Med J.* 2000; 321: 990–2.

4. Bailey IL, Lovie JE. New design principles for visual acuity letter charts. *Am J Optom Physiol Opt.* 1976; 53: 740.

5. Donderi DC. Visual acuity, color vision and visual search performance at sea. *Hum Factors.* 1994; 36: 129–44.

6. Dain SJ. Sunglasses and sunglass standards. *Clin Exp Optom.* 2003; 86(2): 77–90.

7. de Fez MD, Luque MJ, Viqueira V. Enhancement of contrast sensitivity and losses of chromatic discrimination with tinted lenses. *Optom Vis Sci.* 2002; 79: 590–7.

8. Kelly SA, Goldberg SE, Banton TA. Effects of yellow tinted lenses on contrast sensitivity. *Am J Optom Physiol Opt.* 1984; 61: 657–62.

9. Lee JE, Stein JJ, Prevor MB, Seiple WH, Hlopigian K, Greenstein VC, Stenson SM. Effect of variable tinted spectacle lenses on visual performance in control subjects. *CLAO J.* 2002; 28: 80–2.

10. Rabin JC, Wiley RW, Levine RR, Wicks JP, Rivers AG. U.S. Army sunglasses: Issues and solutions. *J Am Optom Assoc.* 1996; 67: 215–22.

11. Wolffsohn JS, Cochrane AL, Khoo H, Yoshimitsu Y, Wu S. Contract is enhanced by yellow lenses because of selective reduction of short-wavelength light. *Optom Vis Sci.* 2000; 77: 73–81.

12. Clarke A. Eye health and vision standards for lifeguards. *Proceedings of the US Lifesaving Association meeting on Eye Health & Vision Standards*, Philadelphia, 2001.

13. Clare G, Pitts JA, Edgington K, Alan BD. From beach lifeguard to astronaut: Occupational vision standards and the implications of refractive surgery. *Br J Ophthalmol.* 2009; 94: 400–5.

15

Occupational fitness and strength standards for beach lifeguarding

TARA REILLY AND MIKE TIPTON

INTRODUCTION

Historically, physical employment standards (PES), including those for beach lifeguards (BLGs), were not based on scientific evidence. Occupations with a physical component were often linked to height and weight standards, age or gender, with the assumption that these identifiers were indicative of the ability to perform physical tasks. Over time these assumptions have been challenged; in 1971 the New York City Department of Parks and Recreation was not able to defend why Candy Callery, a female BLG applicant, was denied employment as a lifeguard because of her failure to meet the minimum height and weight requirements (at least 5'7" and 61.2 kg [135 lbs]) [1]. Without doubt, anthropometry can be linked to the ability to perform heavy lifting tasks [2]. In fact, the ability to cross-chest tow an unconscious victim 100 m in 6 minutes has been linked to deltoid circumference [3]. Michniewicz et al. [4] indicate that heavy, muscular victims with a large chest circumference are difficult to encircle and hold by a lifeguard. However, as most physically demanding tasks within an occupation are trainable, it is no longer acceptable to discriminate based on weight or height, and task-related standards should be independent of age or gender [5]. Often those who are smaller will adapt to find ways to safely and successfully accomplish a task.

Establishing occupational fitness standards does involve some degree of subjectivity; the standard is generally based on the physical and physiological components of individual tasks that are considered to be criteria, *generic* and *critical* or *essential* to the safe and successful completion of a job [5]. Different occupations and research institutions use varying criteria for the determination of what constitutes a critical task. Some use the most demanding, frequently occurring tasks, while some identify tasks which, if a minimum standard is not achieved, result in a threat to the safety and well-being of the public, co-workers or the individual [5,6]. After the tasks are identified and a task analysis is performed, there must be agreement on an acceptable minimum level of performance on the critical tasks. This is often not a simple decision and has significant consequences, because such decisions will determine what is required in terms of performance for a pass on the PES.

IDENTIFYING THE CRITICAL TASKS

In the context of developing an occupational fitness standard, task analysis is most frequently used to identify tasks that are physically demanding in nature and representative of those components of a job that are considered to be the most essential or critical [7–10]. The elements of a task analysis are determined through both objective and subjective analysis and require the importance, difficulty, intensity, duration and frequency of the task being considered to be identified and quantified [7,8,11–16].

Objective measurement involves measuring the physical demands of tasks and the physiological responses and capacities required to undertake them at an agreed intensity. Subjective analysis involves the gathering of perceptual data of current and experienced employees and subject-matter experts within the field. This can be achieved through interview, survey and questionnaire or a combination of all three [7,9,10,13,15,17–21]. On the basis of structured interviews with 91 BLG (male and female) from every region operated by the RNLI in the United Kingdom, the most demanding physical tasks undertaken by UK BLG were identified as towing a casualty at sea, paddling with a casualty on the rescue board and casualty handling [3]. The physical demand of these tasks was then assessed in the lab, on the beach and at sea [3].

Similar methods were used in the UK to establish the physical demands of operating an inshore rescue boat (IRB) or rescue watercraft (RWC) [22]. Experienced BLG indicated that the most demanding tasks associated with the IRB included lifting the trailer to launch the IRB, pulling the IRB off of the trailer, pulling and lifting the IRB, pulling and lifting the trailer and dragging the IRB on the beach to launch it. The most demanding tasks associated with the RWC included riding the rescue sled, lifting a patient, moving the trailer with the RWC, pulling the RWC from the trailer, recovering the RWC and dragging the RWC. The RWC used by the RNLI at the time was the Yamaha Waverunner XL700, 80 hp and 310 kg with sled. The IRB was the Arancia 380, 68 kg with a 30 hp engine, 70 kg. Of course, as equipment changes so may the demands of the tasks associated with them. Indeed, one of the functions of setting a physical standard is to determine if other ways or equipment can be used to complete a task and thereby make it easier, i.e. fitting the task to the person, rather than *vice versa*.

ESTABLISHING MINIMUM STANDARDS OF THE CRITICAL TASKS

Some BLG organizations have attempted to link the standards of the PES to the maximum predicted survival time for a victim in the sea, as rescuing the victim obviously qualifies as the most critical task. Martinez [23] indicates that in the BLG pre-employment PES in Staten Island, New York, passing performance is based on the acceptable duration from the start of the rescue simulation component of the test until cardiopulmonary resuscitation (CPR) is administered; the time elapsed must be no more than 2 minutes 45 seconds. In this timeframe, BLG are required to perform a simulation consisting of swimming 50 yards through a pool to a passive victim (manikin), performing a cross-chest carry tow back 50 yards, exiting the pool, walking 5 feet to a different manikin and commencing CPR. In addition, a prospective BLG must be capable of running 1.5 miles on a track in less than 12 minutes; and swimming 600 yards in a 25 yard pool in less than 10 minutes (front stroke only). The task-related reasons for these aerobic fitness components are not clear.

Martinez [24] discusses the window of opportunity for successful recovery of a submerged victim, citing the 2003 US Lifesaving Association (USLA) 'Manual of Open Water Lifesaving', which indicates that 'based on the experience of professional open water lifeguards, USLA believes there is a 2-minute window of enhanced opportunity for successful recovery and resuscitation of submerged victims. Thereafter, the chances of successful recovery decline very quickly'. USLA lifeguards should be prepared to respond immediately to life-threatening emergencies without motorized equipment, as it may not always be where needed, when needed. Martinez [23] indicates that the standards (run and swim times) contain all three of the following elements:

1. Task: Describe what is to be done. What is to be shown to, and seen by, the observer?
2. Conditions: Describe what particular conditions the task is to be executed under.
3. Criteria: Describe what the threshold is for acceptable versus unacceptable performance.

There is no accommodation for age or gender, as the surf lifeguard work environment makes no accommodation for one's age, gender, race or status as a non-supervisor or supervisor. In terms of adverse impact, there is no objective or measurable data that demonstrate that use of this test has negatively affected workforce diversity: The test has not prevented the employment of one chief lifeguard in his 60s, two chief lifeguards who are minority group members and three other chief lifeguards who are women [23].

In Poland, the *WOPR* (*Wodne Ochotnicze Pogotowie Ratunkowe* ['Water rescue teams and lifeguards', 1993]), a publication about water rescue, suggests that loss of consciousness occurs 95–165 seconds after the first signs of the drowning victim panicking, choking or momentarily swallowing water [4]. This reference point was used to formulate the performance standards for Polish BLG and stems from US work originally published in 'On the Guard II (2001)', a YMCA publication that indicates that this time is between 70 and 150 seconds.

When examining medical research to estimate survival time, 61 drowning/near-drowning victims (40 males and 26 children <16 years; average water temperature was 17°C with a range of 0°C to 33°C) were reviewed. It was determined that the median submersion time for the survivors (n = 43) was 10 minutes; those with mild neurological disability (n = 26) were submerged for 5 minutes [25]. Submersion time was the only independent predictor of survival in a linear regression analysis ($p < 0.01$); age, water temperature and rectal temperature (in the emergency room) were not.

Claesson et al. [26] discuss the need to reach the drowning victim relative to the exposure to hypoxia and reference other work [25,27] to conclude that submersion times longer than 9–16 minutes have a poor outcome. Modell and Moya [28] and Modell et al. [29] concluded that submersion of 3–5 minutes could result in survival. Most recently, Quan et al. [30] reported that victims with good outcomes were 61% less likely to be submerged for 6–10 minutes and 98% less likely to be submerged for 11 minutes or longer. This supports the maximum permissible time of anoxia of about 10 minutes.

Reilly et al. [6], having reviewed this relevant research, concluded that the surf lifeguard should reach the victim as soon as possible or, at worst, within 3.5 minutes because of hypoxia, and then return the victim to the beach within 6.5 minutes (total of 10 minutes to basic life support). A casualty face down in water will begin to aspirate seawater immediately and death will usually ensue within about 2 minutes [31–33]. Should the casualty be observed experiencing difficulties, aspiration may be absent initially, thereby increasing the potential rescue time. However, panic and fatigue will limit the length of time available to effect a rescue before aspiration commences. Therefore, it was concluded that in this scenario there is a 3–4 minute rescue window.

A survey of beaches supervised by the RNLI established that the median distance to be covered on land was 170 m and the median patrolled area out to sea was 400 m, with a maximum distance offshore that a rescue would be attempted by swimming being 200 m [6]. Therefore, the RNLI BLG in the United Kingdom must be capable of a sea swim of 200 m in 3.5 minutes (210 seconds). As the above review indicated, the task performance standard was determined as the total transit time of the rescue with the victim returned to the beach, a maximum of 10 minutes. This approach, determining minimum acceptable performance, established independently of the consideration of subgroups, makes the resulting standard age and sex 'free' [6,34,35].

To what degree a BLG would attempt an offshore rescue by swimming was compared globally to BLG expectations. The International Life Saving Federation states that an international surf lifeguard should be able to perform the rescue of a conscious victim who is a minimum of 100 m away from the shore. However, Claesson et al. [26] indicate that both Australian [36] and UK surf lifesaving organizations report that most drowning incidents are likely to occur within 100 m of the shore. In 2002, the UK Royal Lifesaving Society reported on 230/503 drowning incidents where the distance had been measured; 181/230 (79%) occurred within 50 m of the shoreline [37]. Circumstances in the UK correspond to those in Australia, where the majority of rescues undertaken by BLG also occur within 50 m of the shore [36]. For this reason, the distance of 200 m was flexible, dependent on the current abilities of incumbents, which were yet to be determined by Reilly et al. [6].

MEASURING THE DEMANDS OF THE CRITICAL TASKS

Once the critical and essential tasks are established, their physical and physiological demands must be measured to determine which tasks are most demanding and what degree and type of physical fitness is required for safe and efficient performance. In order to quantify the physical and physiological demands of the critical tasks, the 'method of best practice' for each task should be determined [15]. This is the standardized, agreed method by which a task should be performed and is specified and quantified in terms of task duration, rate, load and technique. It can be established in conjunction with a task analysis; the process of establishing a method of best practice may involve the biomechanical and physiological assessments of a task to determine the most efficient way of undertaking it [5]. It also includes consideration of other methods and equipment.

To determine the physiological demands of the critical and essential tasks of BLG in the UK, testing was performed on beaches with varying sea conditions and wave heights of 0.5, 0.5–1 and 0.5–2 m, respectively. Twenty-eight BLG (22 males, 6 females) between the ages of 18 and 45 years were tested on the following outdoor tasks at maximum effort (confirmed by post-test blood lactate measurement):

1. Time to run 200 m on the beach parallel to the sea, immediately followed by an offshore swim in the sea to a buoy secured at 200 m.
2. Time to run 200 m on the beach parallel to the sea, immediately followed by a 400 m prone paddle on a rescue board (Gaisford Surf Equipment, Redruth, UK).

Two self-paced tasks were performed continuously for a minimum of 4 minutes at sea while the aerobic metabolic demands were measured:

1. Cross-chest tow: The volunteer BLG towed a 50 kg marine anthropometric manikin (designed to float in the sea as an unconscious 50th percentile male) using a rescue tube secured around the chest of the manikin.
2. Paddle (prone): The manikin was placed on the rescue board and the subject paddled the rescue board. The manikin and BLG were prone.

In both tests, the BLG were asked to work at the pace they would choose if they were with a casualty, had secured the airway and were returning to shore. The tests were undertaken parallel to the shore beyond the break to minimize the influence of waves and tide. Sea temperature was 17°C–18°C. BLG wore lifeguard-issue swimming costumes or wetsuits and a nose clip; they breathed through a mouthpiece into a bag that collected their expired air for the determination of metabolic rate. To the authors' knowledge, these are the only data resulting from the directly measured physiological demands of surf rescue in the sea. The mean aerobic demands measured for towing and paddling are shown in Table 15.1 and are approximately equivalent to those when running at 11 km h^{-1} (towing) and walking at 7.5 km h^{-1} (paddling).

As stated, a BLG in the RNLI must be capable of returning the casualty to the beach in 6.5 minutes. Given that a BLG should not reach the beach exhausted and should be able to assist in casualty handling and resuscitation, the demands of towing or paddling should not exceed 70% of BLG maximum oxygen consumption (VO$_{2max}$). In fit, trained but non-elite athletes, this is as high a percentage

Table 15.1 Mean (SD) oxygen consumption while beach lifeguard tows a manikin representing a casualty and paddles in the sea

	Towing		Paddling	
	VO$_2$ (L min^{-1})	VO$_2$ (mL kg^{-1} min^{-1})	VO$_2$ (L min^{-1})	VO$_2$ (mL kg^{-1} min^{-1})
Mean	3.2 (0.6)	40.4 (7.3)	2.1 (0.4)	25.8 (4.9)
5th percentile	2.2	30.2	1.4	20.3
95th percentile	4.0	51.2	2.6	32.9

Note: n = 23.

as is recommended to work to avoid excessive anaerobic metabolism and fatigue [38–41].

Saborit et al. [42] investigated the cardiovascular demands of aquatic rescue simulations in simulated adverse sea conditions in a pool, indirectly. The conditions were simulated and only heart rate (HR) was measured, as the authors suggest that measuring oxygen uptake (VO_2, aerobic demand) while performing rescues in water is difficult and the use of a portable gas analyzer would considerably affect progress and modify the position of the lifeguard's body. They chose to estimate VO_2 from the relationship between individual VO_2 and HR obtained during a running treadmill test. Saborit et al. [42] assume a relationship between VO_{2max} while harnessed swimming in a pool and when running on a treadmill. HR was measured during the rescue simulations, and values were modified due to the following factors associated with swimming in the sea and known to affect the HR response: (1) body submersion (subtract 5–8 bpm) and (2) facial submersion (measured on each individual for their specific drop in HR as a response to cool water, on average an 8 bpm fall).

The simulations occurred in a pool capable of making different types of surf waves up to 1.7 m high. The rescue simulation included a swim of 55 m to reach a volunteer simulating an unconscious state, then towing the victim back 55 m. This distance was chosen as it was considered the maximum distance that a lifeguard needs to cover on a well-organized beach as reported in the study of Michniewicz et al. [4]. It is not clear if the 55 m only applies to Spanish beaches. The simulations included rescues with and without equipment. The average (SD) estimated rate of oxygen consumption during the rescue was 3.4 (0.8) L min^{-1}, which represents 85.5% of the participants' VO_{2max} with equipment and 84.6% without equipment. Maximum HR was 184 bpm without equipment and 180 bpm with equipment, and average HR was 177 and 175.5 bpm, respectively. Saborit et al. [42] argue that the HR in the rescue was near maximal and is the result of the mental stress associated with high waves, despite swimming being slow or interrupted.

The research for the RNLI [6] also required each BLG to perform a casualty evacuation, by approaching a 41-kg head and torso manikin from the rear, grasping it under the arms, lifting it and carrying it backwards for 10 m across the beach. This task was used to simulate the individual contribution to a two-man casualty lift. Forty-one kilograms represents 60% of the 50th percentile body mass of the combined male and female British adult aged 19–65 years [43]. On average, the individual at the head end of a casualty carries 60% of the mass of the casualty [44]. The chest circumference of the manikin was 91 cm to match the mean of the 50th percentile British male and female [43].

Daniel and Klauck [45] investigated the demands of casualty rescue with 17 lifeguards who performed a simulated rescue involving a sprint swim of 25 m, a 2 m dive to retrieve a dummy and a tow of 25 m. They concluded that lifesaving training and events are predominantly endurance-based and require training similar to competitive swimming, the major difference being the requirement to tow a casualty during lifesaving. The addition of passive drag while towing requires a contribution from anaerobic energy sources with consequent earlier fatigue.

One difficulty with setting PES for BLG arises from the differences in the environmental demands associated with rescues; these demands can be very specific to a given beach and environment and can vary significantly with time of year. Gifford [46] indicates that on the Hawaiian North Shore rip currents could lead to a victim being swept out to 800 yards offshore and a typical North Shore rescue takes as long as 45 minutes.

The RNLI and University of Portsmouth (UK) also developed a fitness test for IRB or RWC operations. To measure the demands of using an IRB or a RWC, a method of best practice was established and, working with BLG on the beach, these tasks were quantified using load cells in terms of the force required to lift, pull, launch (pull, pivot, drag) on dry and wet sand. Manoeuvring both the IRB and RWC in the sea was quantified as was the force required to operate equipment, such as winching the RWC onto the trailer. Tasks were repeated two to five times to ensure reproducibility [22]. Figure 15.1 is a photo of a BLG lifting the engine on the IRB. The graph demonstrates the load measured (kg) at the prop. The second photo (Figure 15.2) is of a pivot and drag of an IRB in wet sand with the prop up on tilt lock (engine dragging in sand). This is a two-person job and here in the graph the load for each subject was measured for 10 m. The green line represents the subject inside the turning circle during pivot.

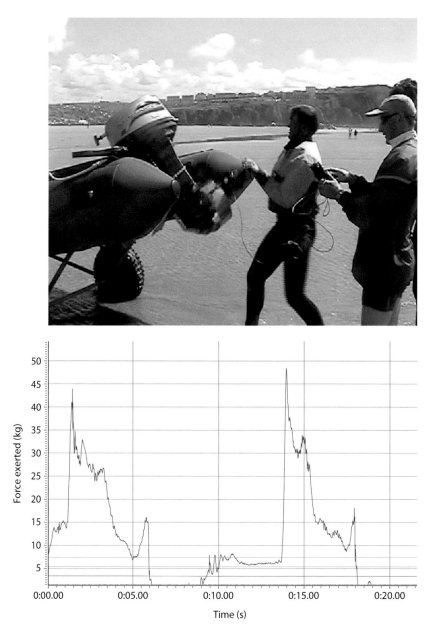

Figure 15.1 A photo of one beach lifeguard lifting the engine on an inshore rescue boat. The graph demonstrates load measured (kg) at the prop.

DEMANDS OF CPR

One of the potential job demands of a BLG is the performance of CPR. Miles et al. [47] reported that the provision of one-man CPR under non-stressful conditions represents only a moderate physiological demand requiring a HR of 50% of maximum and an oxygen consumption of 1.24 L min⁻¹ (18 ml kg⁻¹ min⁻¹). Similar metabolic demands while performing CPR have been reported by other authors [48–50]. Bridgewater et al. [51] also sought to identify whether the ability to perform CPR should be used to determine a standard of fitness. As previous research had employed young participants, these authors sought to identify whether the demands of performing CPR for 10 minutes were significantly higher with an older cohort. Their findings indicated that regardless

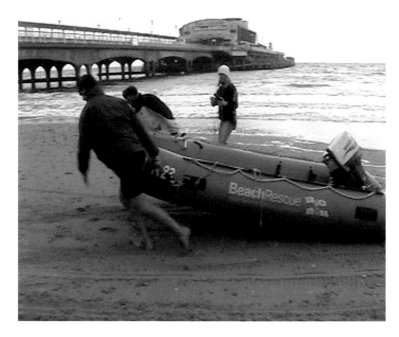

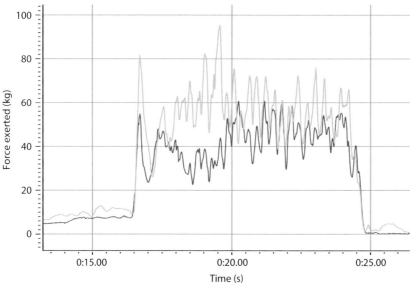

Figure 15.2 A pivot and drag of an inshore rescue boat in wet sand with prop up on tilt lock (engine dragging in sand). This is a two-person job; the graph shows the load measured for each subject for 10 m. The green line represents the subject inside the turning circle during the pivot.

of age, the demands of CPR are relatively low, with absolute peak HR of 116–129 bpm (63%–69% Max HR).

It has been debated whether the demands of CPR are such that they require a 'minimum level of fitness'. The BLG population is predominantly young and aerobically fit with a healthy lung capacity [52]. Reilly et al. [6] reported that the VO$_{2max}$ and other fitness characteristics of British BLG demonstrated that, if they are capable of performing the victim rescue tasks, they possess the necessary fitness to perform CPR after a strenuous rescue. Similar research measured the aerobic capacities among 42 Swedish BLG and found that CPR performance was unaffected following a 100 m rescue and tow/carry [26].

Moran and Webber [52] and Claesson et al. [26] found that both rested and exercised/fatigued surf lifeguards, if anything, tended to over-inflate the lungs during rescue breathing. However, Barcala-Furelos et al. [53] studied the effect of physical fatigue caused by a water rescue on the quality of CPR with 60 lifeguards from Spain. They report that the accumulated fatigue during a water rescue reduced the quality of chest compressions and ventilations of CPR for 5 minutes following a water rescue. This provided evidence for the authors to recommend a 15% increase in maximum aerobic capacity above the measured demands of the rescue task, to prevent accumulation of lactic acid and to reduce the influence of fatigue on CPR. However, this is still a relatively low level of aerobic fitness and so it is concluded that a BLG who has sufficient fitness to satisfactorily swim and tow/paddle with a casualty should possess the necessary fitness to undertake CPR, even after a rescue.

TYPES OF STANDARDS

There are generally three types of physical employment tests: (1) task simulation, (2) predictive fitness tests and (3) profiling the incumbents or norm referencing.

Historically, to develop a fitness standard, norm referencing or profiling of incumbents was performed in which the fitness levels of current BLG were measured. This was then used to set a standard for future applicants. Gulbin et al. [36] provide a physiological profile of 55 Australian elite surf iron men, full-time lifeguards and patrolling volunteer surf lifesavers. They conclude that not all of the latter group would be capable of undertaking all modes of rescue in all surf conditions and that lifesavers should have 'good' aerobic fitness (3.55 L min^{-1} for 20-year-old males, 2.3 L min^{-1} for 20-year-old females). However, these authors did not determine the physical demands of the tasks associated with surf lifesaving as a basis for these conclusions. This method is therefore discouraged as it would not be legally defensible: it in no way reflects the actual demands of the job.

Profiling incumbents is not recommended for developing PES but can be useful to determine if current job-related standards are reasonable. The RNLI BLG were required to patrol up to 400 m out to sea on the paddle board; however, after testing it was identified that only 30% of the BLG were able

to paddle 400 m in 3.5 minutes. The 5th percentile paddling speed was 1.38 m/s; therefore, 95% of the BLG tested had the ability to paddle 289 m in 3.5 minutes. Based on this evidence of the ability of current incumbents, the area patrolled by rescue board was reduced to the 5th percentile paddling speed of 1.38 m/s, achievable by 95% of BLG in 3.5 minutes. As a consequence, it was recommended that on beaches with rescue boards but no IRB or RWC, the patrolled area be reduced from 400 to 300 m.

In its final form, an objectively developed PES can be presented as a requirement for candidates to demonstrate their ability to do different aspects of a job; it can be a direct simulation of the job which has high levels of validity but is difficult to administer. Or it can be based on simple-to-administer tests that predict, based on statistical relationships, an individual's capacity to undertake critical tasks. Each of these approaches has its pros and cons [5]. For example, the most valid and easily defended approach is to ask the candidate to do the job or a valid simulation of it. One problem with this approach is that it is impossible to know how hard the candidate is working to complete the task; it could be at 100% with no spare capacity. The predictive tests are much easier to administer; it is possible to establish how much spare capacity a candidate has. However, because they are based on predictive equations that contain some degree of error, there must be a strategic approach to minimize false positives (predict someone can do the job when they cannot) and negatives (predict someone cannot do the job when they can).

Because results obtained on a beach or in the sea will be influenced by environmental conditions, a predictive fitness test which can be performed in a gym/pool is an ideal design for a BLG PES, but will rely on predictive relationships (e.g. between pool swimming and sea swimming). In addition, if an applicant is not a skilled swimmer, an open water test poses the potential for accidents or injury.

TOWARDS A FITNESS STANDARD FOR BLG

The most researched areas which can be applied to performance standard setting for BLG are survival times in the sea, the demands of CPR and the documented physical demands of manually handling equipment such as rescue craft. This chapter has presented information on each of these areas, which can be used as a reference for those trying to develop a rational and defensible BLG PES. In the United Kingdom, the BLG fitness test was specifically designed based on the following rational steps:

- Task analysis to determine the critical and essential tasks
- Establishment of a method of best practice
- Establishment of a minimum acceptable standard on the basis of evidence and subject matter experts
- Measurement of the physical and physiological demands of the critical and essential tasks
- Design of potential tests
- Administration of potential tests to a group of incumbents at maximum effort
- Validation

The resulting tests were as follows:

Task-related tests (task prediction)

- **Pool swim of 400 m in less than 7.5 minutes.** The ability to paddle 300 m in the sea in 3.5 minutes correlated well ($r = -0.82$) with the ability to complete a 400-m front crawl swim in a pool in less than 7.5 minutes.
- **Pool swim of 200 m in less than 3.5 minutes.** This can be undertaken as part of the 400-m swim, the first or second 200 m of which should take less than 3.5 minutes. Pool swimming predicted moving 200 m out to sea when the sea swim included running into the sea.
- **25-m underwater swim immediately followed by 25-m surface swim. Complete in less than 50 seconds.** This test is not predictive but ensures the applicant can demonstrate swimming efficiency and comfort in undertaking submersions.
- **Lift 41-kg torso manikin by grabbing around the circumference with both arms and move backwards 10 m.** This test is a direct simulation of a casualty rescue, simulating one-half of a two-man manual handle of a casualty on the beach.

In addition, the relationship between the anthropometric measurement of shoulder circumference and ability to tow a casualty was included for guidance only.

- **Candidate's deltoid (shoulder) circumference (cm) to be measured and divided by the $\log_{10}$ of his/her 400-m front crawl swim time.** The resulting number, if it exceeds 41, predicts the ability to tow a casualty. This point is included for guidance only at this time.
- **200-m beach run as fast as possible, complete in less than 40 s.**

Non-task-related targets – Not to be used as a reason for exclusion

The following tests should not be used for selection. Rather they represent a recognition of the importance of upper body strength and aerobic capacity in the role of BLG. They are easy targets to train towards and could be sent to potential BLG with their application form, along with details of the task-related tests.

Push-ups, body straight, knees off floor, chest lowered until it touches the clenched fist of the tester. Males to achieve 37, females 15 in 1 minute, resting permitted during the minute.

A 2.4-km (1.5 mile) run to achieve 'good' or above according to population norms.

Potential male recruits should train so that they can run 1.5 miles in 10 minutes 15 seconds and no slower than 11 minutes 44 seconds. Potential female recruits should train so that they can run 1.5 miles in 11 minutes 56 seconds and no slower than 14 minutes 24 seconds.

In addition, for UK BLG the recommended fitness tests for qualification to crew a RWC and IRB were established in Table 15.2. It is important to note the following:

1. It is strongly recommended that BLG receive manual handling training before undertaking the tests, as loads required to operate RWC and IRB exceed the maximum limits recommended by the US National Institute for Occupational Safety and Health.
2. The tests are not simulations of actual tasks, but test whether BLG have the necessary strength to undertake the generic tasks associated with operating RWC and IRBs.
3. Successful completion of these tests does not guarantee that a BLG has the skills necessary to operate an RWC or IRB.

Table 15.2 Physical requirements of BLG in the UK to crew an IRB or RWC

Requirement	Individual load	Test
RWC		
Pivot 180 (two-person)	72 kg initiate 56 kg mean	Pull IRB at lower bow handle using top handle across wet sand, parallel to sea (without engine or fuel bladder) for 5 m, once with each hand
Hand crank onto trailer with winch (one-person)	15–22 kg	Perform task on beach
Lift to load onto trailer (two-person)	55 kg lift of 30 cm	Lift two suitable 25 kg containers, underhand grip, one in each hand, hold for 3 seconds
IRB		
Pivot 180 and pull 10 m (two-person)	62–83 kg initiate 42–53 kg mean	Pull IRB at lower bow handle using top handle across wet sand, parallel to sea (without engine or fuel bladder) for 5 m, once with each hand
Lift overhead to load onto trailer (two-person lift, one-person hold)	50 kg	Perform task on beach; two BLG lift the IRB, candidate then supports it overhead for 10 seconds

Note: BLG, beach lifeguard; IRB, inshore rescue boat; RWC, rescue watercraft.

In addition, it is recommended that the BLG demonstrate the necessary range of motion to operate the outboard motor, to ensure that their anthropometrics do not restrict their ability to control the vessel.

CONCLUSION

It has been beyond the scope of this chapter to detail all existing fitness standards of BLG worldwide; they often vary from organization to organization. However, the approach for achieving a rational and defensible performance standard for BLG has been described. The standard will vary depending on sea state, environmental conditions, beach topography and user population as well as the expectations of different lifesaving organizations. Many standards are available on regional websites, but the scientific rationale underpinning them is usually not presented or does not exist. In many cases, standards are developed based on history or past standards, which at best may be the result of incumbent profiling or norm referencing. At present, very few standards are based on scientific methods established within the occupational physiology research community.

REFERENCES

1. Division of Human Rights on the Complaint of Candy Callery, Complainant, vs. New York City Department of Parks and Recreation, Respondent. New York City Department of Parks and Recreation, Petitioner, 9 December 1971.
2. Reilly T, Prayal-Brown A, Spivock M, Stockbrugger B, Blacklock R. The influence of anthropometrics on physical employment standard performance. *Occup Med.* In Press.
3. Reilly T, Iggleden C, Gennser M, Tipton M. Occupational fitness standards for beach lifeguards. Phase 2: The development of an easily administered fitness test. *Occup Med.* 2006; 56: 12–17.
4. Michniewicz R, Walczuk T, Rostkowska E. An assessment of the effectiveness of various variants of water rescue. *Kinesiology.* 2008; 40: 96–106.
5. Tipton M, Milligan G, Reilly T. Physiological employment standards I. Occupational fitness standards: Objectively subjective? *Eur J Appl Physiol.* 2013; 113(10): 2435–46.

6. Reilly T, Wooler A, Tipton M. Occupational fitness standards for beach lifeguards. Phase 1: The physiological demands of beach lifeguarding. *Occup Med.* 2006; 56: 6–11.

7. Greenberg G, Berger R. A model to assess one's ability to apprehend and restrain a resisting suspect in police work. *J Occup Med.* 1983; 25(11): 809–13.

8. Rayson M. Fitness for work: The need for conducting a job analysis. *J Occup Med.* 2000; 50(6): 434–6.

9. Shephard R, Bonneau J. Assuring gender equity in recruitment standards for police officers. *Can J Sports Sci.* 2002; 27(3): 263–95.

10. Payne W, Harvey J. A framework for the design of physical employment tests and standards. *Ergonomics.* 2010; 53(7): 858–71.

11. Gledhill N, Jamnik V. Development of fitness screening protocols for physically demanding occupations. *Can J Sports Sci.* 1992; 17(3): 222–7.

12. Anderson G, Plecas D, Segger T. Police officer physical ability testing: Re-validating a selection criteria. *Policing Int J Police Strategies Manag.* 2001; 24(1): 8–31.

13. Taylor NAS, Groeller H. Work-based physio-logical assessment of physically-demanding trades: A methodological overview. *J Physiol Anthropol.* 2003; 22: 73–81.

14. Reilly T. *Fitness Standards for the Royal National Life Boat Institution (RNLI) Lifeboat Crew.* PhD Dissertation, University of Portsmouth, 2007.

15. Gumieniak R, Jamnik V, Gledhill N. Physical fitness bona fide occupational requirements for safety-related physically demanding occupations; development considerations. *Health Fit J Can.* 2011; 4(2): 47–52.

16. Milligan G, Reilly T, Tipton M. Validity of tests and standards: The transition from task analysis to test and standard devel-opment. *To be Presented at the Second International Conference on Physical Employment Standards*, Canmore, AB, Canada, August 23–26, 2015.

17. Rodgers S. Job evaluation in worker fitness determination. *Occup Med.* 1988; 3(2): 219–39.

18. Reilly R, Zedeck S, Tenopyr M. Validity and fairness of physical ability tests for pre-dicting performance in craft jobs. *J Appl Psychol.* 1979; 64: 262–74.

19. Jackson A, Osburn H. Validity of isometric strength test for predicting performance in physically demanding tasks. *Proceedings of the Human Factors Society—28th Annual Meeting*, 1984. 1984, pp. 452–4.

20. Jamnik V, Thomas S, Shaw J, Gledhill N. Identification and characterization of the critical physically demanding tasks encountered by correctional officers. *Appl Physiol Nutr Metab.* 2010; 35(1): 45–58.

21. Jamnik V, Gumienak R, Gledhill N. Developing legally defensible physiological employment standards for prominent physi-cally demanding public safety occupations; a Canadian perspective. *Eur J Appl Physiol.* 2013; 113(10): 2447–57.

22. Reilly T, Wallace S, Carter P, Tipton M. *Technical Report. Fitness Requirements for RNLI Beach Lifeguards to Operate Rescue Watercraft and Inshore Rescue Boats.* University of Portsmouth, UK; 2004.

23. Martinez, C. *Surf lifeguard pre-employment test.* United States Department of the Interior. National Park Service. Gateway National Recreation Area, Washington, DC; 2010.

24. Martinez C. Near drowning at Jacobs Riss Park: A case study of physical fitness needed by oceanfront lifeguards. *World Conference on Drowning Prevention*, Da Nang, Vietnam, 2011.

25. Suominen P, Baillie C, Korpela R, Rautanen S, Ranta S, Olkkola K. Impact of age, submer-sion time and water temperature on outcome in near-drowning. *Resuscitation.* 2002; 52(3): 247–54.

26. Claesson A, Karlsson T, Thoren A, Herlitz J. Delay and performance of cardio pulmonary resuscitation in surf lifeguards after simulated cardiac arrest due to drowning. *Am J Emerg Med.* 2011; 29: 1044–50.

27. Quan L, Went K, Gore E, Copass M. Outcome and predictors of outcome in pediatric submersion victims receiving prehospital care in King Co. Washington. *Pediatrics.* 1990; 86(4): 586–93.

28. Modell J, Moya F. Effects of volume of aspi-rated fluid during chlorinated fresh water drowning. *Anesthesiology.* 1966; 27(5): 666–72.

29. Modells J, Moya, F, Newby E, Ruiz B, Showers A. The effects of fluid volume in seawater drowning. *Ann Intern Med.* 1967; 67(1): 68–80.

30. Quan L, Mack C, Schiff M. Association of water temperature and submersion duration and drowning outcome. *Resuscitation.* 2014; 85(6): 790–4.

31. Conn A, Miyassaka K, Katayama M, Fujita M, Orima H, Baker G, Bohn D. A canine study of cold water drowning in fresh vs salt water. *Crit Care Med.* 1995; 23: 2029–36.

32. Fainer D, Martin C, Ivy A. Resuscitation of dogs from freshwater drowning. *J Appl Physiol.* 1951; 3: 417–26.

33. Golden F, Tipton M. *Essentials of Sea Survival.* Champaign, IL: Human Kinetics; 2002.

34. Reilly T, Tipton M. *Fitness Standards for the Royal National Lifeboat Institution Lifeboat Crew.* Report to the RNLI. Portsmouth, UK: University of Portsmouth; 2005.

35. Milligan G, House J, Long G, Tipton M. *A Recommended Minimum Fitness Standard for the Oil and Gas Industry.* Energy Institute Report, University of Portsmouth, UK; 2010.

36. Gulbin J, Fell J, Gaffney P. A physiological profile of elite surf ironmen, full time lifeguards and patrolling surf life savers. *Aust J Sci Med Sport.* 1996; 28: 86–90.

37. The Royal Life Saving Society. *Lifesavers.* Report #47. UK: Royal Lifesaving Society, Alcester, UK; 2003.

38. Wilber R, Zawadzki K, Kearney J, Shannon M, Disalvo D. Physiological profiles of elite off-road and road cyclists. *Med Sci Sports Exerc.* 1997; 29: 1090.

39. Wasserman K, Whipp B, Davis J. Respiratory physiology of exercise: Metabolism gas exchange and ventilator control. *Int Rev Respir Phyiology.* 1981; 23: 149–211.

40. Whipp B. The slow component of O_2 uptake kinetics during heavy exercise. *Med Sci Sports Exerc.* 1994; 23: 149–211.

41. Tschakovsky ME, Hughson RL. Interaction of factors determining oxygen uptake at the beginning of exercise. *J Appl Physiol.* 1999; 86: 1011.

42. Saborit J, Soto M, Diez V, Sanclement M, Hernandez P, Rodriguez J, Rodriguez L. Physiological response of beach lifeguards in a rescue simulation with surf. *Ergonomics.* 2010; 53(9): 1140–50.

43. Pheasant S. *Bodyspace.* UK: Taylor and Francis, Abingdon, UK; 1996.

44. Scarpello E, Bilzon J, Rayson M. *Development of Job-Related Physical Fitness Tests for Royal Navy Personnel.* INM MOD Report No. 2000.044. Institute of Naval Medicine, Ministry of Defence, Gosport, UK; 2000.

45. Daniel K, Klauck J. Physiological and biomechanical load parameters in life saving. In McLaren D (ed.). *Biomechanics and Medicine in Swimming.* London: E & FN Spon; 1992, pp. 321–5.

46. Gifford B. Tipped abs … to the rescue! *Men's Health.* 2014; 23(9).

47. Miles D, Underwood P, Nolan D, Frey M, Gotshall R. Metabolic, hemodynamic and respiratory responses to performing cardiopulmonary resuscitation. *Can J Sport Sci.* 1984; 9: 141–7.

48. Buono M, Golding L. The energy cost of performing cardiopulmonary resuscitation. *Arizona J Health Phys Educ Recreat.* 1981; 3: 10–11.

49. Johnson S, Bernstein M, Franklin B, Vander L, Rubenfire M. Cardiopulmonary training: Feasibility for cardiac patients. *Med Sci Sports Exercise.* 1983; 15: 120.

50. Squires W, Hartung G, Pratt C, Miller R. Metabolic cost and electrocardiograph changes in cardiac patients during cardiopulmonary resuscitation practice. *J Cardiac Rehabil.* 1982; 2: 313–17.

51. Bridgewater F, Bridgewater K, Zeitz C. Using the ability to perform CPR as a standard of fitness: A consideration of the influence of aging on the physiological responses of a select group of first aiders performing cardiopulmonary resuscitation. *Resuscitation.* 2000; 45: 97–103.

52. Moran K, Webber J. Too much puff, not enough push? Surf lifeguard simulated CPR performance. *Int J Aquat Res Educ.* 2012; 6: 13–23.

53. Barcala-Furelos R, Abelairas-Gomez C, Romo-Perez V, Palacios-Aguilar J. Effect of physical fatigue on the quality CPR: A water rescue study of lifeguards. *Am J Emerg Med.* 2013; 31(3): 473–7.

PART 6

Safety Education

16

Beach safety education: A behavioural change approach

MICHAEL WRIGHT

INTRODUCTION

There is evidence from many areas of public safety, such as road safety, fire safety, food safety and water safety, that the provision of information and advice, while important, is by itself ineffectual in changing safety behaviour. Knowledge of recommended safety practices, while essential, does not necessarily lead to self-protective behaviour. There are numerous studies across many fields of safety (fire, food, road, water) that show that public awareness of risks, or lack of it, is a major factor in failing to adopt safety practices. Research [1] has found that the majority of drowning casualties in Australia tended to be engaged in recreational and everyday activities (such as walking home) rather than commercial activities. A similar profile can be found in other countries. This leads to the question of how safety practitioners can change attitudes and behaviours of members of the public, particularly that of adult men, who make up the vast majority of fatal drowning casualties. This chapter focuses on how education can be applied to influence the safety behaviour of the public in open water environments.

Research indicates that people often lack understanding of the hazards, perceive them to be low and overestimate their ability to manage the risks. For example, the following reasons were cited [2] by leisure marine participants in the United Kingdom for not wearing a life jacket:

- A belief there was not a high risk of falling into the water
- Not perceiving falling into water as a threat, because they believed they would be able to climb out or survive for a long time
- Belief that life jackets would not save their lives, because hypothermia was a greater risk

The latter study [2] suggested these findings indicate a lack of awareness of the early phases of cold-water immersion, especially cold-water shock associated with the low water temperatures around the United Kingdom [3]. It has been suggested that by using a life jacket people could prevent the majority of boating fatalities [4]. The US Coastguard reported [5] wear rates of 4.9% among adults in open motorboats in 2013 and 17.7% for all boaters excluding jet skiers (personal watercraft).

Clearly the low level of risk awareness and other behavioural factors remain a common factor in water safety behaviour.

A Canadian report [6] suggested that boaters tend to engage in the following careless behaviours:

- Not checking weather and water conditions prior to using their boats, despite checking weather and road conditions prior to driving to their boat
- Not ensuring that their boats are fit for purpose, many having limited information on how to do so
- Being more likely to load up their boat with alcohol supplies than a personal flotation device

A study of 1,200 US beachgoers in New Jersey found that, while the majority were aware of rip currents, only 26% knew what proportion of lifeguard rescues involved rip currents, 40% knew how many people drowned due to rip currents and only 21% knew how long a rip current can last [7]. Thus, respondents, although aware of rip currents, had a low understanding of their risks and hazardous nature.

A 2009 report [8] suggests that risk of drowning may be increased by the following:

- Perception of a low threat of experiencing difficulty while swimming
- Low belief in the efficacy of drowning prevention measures

Males and young adults were particularly found to overestimate their ability and underestimate their risk of drowning.

There is also evidence that some people knowingly disregard safety advice, for example, swimming outside the area patrolled by lifeguards despite awareness of hazards such as rip currents. For example, interviews of rip current survivors found that despite being aware of rip currents, being able to spot rip currents in photographs and recall rip current safety messages, they were more likely to swim outside of the lifeguarded flagged areas [9]. The survivors tended to be regular and able swimmers. Finally, younger respondents were reported to be more likely to swim at unpatrolled spots and not signal for help when caught in a rip current. These findings suggested overconfidence among the respondents. The Australian drowning

prevention strategy of 2012 [10] cites a recent Australian report noting that more than 42% of people surveyed had swum outside of the red and yellow flags at some point during a year.

EXPLAINING SAFETY BEHAVIOUR

Why might people disregard safety advice even when aware of a hazard? We have already alluded to low awareness of the risks and overconfidence. Safety behaviour is influenced by a rich combination of risk perceptions, peer attitudes, social values and norms.

Understanding behaviour: Models of behaviour

Social cognition models, such as the theory of planned behaviour, help in understanding the discontinuity between knowledge and behaviour. They have also been used to help design educational initiatives that target attitudes, beliefs and knowledge. Cognition refers to the process of thinking. The social aspect refers to the influence of other people's behaviours and their opinions on your thoughts. These models and empirical research findings indicate that it is essential to understand people's attitudes, norms, values and perceptions in order to be able to influence them through education.

Three key social cognition models are the health belief, the theory of planned behaviour and the health action model. These models have been developed and applied to health behaviour in general and are not unique to water safety. The models indicate that the application of knowledge of recommended safety practices would be influenced by a person's observation of how other people behave, other peoples' attitudes and their own experience of water safety. Each of these approaches has value in that they help to explain elements of safety behaviour. Key aspects of these approaches are noted in Table 16.1.

Turner et al. [2] applied a variant to the transtheoretical stages of change model to the assessment of life jacket use. The variant, a combination of protection motivation theory (PMT) [11] and the stages of change approach, was used. PMT focuses on how people perceive threats and how to respond to them; thus PMT is very relevant to the issue of risks being underestimated by the public.

Table 16.1 Summary of behavioural models

Health belief model

The health belief model [12] has six central constructs: *perceived susceptibility, severity, benefits, barriers, self-efficacy* (a person's belief about his or her capability) and *cues to action*. For example, if people believe they are susceptible and the consequences are severe, then the costs (such as time and effort) of engaging in unsafe behaviour are outweighed by the benefits. Cues to action may include advertising and alerting people to a risk.

Theory of planned behaviour [13]

The theory of planned behaviour assumes that while behaviour is rational, decision-making is influenced by motivation, social norms and beliefs. Beliefs may include perceptions of the risk. Norms may include the influence of how 'significant others' view an activity. It also introduces the idea of *perceived behavioural control*, i.e. whether individuals believe they have control over an issue and are capable of a behaviour.

Health action model [14]

The health action model was developed as a combination of the health belief model and the theory of reasoned action. This model cites social pressure as an influence on behavioural intention and presents a stages of change model. Previous research [15] suggests the following:

- The approach to behaviour change should be split into two phases – the 'motivation' phase in which people develop their intentions and then the 'volition' phase.
- There are two groups of individuals: those who have not yet translated their intentions into action and those who have.
- People are motivated to change, but need to plan a strategy and may need to acquire the right skills to translate their intention into action.
- Planning can be divided into action planning and coping planning. Coping planning includes overcoming barriers to change.
- Perceived self-efficacy (self-belief in one's capabilities) is required throughout the entire process.

Transtheoretical model [16]

This model presents behaviour change as a set of stages, namely the following:

1. Pre-contemplation: people are not intending to take action in the foreseeable future
2. Contemplation: raising consciousness and awareness of the issue, with consideration to take action in the future
3. Preparation: self-evaluation and advanced planning in order to take action in the near future
4. Action: people are making changes to behaviours
5. Maintenance: continuing behavioural changes made and working to prevent relapse
6. Termination: complete behavioural change whereby individuals are sure they will not return to their old behaviours

For an individual to move from the pre-contemplation stage to the contemplation stage, they must first become aware of the hazard. As with other models, this one asserts that people make behavioural decisions by balancing pros and cons, and these decisions are influenced by self-confidence. People with more self-confidence are more likely to adopt recommended behaviours.

PMT asserts that we protect ourselves based on the following:

- The perceived severity of a threatening event
- The perceived probability of the occurrence
- The efficacy (effectiveness and 'costs' such as discomfort) of the preventive behaviour
- The perceived self-efficacy of the preventive behaviour (can it be enacted properly)

As noted by Turner et al. [2], PMT asserts 'if a threat is perceived to be significant, relevant to the self and the threat can be avoided effectively with a safe behaviour, that behaviour will be adopted'. The study [2] had a sample of 68 leisure marine participants. Their main findings were 'that participants did not believe there was a high risk of falling into the water. If they did, they did not necessarily view it as a threat because many expect to be able to climb out easily or survive for a long time'. Participants also said they would not go out in rough conditions and would don a life jacket if conditions got rough. Moreover respondents lacked confidence in life jackets, preferring to harness themselves and/or move carefully around the boat. Among other findings, respondents said that they viewed hypothermia as the most prominent threat, possibly betraying a lack of awareness of the debilitating effects of cold water shock.

The results were interpreted in respect of the stages of change model and the PMT model [2]. In respect of the stages of change model, the results were said to indicate that participants were in what they termed the 'decision-making' and 'hazard appraisal' stages of change, which fall within contemplation of the need to change. With respect to PMT, the authors concluded that it was necessary to enhance perception of the severity of the threat and beliefs of personal susceptibility as well as increase confidence in life jackets.

The models in Table 16.1 suggest that safety behaviour is influenced by a combination of knowledge of recommended safety practices, awareness of the risk, social pressure, normative values and motivation. They provide a framework for explaining how these factors may interact and how to influence these behaviours. In aggregate the models would suggest that it is important to take the following actions:

- Help people recognize unsafe behaviours and their consequences
- Recognize if people feel they are not susceptible and raise the profile of (underestimated) risks

- Address any misconceptions of risks and behaviours, as well as social pressures and norms
- Demonstrate the benefits of changing behaviours, as well as the severity of harm if they do not
- Ensure people feel confident and able to implement the suggested behaviours
- Cite credible behaviours when trying to change behaviours
- Ensure the source of advice is credible

Risk awareness and perception

The models in Table 16.1 and research into water safety behaviour highlight the role of risk perceptions. This leads to the question of how to characterize risk perceptions, such as what factors distinguish and influence perceptions of different water safety risks. There have been many studies regarding public risk perceptions, summarized in Ref. [17]. Indeed, the psychology of risk communication is a subject in its own right. Risk perception work builds on these models by helping to explain how people perceive risks and how these risk perceptions may be influenced. The research indicates that people do not comprehend risk according to fatality estimates.

People have more elaborate conceptualizations that include considerations such as the following:

- Immediacy of effect
- Voluntariness of risk
- Self-control over risk
- Newness (familiarity)
- Vulnerability of the casualty
- Perceived 'dreadfulness'

People tend to be averse to risks that can be readily imagined, seem unfamiliar and a 'dreadful' form of harm. Risks that are perceived as 'old', that they have control over and are not severe are regarded as lower risk. If people feel they understand a risk and can control it, it may be judged as lower. Awareness of risks is important, as this would influence perceived severity. Issues such as trustworthiness and credibility of sources of information also influence the impact of risk communication. If people trust the source of information it will be more readily accepted along with the risk message.

The aforementioned research into risk perception highlights that it can be necessary to go beyond perceived likelihood and severity to consider other factors, such as voluntariness, familiarity and perceived self-control. Risk perceptions are subjective and reflect how people 'feel' about a hazard and its risk. In the context of water safety, to raise risk perceptions, it is necessary to increase the sense of dread while reducing the sense of familiarity and self-control and raising perceptions of personal vulnerability.

GETTING THE EDUCATIONAL MESSAGE ACROSS

This topic leads to the question of how the safety message can be effectively communicated to the target audience. There are a number of dimensions to this, including the following:

- Understanding the audience and how to reach them
- Designing an effective 'risk' message

Understanding the audience

Advice and information should be specific to each target group, address their particular attitudes and be presented in a way that they can identify with. A key contemporary example of this approach is what is termed *social marketing*, as advocated by the UK Department of Health [18]. The six key features and concepts underpinning social marketing are summarized in Table 16.2.

The approach aims to ensure safety education and is designed on the basis of an understanding of people's attitudes and beliefs, such as about whether life jackets are effective and what the main risks are from falling into cold water. As attitudes vary across people, it is essential to segment people by their attitudes and tailor educational messages to each segment. In addition, a fundamental implication of behavioural change models is that people will not respond to safety advice if they do not recognize the hazard or the risk of harm.

Accordingly it is important to understand the current risk perceptions and hazard awareness of the target audience, as well as their attitudes towards safety practices. An experienced swimmer who is already aware of rip currents may welcome the latest advice on how to respond to being caught in a rip current. A novice swimmer who is unaware of rip currents may welcome being shown examples of rip currents and their risks and, indeed, may need to be convinced of the risk from rip currents before they accept safety advice such as swimming between lifeguard flags.

However, it must also be noted that if the audience perceive that the educational message is

Table 16.2 Key features of social marketing

Feature of social marketing	Summary
Consumer orientation	Gaining deep insight and understanding about the target audience; their knowledge, attitudes and beliefs; and the social context in which they live and work.
Behaviour and behavioural goals	Understanding existing behaviour and key influences on behaviour in order to develop behavioural goals.
'Intervention mix' and 'marketing mix'	Using a range of methods to achieve behavioural goals – an 'intervention mix', such as mass media and face-to-face engagement with the target audience.
Audience segmentation	Segmenting the audience in order to target effectively.
Exchange	Understanding what people must give up or pay in order to receive the benefit from changes in behaviour. Understanding the real cost to people to enable a more effective exchange, whereby the potential benefit from behaviour change can be optimized and the 'cost' (such as discomfort from wearing protective equipment) minimized.
Competition	Understanding all the demands on people's attention and willingness to change behaviour (e.g. the influence of other people, the internal drivers of pleasure or habit).

directed at other people, perhaps a more vulnerable group of people, they may not perceive it to apply to them and it may reinforce their own 'optimism bias'. One study [19] came to the following conclusion:

> Optimistic bias may represent one of the biggest barriers to the impact of effective risk communication if people believe that the information is directed towards a vulnerable other person, rather than the self, they are unlikely to pay attention to the risk information. (p. 768)

Thus, while personalized information is advocated, it may lead to a 'narrow' impact. Accordingly, targeted approaches should be complemented by general messaging through mass media, such as television and schools, to ensure that targeted messages do not lead other people to believe they are not at risk.

Designing messages

The field of risk communication offers many pointers on how to design messages geared to changing perceptions and hence behaviour. Given the importance of risk perceptions in public safety behaviour, this is a key aspect to safety education. Some key points are summarized in the remainder of this section.

The credibility of the source of information influences whether people will believe the message. As per social marketing, a key step is to understand who the target audience considers to be credible sources. In the context of drowning prevention this might be well-known sportspeople, who the audience might recognize as independent 'experts' and enthusiasts for the sport that they can trust. In the context of activities such as coastal walking this might be people who survived a fall into the sea, someone that the audience recognize as being like them, someone they can identify with and trust.

The UK Royal National Lifeboat Institution (RNLI) has adopted this approach in their Respect the Water campaign.* For example, they promote James's story, a sympathetic real life story about a student

drowning after accidentally falling into a tidal river after a night out socializing. The casualty was similar to a key target audience – young men – and the message emphasized that he was a strong swimmer. A similar approach can also be found in the work of other safety agencies, such as the use of survivor stories by the US National Oceanic and Atmospheric Administration Rip Current Resources.† The stories are real and expressed with emotion, again enabling the audience to subjectively and emotionally connect with the message and messenger.

'Persuasive content' is equally important. In the context of risk, typical features of persuasive content include:

- Making it possible to imagine the hazard – such as by use of visual imagery
- Conveying the nature of the hazard – such as concise statements about the way the hazard can cause harm
- Communicating vulnerability
- Being clear and memorable – typically limiting each message to one or two key points

Some examples of risk message design can be seen in the RNLI's Respect the Water campaign:

> Rip current flow speeds are typically 1–2 mph but they can reach 4.5 mph. That's faster than an Olympic swimmer.
> This can all happen very quickly: it only takes half a pint of sea water to enter the lungs for a fully grown man to start drowning.
> Cold water shock can cause heart attacks, even in the relatively young and healthy.

The three examples are concise, informative and they convey the nature of the hazard and demonstrate vulnerability. The RNLI also quotes as follows:

> In 2013, 167 people died in water-related incidents around the UK coast. More than two thirds of them were men. That's more than the number killed in cycling accidents.

* Royal National Lifeboat Institution. http://rnli.org/safety/respect-the-water/Pages/respect-the-water.aspx?utm_source=rnli-website-redirect&utm_medium=vanity-urls&utm_campaign=safety [accessed December 2014].

† United States National Oceanic and Atmospheric Administration. http://www.ripcurrents.noaa.gov/real_life.shtml [accessed December 2014].

In the United Kingdom, cycling is perceived to have a high rate of fatal accidents, with a popular national campaign to improve cycling safety. Comparing the number of drownings with the number of deaths in an activity people are already familiar with helps people understand the relative risk within their own framework of beliefs. Also the quote of 167 deaths is, subjectively, a large number. Quoting the number of deaths is designed to prompt people to think that the risk is high.

The latter examples are text-based. However, research also indicates that visual imagery is highly effective, transparent, quick to present and memorable. Most examples of successful public safety education campaigns involve vivid imagery. The Canadian Safe Boating Council produced a Cold Water Poster* which shows the image of a (imaginary) drowning man in cold water and emphasizes its fatal effects. There are numerous examples of imagery of rip currents designed to communicate how they look and their effects, with the Australian Surf Life Saving BeachSafe website† being a good source of examples.

For the message to be considered relevant to you and your activity, it needs to be 'framed'. Framing includes using images that are typical – settings and people that the audience identify with (usually people like them). Taking another example from the RNLI's Respect the Water campaign, an online video titled 'Think or Sink Checklist' targeting people angling from boats has a middle-aged man (typical of the target audience) on a small motorboat (a typical day angler), set in a small sea side harbour. The angler, dressed casually, speaks through the recommended safety practices in a considered yet 'everyday' presentational manner rather than speaking as a professional presenter. All these features help frame the message such that the target audience can identify with the presenter and the message.

Another element of framing is whether to emphasize the potential 'loss' from unsafe behaviour, such as death, or the 'gain' to be achieved from changing behaviour, such as greater confidence when participating in a sport. Research [20] indicates that loss

messages are more persuasive when the behaviour could result in a high risk, such as death. A cursory review of public safety education in fields such as road safety, fire safety and health behaviours (such as smoking cessation) reveals that loss messages are commonly used, typically highlighting the risk of death or serious life-changing injury or disease. Rather than stating that changing behaviour may increase your life span, a loss message will state that unsafe behaviour will shorten your life span.

However, it is also important to note that the loss message should be accompanied by a recommended positive action, such as swimming between the flags, rather than a negative recommendation, such as not swimming outside of the flagged area. A positive message should highlight a credible and practical safe behaviour, something that people can believe is possible and effective. This reflects the self-efficacy element of behaviour change, believing that it is possible to adopt a safe behaviour.

Gain messages are advocated where the behaviour is perceived to pose less risk and for behaviours related to health, such as exercise and diet, where the harm from unsafe behaviour is remote in time and uncertain, although evidence is mixed on this point.

Messages should also address some of the main social or perceptual barriers to accepting a safety message. Some common tactics include (again) using messengers the audience identify with, stating that many people (like you) are already changing their behaviour (appealing to peer reference points) and directly contesting perceived barriers such as being unable to find lifeguarded beaches. Referring back to the models of behaviour change, these elements of messaging are helping to overcome social and perceptual barriers to behaviour change. Highlighting the large number of people using lifeguarded beaches, for example, helps engender the idea that this is now the norm.

Examples

There are many examples of safety education exemplifying the psychological principles of behaviour change and risk communication. Some publicly reported examples are noted below.

A New Zealand [21] project was initiated in 2006 by Surf Life Saving New Zealand to improve the safety of rock fishers from minority communities. They identified the majority of fishers as male and of Asian origin and ascertained that only

---

* Canadian Safe Boating Council. http://www.coldwaterbootcamp.com/pages/safety_partners/life_savev2.html [accessed December 2014].

† Australian Surf Life Saving BeachSafe website. http://beachsafe.org.au/surf-ed/ripcurrents [accessed December 2014].

27.6% wore a life jacket. A survey gathered data on fisher perceptions of risk of drowning and their knowledge and practice of fishing safety. Part-time safety advisors provided tailored safety advice. Afterwards 65.6% fishers were reported to wear a life jacket or other flotation device 'sometimes' or 'often' when rock fishing. Also the rock fishers had a 'heightened awareness of the severity of risk of drowning' and 'increased awareness of safety signage'. However, resistance to behaviour change in relation to other unsafe behaviours remains, namely alcohol consumption and going down the rock face to retrieve snagged lines.

In Sydney, Australia, a community outreach programme (Science of Surf) was initiated in 2011. The campaign provided beachgoers with basic scientific knowledge of how beaches, waves and rip currents work. The campaign had two main parts, firstly a mass media campaign and secondly poster, postcards and brochures were placed in local retail outlets. An evaluation of the campaign at the 2011 World Drowning Conference has been reported [22]. The results 'showed significant improvements in beach safety knowledge immediately after the presentations which remained high at a one-month follow-up survey'. Specific elements recalled included greater knowledge in identifying rips, responses to being caught in a rip, etc.

It has been reported by Surf Life Saving Australia that the percentage of rip-current-related incidents has decreased from 34% to 17% over the period 2004–2013 in Australia [23]. The 2011 survey of survivors shows awareness of rip current safety message was high among survivors [9]. However, the 2011 evaluation [19] also reported that the increased confidence gained from attending courses meant some recipients were more likely to 'choose swimming outside lifeguard-patrolled areas at follow-up compared to pre-intervention'. This highlights the importance of evaluation to verify the impact of education on behaviour.

SUMMARY OF KEY POINTS

This chapter has focused on changing water-related safety behaviour, particularly among adults. The key points regarding effective safety education include the following:

- Effective education requires that the behavioural causes of incidents be assessed,

profiled and understood. Safety messages need to be tailored to the attitudes and behaviours of each segment of the target population – which in turn requires that the target population be segmented and their respective attitudes and behaviours profiled.
- For education to prompt behaviour change, awareness of risks and understanding of hazards needs to be raised by using visual and auditory illustrations as well as concise information, prompting people to contemplate behaviour change.
- Effective educational messages are clear and memorable; the audience identifies with the message and the messenger.
- Education also needs to empower people by stating practical safety actions as well as raising awareness (and concern) about a risk by using visual and auditory illustrations of the hazard. Effective messages advise people what to do, rather than telling them what *not* to do.

These points draw on the psychology of behaviour change, which highlights the need to prompt people to want to change their behaviour (by alerting them to the risk) and to indicate practical safe behaviours and show that the effort required to practically control the risk is justified by the safety benefit. There is also a body of psychology research regarding risk communication that indicates how people can perceive the risk to be low, such as due to familiarity (complacency), and how these misperceptions need to be countered by (for example) provision of risk information. This leads to the issue of behavioural norms and how it may be necessary to recognize and change behavioural norms through a concerted awareness-raising campaign – to alert people to the risk and to challenge 'accepted behavioural norms' (as was achieved with drink driving).

There is always a possibility that safety education will have unintended consequences, such as people developing false self-confidence or thinking that they are not part of the 'at risk' population. Evaluation is an essential part of safety education, verifying that education has had the intended effect and lessons for future safety education have been learnt.

CONCLUSION

Recalling that the majority of fatal drownings involve male adults in many countries, water safety needs to incorporate an approach aligned to the needs of adults as well as young people. The reported role of low risk awareness and overconfidence in drownings highlights the need to change people's perceptions and understanding of water hazards. An educational approach that focuses on communicating the magnitude of risk and the nature of the hazards enables people to make more informed and appropriate decisions on how to behave. The psychology of risk and behaviour change can be drawn on to help develop effective safety education aimed at behaviour change.

REFERENCES

1. O'Conner PJ, O'Conner N. Causes and prevention of boating fatalities. *Accid Anal Prev.* 2005; 37: 689–98.
2. Turner S, Wylde J, Langham M, Sharpe S, and Jackson K. *MCA Lifejacket Wear—Behavioural Change.* Maritime Coastguard Agency and the RNLI; 2009. Available at https://www.gov.uk/government/uploads/system/uploads/attachment_data/file/302769/lifejacket_wear_behavioural_change_submitted_final_no_copyright-2.pdf (accessed December 2014).
3. Tipton MJ. The initial responses to cold-water immersion in man. *Edit Rev Clin Sci.* 1989; 77: 581–8.
4. Norman N, Vincenten J. *Protecting Children and Youths in Water Recreation: Safety Guidelines for Service Providers.* Amsterdam, The Netherlands: European Child Safety Alliance, Eurosafe; 2008.
5. Mangione TW, Imre M, Heitz E, Chow W, and Lisinski HE. *2013 Lifejacket Wear Rate Observation Study Featuring. National Wear Rate Data from 1999 to 2013.* Boston, MA: JSI Research & Training Institute; 2014.
6. The Canadian Red Cross. *Boating Immersion and Trauma Deaths in Canada: 16 Years of Research—A Report on Boating-Related Deaths across Canada for 1991–2006.* Ottawa, Canada: The Canadian Red Cross and Transport Canada; 2010.
7. Brummer L, Dunphey R, Koppa D, and Kubricki K. Rip Current Awareness & Knowledge. *A Study of What Beachgoers know about Rip Currents & Knowledge.* The Effectiveness of the NOAA, Sea Grant and LAA Outreach and Education Program. A Study Conducted on Long Beach Island, New Jersey; 2006. Available at http://www.amstat.org/education/posterprojects/projects/2008/4-Grades7-9-ThirdPlace.pdf (accessed December 2014).
8. McCool J, Ameratunga S, Moran K, and Robinson E. Taking a risk perception approach to improving beach swimming safety. *Int J Behav Med.* 2009; 16: 360–6.
9. Drozdzewski D, Shaw W, Dominey-Howes D, Brander R, Walton T, Gero A, Sherker Goff SJ, and Edwick B. Surveying rip current survivors: Preliminary insights into the experiences of being caught in rip currents. *Nat Hazards Earth Syst Sci.* 2012; 12: 1201–11.
10. Australian Water Safety Council. Australian Water Safety Strategy 2012–15. 2012. Available at http://www.royallifesaving.com.au/__data/assets/pdf_file/0011/4016/AWSC_Strategy2012_Brochure-Lowres.pdf (accessed December 2014).
11. Rogers RW. Cognitive and physiological processes in fear appeals and attitude change: A Revised theory of protection motivation. In Cacioppo J and Petty R (eds.). *Social Psychophysiology.* New York: Guilford; 1983; 153–177.
12. Rosenstock IM. Historical origins of the health belief model. *Health Educ Monogr.* 1974; 2: 328–55.
13. Ajzen I. From intentions to actions: A theory of planned behavior. In Kuhl J and Beckmann J (eds.). *Action Control: From Cognition to Behavior.* Berlin: Springer-Verlag; 1985, pp. 11–39.
14. Schwarzer R. Modeling health behavior change: How to predict and modify the adoption and maintenance of health behaviors. *Appl Psychol Int Rev.* 2008; 57(1): 1–29.
15. Nieto-Montenegro S, Lynne Brown J, and LaBorde L. Using the Health Action Model to plan food safety educational materials for Hispanic workers in the mushroom industry. *Food Contr.* 2006; 17: 757–67.

16. Prochaska JO, and DiClemente CC. The transtheoretical approach. In Norcross JC and Goldfried MR (eds.). *Handbook of Psychotherapy Integration.* 2nd ed. New York: Oxford University Press; 2005, pp. 147–71.

17. Schmidt M. Investigating risk perception. A short introduction. 2004. Available at http://www.markusschmidt.eu/pdf/Intro_risk_perception_Schmidt.pdf (accessed December 2014).

18. Department of Health. Changing behaviours, improving outcomes. A new social marketing strategy for public health. 2011. Available at https://www.gov.uk/government/uploads/system/uploads/attachment_data/file/215610/dh_126449.pdf (accessed December 2014).

19. Frewer L, Howard C, and Shepherd R. Public concerns in the United Kingdom about general and specific applications of genetic engineering: Risk, benefit and ethics. *Sci Technol Hum Values.* 1997; 22: 98–124.

20. Rothman AJ, and Salovey P. Shaping perceptions to motivate healthy behavior: The role of message framing. *Psychol Bull.* 1997; 121: 3–19.

21. Moran K. Rock fisher safety in Auckland, New Zealand: Five years on, University of Auckland. *Int J Aquat Res Educ.* 2011; 5(2): 164–73.

22. Brander R, Hatfield J, Sherker S, and Williamson A. An evaluation of a community knowledge-based intervention on beach safety: The Science of the Surf (SOS) presentations. *World Drowning Conference 2011*, Vietnam, 2011.

23. Surf Life Saving, Australia, Research News. Issue 8, July 2014. Available at http://sls.com.au/sites/sls.com.au/files/downloads/Publications/SLSA%20Research%20News%20-%20Issue%208.pdf (accessed December 2014).

FURTHER READING

Breakwell GM. *The Psychology of Risk: An Introduction.* Cambridge: Cambridge University Press; 2007.

COI (Central Office of Information). *Communications and Behaviour Change.* London: COI; 2009.

Conner M, and Norman P (eds.). *Predicting Health Behavior: Research and Practice with Social Cognition Models.* 2nd ed. Buckingham, England: Open University Press; 2005.

Corvello VT. Risk comparison and risk communication: Issues and problems in comparing health and environmental risk. In Kasperson RE and Stallen PJM (eds.). *Communicating Risks to the Public.* Dordrecht: Kluwer; 1991, pp. 79–118.

Corvello VT. Risk communication. In Callow P (ed.). *Handbook of Environmental Risk Assessment and Management.* Oxford: Blackwell Science; 1998, pp. 520–41.

Darnton A. *Practical Guide: An Overview of Behaviour Change Models and Their Uses.* London: Government Social Research Service (GSR); 2008.

Maibach E and Parrott RL. *Designing Health Messages: Approaches from Communication, Theory and Public Health Practice.* Thousand Oaks, CA: Sage; 1995.

NICE (National Institute for Health and Clinical Excellence). *NICE Public Health Guidance 6 'Behaviour Change at Population, Community and Individual Levels'.* London: NICE; 2007.

Petty RE, and Cacioppo JT. *Communication and Persuasion: Central and Peripheral Routes to Attitude Change.* New York: Springer-Verlag; 1986.

Slovic P (ed.). *The Perception of Risk.* London: Earthscan, VA; 2000.

Sniehotta FF. Towards a theory of intentional behaviour change: Plans, planning, and self-regulation. *Br J Health Psychol.* 2009; 14: 261–73.

17

Beach safety education

KEVIN MORAN

INTRODUCTION

Many beach lifeguarding organizations recognize that, as providers of public safety, their primary role of drowning prevention through rescue is invariably underpinned by promotion of water and non-water beach injury prevention. In keeping with the axiom (attributed to Benjamin Franklin in relation to fire safety) that an ounce of prevention is worth a pound of cure, many organizations have engaged in public education programmes that promote beach safety. While the public and media perception of a beach lifeguard's role invariably focuses on the emergency response capacity at the beach, the role of prevention has become institutionalized in many organizations with the establishment of public beach safety education strategies and programmes. This has not always been an easy process, especially where resources are limited and rescue/sport functions appear to some to be compromised by the diversion of much-needed funds to beach safety promotion. Such internal tensions within organizations are sometimes ameliorated by the resultant high profile of beach lifeguards in the community, the possibilities of employment of lifeguards in an instructional capacity and the provision of commercial sponsorship for beach safety promotion. It is the purpose of this chapter to examine the provision of beach safety programmes in selected countries so as to provide examples of the various forms of beach safety education that are currently promoted. Extensive web links are provided to guide the reader to the sites for further information on the available beach safety programmes.

NEW ZEALAND

Surf Life Saving New Zealand (SLSNZ) offers a range of surf safety courses and resources for both the school sector and the public at large [1]. Courses are organized at a national level via a designated education development officer and run regionally by lifeguards employed as part-time instructors during the summer season. Courses are available at the beach (Beach Ed) and in the classroom (Surf to School). The programmes are curriculum-based and designed for primary school children aged 5–13 years. Beach Ed is taught at surf clubs in a day-long programme; it caters to groups of 25–70 students and costs under $10 per student [2]. The programme is structured across four groups: Year 0–2 (Surf Aware), Year 3–4 (Surf Smart), Year 5–6 (Surf Sense) and Year 7–8 (Surf Safety). Some high schools also take part in modified Beach Ed programmes. This scaffolds learning opportunities and allows schools to attend and receive a different programme every second year. It includes education on rip currents; wading, duck diving, swimming, games and relays; age-appropriate learning from school years 0–8; and sun smart awareness. Approximately 35,000 students enrolled in this programme in 2013–2014.

A more recent development is the Surf to School programme that is school-based where lifeguard instructors teach children beach safety and survival skills [3]. It is designed for schools that have difficulty getting their students to the beach and costs between $2 and $5 per student. A Surf to School trailer brings resources such as rescue equipment to the school and, where a swimming pool is available, children are taught practical water competencies. A typical 60–90 minute session includes the following: how to recognize rips and dangers at the beach; how to be sun smart; instruction on rescue equipment and how it is used; the role of the lifeguard; and how to join a surf lifesaving club. As a follow-up to the school visit, beach education fact sheets and quizzes are available online to reinforce student learning. Approximately 6,000 students enrolled in this programme in 2013–2014.

In addition to the formal school programmes, SLSNZ also promotes surf and beach safety via its public education website [4]. Resources include beach safety tips, information on rip currents and rock-based fishing safety. A beach-specific database called *Find a Beach* is also available to the public providing important information on water and weather conditions, patrol hours, hazards and suitability for activities such as surfing and fishing [5]. Generic beach/water safety information with supporting videos (such as the 'New Zealand Water Safety Code' and 'SunSmart') are also available online.

Collaborating organizations also contribute to beach safety, especially where research suggests that educational interventions are necessary. For example, rock-based fishing has been identified as a high-risk activity in the Auckland region where easy access to the rugged west coast makes rescue problematic and prevention a priority [6]. Based on an annual evaluation of fishers' knowledge, attitudes and behaviours, Watersafe Auckland Inc. has developed multilingual resources available electronically (including booklets, brochures, posters, DVDs, CDs and videos) aimed at new migrant fishers, who make up the majority of fishers [7]. Other organizations also offer public safety advice on beaches on their websites including Water Safety New Zealand [8] and New Zealand Search and Rescue through its Adventure Smart branding [9].

AUSTRALIA

Surf Life Saving Australia (SLSA) has committed extensive resources in both school and community beach safety education with over 100 surf education programmes delivered nationwide [10]. The youngest age group targeted are preschool children with programmes called *Surf Babies* and *Little Lifesavers*. In the school domain, SLSA developed a cross-curricula resource for primary schools in 2007 called *Surf's Up* [11]. A second edition in 2009 contains worksheets, lesson plans and activities for use by primary school teachers to teach about surf safety. Primary age children are provided with two programmes entitled *Surf Awareness* and *Beach to Bush*. Rural children, perhaps not familiar with the beach environment, are included via the Beach to Bush programme [12]. It involves lifeguard instructors who travel to regional and remote schools to teach about beach and aquatic safety. Since it began in 2004, the Beach to Bush programme has travelled more than 100,000 km and addressed 250,000 students in over 1,000 schools. The skills and safety lessons focus on surf conditions and how to stay safe when visiting the beach, with the water safety principles taught being equally applicable to other aquatic environments, including rivers, dams, creeks, pools or other waterways. A programme called *Surf Survival* is available for high school students while minority groups such as new migrants have a programme entitled *On the Same Wave* to introduce new residents to the surf beach lifestyle and its vagaries.

In the public domain, SLSA provides extensive electronic resources under its branding of BeachSafe via two sites entitled *Beach Safety* [13] and *Find a Beach* [14]. The Beach Safety site offers advice on topics such as flags and signs, rip currents, marine stingers and first aid. Many of the resources include video clips that help demonstrate beach hazards (such as rip currents) and safety features (such as cardiopulmonary resuscitation). Beach safety brochures and videos are available in several languages, including English, Arabic, Malay, Chinese and Korean.

SLSA also has a very comprehensive electronic database on beaches available to the public via its Find a Beach portal. Its primary source of information is the Australian Beach Safety and Management Programme database, which provides summaries of all of a beach's unique qualities – its hazards, geographic location and facilities as well as large photos which head up every beach's page. This is complemented by current weather conditions and warning advisories for each beach (supplied by the Bureau of Meteorology), live patrol data (taken from Surfguard and Surfcom information via SLSA), live news (taken from organization Twitter feeds) and even ongoing events which can be managed by surf club administrators and members of the public alike. The beach data are available as a free Beachsafe application that can be downloaded for smartphone devices at the App Store for iPhone and iPad and Google Play for all Android devices.

UNITED KINGDOM

Several organizations offer surf and beach safety programmes to schools. The Royal National Lifeboat Institution (RNLI) resources for schools and youth groups are available online and include lesson plans, whiteboard activities, fact/activity sheets, assembly packs, youth group activities, multimedia and other interactive resources [15]. The Royal Life Saving Society United Kingdom offers a range of certificated awards under its Survive and Save scheme entitled the *Beach Lifesaving Awards* (bronze, silver and gold), which include rescue and survival skills in the surf as well as skills and information relating to identifying and surviving rip currents, tides and sandbars [16].

Surf Life Saving Great Britain offers a programme entitled *Junior Lifeguard* that is designed to teach 7- to 14-year-olds about beach and water safety [17]. During the Junior Lifeguard session, children learn to bodysurf, dolphin dive, paddle a rescue board and identify waves, rip currents and other dangers. A prerequisite of the programme is that children are able to swim 50 m unaided. The programme aims to improve children's confidence, teamwork and social skills while giving them the opportunity to develop a new sporting interest for life.

In the public safety domain, the RNLI provides online resources related to beach safety that include advice on rip currents, flags/warning signs and hazards/dangers [18,19]. Among the dangers highlighted are tombstoning, a high-risk activity that involves jumping or diving from a height into water, coasteering (which involves traversing coastal cliff scenery) and more standard surf-related activities such as surfing and body boarding. A current water safety promotion taking place at three popular beaches entitled *Swim Safe* involves collaboration between the RNLI and the Amateur Swimming Association [20]. The programme is aimed at 7- to 14-year-olds. Each session consists of a 10-minute talk with the lifeguards, followed by 30 minutes of in-water tuition from the swimming instructors. A pilot test of the programme in one location reached 2,300 children in a six-week period in 2013, and Swim Safe has since been rolled out at four locations in 2014, including an inland lake.

As part of the RNLI public beach safety promotion, a Beach Finder app is available at no cost for Apple and Android devices; the app also gives real-time weather and tide information as well as five-day forecasts [21]. The programme includes 214 beaches that are patrolled by lifeguards in the United Kingdom. In addition, information on lifeguard patrol hours and water quality supplied by the Marine Conservation Society are also available. To date, the promotion has had 39,500 downloads.

In 2013, the RNLI piloted a new campaign entitled 'Respect the Water'. This was based on a detailed analysis of the key risks that people were taking, and the evidence suggested that a campaign targeting adult males was required. The Respect the Water promotion used a series of media opportunities to emphasize the folly of male underestimation of risk and overestimation of ability characteristic of many drowning situations. James Haskell, a high-profile England Rugby player, is shown attempting to push a tonne of water to illustrate that while many males may think they are capable of coping with the risk of drowning in open water, many are ill-equipped to manage that risk.

An interesting example of a multilateral approach to beach and coastal safety was the development of a safety policy around coasteering. A joint project involving lead agencies such as the RNLI, the Maritime and Coastguard Agency and the Royal Life Saving Society was established via the National Water Safety Forum beach advisory group [22]. Under their direction, an industry working group was established involving around 120 organizations and individuals to develop industry and commercial standards of practice and guidelines for risk management. These guidelines – which include such topics as risk management approaches, understanding the hazards involved, competency of groups/guides, route planning, weather, emergency response and liaison with coastguards – are currently overseen by the National Coasteering Charter established in 2011, which includes the majority of providers and training bodies.

UNITED STATES

The United States Lifesaving Association (USLA) recognizes the importance of prevention as a primary role of lifeguarding and promotes public safety education through its manual [23] and its website [24]. No formal education programmes are offered to schools by the USLA but USLA chapters and lifeguard agencies presented more than 8,000 public lectures to almost a quarter of a million people in 2013 [25]. Many US beach lifeguard organizations offer junior lifeguard programs, with over 10,000 enrolled each year. These programmes are typically offered for a fee to help offset the cost of assigning lifeguards and assistants to train youth from ages 7 to 17 in safety practices similar to those used by lifeguards. They can last from two to five weeks during the summer months. Some of these junior lifeguards may go on to apply and receive training to work as lifeguards, but most simply learn skills such as basic water safety, understanding rip currents and how lifeguards safely rescue others in distress.

In addition, educational resources are available for teachers online and include information on beach safety topics such as rip current identification and what to do if caught in one; sun and heat safety; and preventing/managing stings, bites and cuts [26]. Public information videos on drowning and rip currents are available in both English and Spanish. These are viewable from the USLA website or via the USLA's YouTube channel. The USLA and the National Oceanic and Atmospheric Administration offer artwork for beach safety signs and brochures at no cost from the USLA and National Oceanic Atmosphere Administration (NOAA) websites.

The USLA offers its top ten safety tips on its website at www.usla.org/safetytips [27]. Other generic safety organizations, such as the Centers for Disease Control [28], also promote beach-related safety messages on their websites.

As part of their public beach safety promotion, the Public Education Committee of the USLA coordinates a National Beach Safety Week through its nine regions. Recently, this has been held in conjunction with a Rip Current Awareness Week. For example, in 2014 several water safety conscious organizations (including the NOAA, the National Sea Grant Program, the USLA and the National Park Service) combined in an effort to heighten public awareness of rip currents at surf beaches, with the catch phrase 'Break the Grip of the Rip!®'. This campaign took place during the first full week of June, which coincides with the traditional start of the summer vacation season [29].

BRAZIL

The Brazilian Life-Saving Society (SOBRASA) [30] is a not-for-profit organization founded in 1995 by a group of professionals with the common objective of drowning prevention. SOBRASA acts as a national coordinator of all the military and civil institutions that participate in rescue services, general public education and projects that promote aquatic awareness, safety and prevention. On its website, SOBRASA has made available online over 6 GB of information on drowning prevention including instructional booklets, for example, a drowning prevention programme for primary/elementary schools that has four different educational tools (a lifeguard presentation, a video, a comic book and a refrigerator magnet) presented during a 30–40 minute session targeted at children aged 5–9 years [31], DVD videos on drowning prevention at beaches [32], recommendations [33] and posters [34].

Among its water safety promotional activities both in the school and public domain, SOBRASA has taken the following actions:

- Distributed 60,000 educational brochures, 35,000 stickers and 1,000 adhesive magnets on drowning prevention topics.
- Made 18 presentations at nautical trade shows and other public events to 9,000 participants.

- Made 84 presentations/exhibitions on rescue and first aid in schools, clubs, condominiums and shopping malls.
- Delivered 499 lectures on drowning in Brazilian schools, clubs, universities, conferences, symposia, courses, gyms, condominiums, hotels and water parks to 16,000 participants.
- Provided instruction on aquatic rescue at the beach to 1,300 children in schools.
- Provided 75 courses on aquatic emergencies to 3,000 students via teachers of physical education and swimming, water sports people and health professionals. The aquatic emergencies course aims to teach simple tips to prevent drowning and how to help save a life without becoming a second victim.
- Delivered 26 first aid courses (12-hour courses) to 780 students [35].
- Organized two national drowning prevention conferences in 2013 and 2014 [36] for lifeguards and swimming teachers.
- Cooperated with ISO to develop Blue Flag status for beach safety.
- Developed an online course [37] on drowning prevention that includes 1,500 questions in a safety quiz on basic life support and aquatic emergencies, to be followed by sections on prevention, first aid and surf lifesaving.

EVALUATION OF EDUCATIONAL INTERVENTIONS

While lifeguard organizations recognize the value of educating the public about beach safety and many have actively developed interventions to promote key safety messages, the evaluation of beach safety programmes is sadly lacking. A recent review of recreational drowning prevention interventions for adults [38] noted that robust data and evaluation of preventative measures was needed to support the development of targeted and tailored prevention interventions. The authors also noted that previous 'interventions have focussed and reported on the proximal or short term effects in the prevention of adult drowning', yet little is known about retention and subsequent application of safety knowledge accrued from such water safety promotion measures. The International Life Saving Federation (ILS) has developed a framework of best practice to assist water safety

organizations [39]. The framework recommended continuous evaluation of interventions, with results being well documented and shared so that results that demonstrate some effectiveness can inform practice and prioritization of interventions. Unfortunately, as Leavy et al. [38] observed, 'To date this approach to the design and delivery of interventions to prevent drowning events has yet to be implemented widely, resulting in a scarcity of clear, theoretically-based relevant information and interventions'.

While acknowledging a lack of consistency in programme evaluation and a lack of robust and uniform measurement, some beach-related interventions have been subject to evaluation. In Australia, the 'Don't get sucked in by the rip' campaign aimed to improve beachgoer recognition of rip currents using posters, postcards and brochures at two intervention areas in New South Wales. A study comparing an intervention and control group at patrolled and unpatrolled beaches of similar hazard rating reported positive changes in understanding of rips [40]. Beachgoers were interviewed one year before and immediately after the intervention using a control and intervention group. Upon completion, intervention respondents demonstrated improvement in intentions to swim away from a calm-looking rip, improved ability and confidence in identifying a rip, better intention never to swim at unpatrolled beaches and more effective responses to being caught in a rip, compared with the control respondents. The authors concluded that 'the relatively brief print-based campaign was effective in warning beachgoers about calm-looking rips'.

A safety project aimed at reducing drowning among rock-based fishers on Auckland's rugged west coast has used a standardized annual self-complete written questionnaire to evaluate the impact of an on-site safety programme promoted by safety advisors and lifeguards [6]. The cyclical nature of the ongoing project meant that the focus of safety changed each year in response to the fisher's perceived safety knowledge and competency. In the first five years of the project, a significant increase in the use of life jackets by fishers was reported; 72% (95% CI 0.66–0.77) in 2010 compared with 34% (95% CI 0.25–0.44) of fishers in 2006. It is anticipated that the project, now in its tenth year of operation, will analyze and report a decade of findings in the near future.

Other programme evaluations currently underway or in the planning stage may offer empirical evidence to substantiate the continuation of beach safety education. In New Zealand, an evaluation of the two programmes currently promoted in primary schools (Beach Ed and Surf to Schools) is about to be initiated and likely to involve a pre/post-intervention evaluation of surf safety knowledge, attitudes and behaviours. In the United Kingdom, a pilot rip current education scheme has been completed and is in the process of reporting.

While such evaluations offer a promissory note of future effective educational interventions, it is critical that organizations investing time and energy in beach safety education build in meaningful evaluations of programme effect that are founded on valid and reliable measures. Robust, standardized evaluations that allow for comparison and universal application are to be encouraged. Furthermore, since many beach safety organizations have limited research capacity and heavy demands on resources for their primary role of lifeguarding, collaborations that share evaluation meanings, methods and measures would be both cost-effective and capacity building. One avenue of collaboration that has demonstrated collective and mutual benefits is the association of lifeguard organizations (such as SLSA, SLSNZ, RNLI) with universities that have the research expertise and capacity to advise/assist evaluation activities and produce publishable results. An excellent example is the International Rip Current Symposium, which brings together both academics and lifeguard practitioners in the common pursuit of understanding rip currents and determining ways to contribute to public safety. To enhance knowledge and avoid duplication of effort, it is further recommended that organizations share evaluation techniques and findings with fellow organizations and that international bodies (such as ILS) take a lead role in dissemination.

A recently published RNLI report [41] on UK lifeguard preventative actions and incident rates has highlighted the importance of another form of safety education intervention – that of direct contact with the public at the beach during operational activity. The Report suggests that this incidental form of intervention has a beneficial effect on public safety behaviour and, in conjunction with other forms of preventative action (such as sign flag changes and tannoy announcements) has a positive effect on incident reduction. Recent research by Woodward [42] has suggested that lifeguards perform an important educative role in their interaction with the public while on duty. When beachgoers (n = 407) were asked to identify how best to educate the public on rip currents, communication from lifeguards was the second highest response (n = 62, 10%) behind signage (n = 148, 24%). Further research on the educational effectiveness of informal safety promotion by on duty lifeguards during their front line guarding at the beach is recommended.

CONCLUSION

Many lifeguard organizations have recognized the value of prevention in saving lives and preventing injury at our beaches. In doing so, many have taken on the mantle of safety educators by providing schools and communities with programmes, promotions and information that inform beachgoers of ways of safely enjoying the beach as a site of leisure and recreation. While not detracting from their primary role of drowning prevention through rescue, many lifeguards actively promote beach safety through prevention informally at the beach when on patrol or formally through educational leadership in the school, community or media. The importance of these latter roles is subject to scrutiny because their value is often more intrinsic and less tangible than the more extrinsic and overt consequences of rescue. It is important therefore that beach safety education is evaluated as part of an ongoing educative process rather than a final product. A future focus on beach safety programme evaluation will hopefully provide evidence of the impact of targeted education interventions and illustrate the worth of institutional investment in prevention to the ongoing safety of beachgoers whose safety under our care demands nothing less.

ACKNOWLEDGEMENTS

My thanks to lifeguard friends and colleagues who contributed to this section; without their guidance and knowledge, I would have had to rely on electronic sources for information – sources that are sometimes idiosyncratic and therefore not always trustworthy.

REFERENCES

1. Surf lifesaving New Zealand. Welcome to education. Available at http://www.surflifesaving.org.nz/education/
2. Surf lifesaving New Zealand. Beach education. Available at http://www.surflifesaving.org.nz/education/school-education/beach-ed/
3. Surf lifesaving New Zealand. Surf to school. Available at http://www.surflifesaving.org.nz/education/school-education/surf-to-school/
4. Surf lifesaving New Zealand. Public education. Available at http://www.surflifesaving.org.nz/education/public-education/welcome/
5. Surf lifesaving New Zealand. Find a Beach. Available at http://www.findabeach.co.nz/
6. Moran K. Rock-based fisher safety promotion: Five years on. *Int J Aquat Res Educ.* 2011; 5(2): 164–73.
7. WaterSafe Auckland Inc. Resources. Available at http://www.watersafe.org.nz/resources.asp?page=149#Rock Fishing
8. Water Safety New Zealand. Beaches. Available at http://www.watersafety.org.nz/education-and-safety/safety-advice-2/beaches/
9. New Zealand Search and Rescue. Water safety code. Available at http://adventuresmart.org.nz/files/water-safety-code.pdf
10. Surf Life Saving Australia. Community education. Available at http://sls.com.au/what-we-do/community-education
11. Surf Life Saving Australia. Surfs up. A cross-curricula resource for primary schools. Available at http://sls.com.au/kids/images/resources/Surf's%20Up%20Cross%20Curicular%20Resource%20for%20Primary%20Schools.pdf
12. Surf Life Saving Australia. Beach to bush. Available at http://sls.com.au/content/water-safety-priority-beach-bush
13. Surf Life Saving Australia. Surf Ed. Available at http://beachsafe.org.au/surf-ed
14. Surf Life Saving Australia. Find a beach. Available at http://beachsafe.org.au/
15. Royal National Lifeboat Institution. Teachers and youth leaders. Available at http://rnli.org/safetyandeducation/teachersandyouthleaders/Pages/teachers-and-youth-leaders.aspx
16. Royal Life Saving Society United Kingdom. Beach lifesaving awards. Available at http://www.rlss.org.uk/index.php/survive-a-save-beach-awards
17. Surf Life Saving Great Britain. Youth development. Available at http://www.slsgb.org.uk/youth-development#fun1
18. Royal National Lifeboat Institution. Safety and education. Available at http://rnli.org/safetyandeducation/Pages/safety-and-education2.aspx
19. Royal National Lifeboat Institution. Beach safety advice. Available at http://rnli.org/safetyandeducation/stayingsafe/beach-safety/Pages/Beach-safety-advice.aspx
20. Royal National Lifeboat Institution. Swim safe. Available at http://rnli.org/safetyandeducation/stayingsafe/beach-safety/Pages/Swim-Safe.aspx
21. Royal National Lifeboat Institution. Beach finder app. Available at http://rnli.org/safetyandeducation/stayingsafe/beach-safety/Pages/Beach-finder-app.aspx
22. Royal Society for the Prevention of Accidents. Staying alive. Coasting safely along. Available at http://www.rospa.com/leisuresafety/Info/PublicationsJournals/staying-alive-coasteering.pdf
23. Brewster BC (ed.). *Open Water Lifesaving. The United States Lifesaving Association Manual.* Upper Saddle River, NJ: Prentice-Hall; 2003.
24. United States Lifesaving Association. USLA beach safety and drowning prevention educational materials. Available at http://www.usla.org/?page=RESOURCES
25. United States Lifesaving Association. 2013 National Lifesaving Statistics. Available at http://arc.usla.org/Statistics/current.asp?Statistics=Current
26. United States Lifesaving Association. Beach and water safety tips for safe day at the beach. Available at http://c.ymcdn.com/sites/www.usla.org/resource/resmgr/docs/uslabrochurefinal.pdf
27. United States Lifesaving Association. USLA's top ten beach and water safety tips. Available at http://www.usla.org/?page=SAFETYTIPS
28. Centers for Disease Control. Drowning risks in natural setting. Available at http://www.cdc.gov/Features/dsDrowningRisks/

29. National Oceanic Atmospheric Administration. Rip current safety. Available at http://www.ripcurrents.noaa.gov/week.shtml

30. Sociedade Brasileira de Salvamento Aquatico. Home page. Available at http://www.sobrasa.org/

31. Sociedade Brasileira de Salvamento Aquatico. Project prevention in primary schools. Available at http://www.sobrasa.org/projeto-de-prevencao-de-afogamento-nas-escolas-de-ensino-primario/

32. Sociedade Brasileira de Salvamento Aquatico. Drowning prevention DVD. Available at http://www.sobrasa.org/doe-ganhe-brindes/

33. Sociedade Brasileira de Salvamento Aquatico. Recommendations. Available at http://www.sobrasa.org/category/recomendacoes-em-salvamento/

34. Sociedade Brasileira de Salvamento Aquatico. Poster folder. Available at http://sobrasa.org/new_sobrasa/wp-content/uploads/2013/01/folder_BLS_frente_2008-copy.jpg

35. Sociedade Brasileira de Salvamento Aquatico. Achievements. Available at http://www.sobrasa.org/realizacoes-2/

36. Sociedade Brasileira de Salvamento Aquatico. 2nd National Drowning Prevention and Lifesaving Pool Conference. Available at http://www.sobrasa.org/ii-simposio-brasileiro-piscinasegura/

37. Sociedade Brasileira de Salvamento Aquatico. Courses. Available at http://www.sobrasa.org/cursos-informativos-gratuitos/

38. Leavy JE, Crawford G, Portsmouth L, Jancey J, Leaversuch F, Nimmo L, Hunt K. Recreational drowning prevention interventions for adults, 1990–2012: A review. *J Community Health.* 2015; 40(4): 725–35. DOI 10.1007/s10900-015-9991-6.

39. International Life Saving Federation. *Drowning Prevention Strategies: A Framework to Reduce Drowning Deaths in the Aquatic Environment for Nations/Regions Engaged in Lifesaving.* Leuven, Belgium: International Life Saving Federation; 2008.

40. Hatfield J, Williamson A, Sherker S, Brander R, Hayen A. Development and evaluation of an intervention to reduce rip current related beach drowning. *Accid Anal Prev.* 2012; 46: 45–51.

41. Royal National Lifeboat Institution (RNLI). Understanding the Relationship between Lifeguard Preventative Actions and Incident Rates. Poole, UK: RNLI; 2015.

42. Woodward E. Rip currents in the UK: Incident analysis, public education and education. Unpublished doctoral dissertation. School of Marine Sciences and Engineering, Plymouth University, UK. 2015.

18

Establishing beach safety and lifesaving programmes in a developing country

NORMAN FARMER AND THOMAS MECROW

INTRODUCTION

The boys, all aged eight and nine, had been playing on the shoreline when they were dragged out to sea by a strong rip current. None of them could swim. By the time the emergency services arrived, it was too late. Had there been a lifeguard service, the children would probably have survived.

This story from Labous [1] is all too familiar in low and middle income countries (LMICs).

However, other than through media there is often very little data on incidents of coastal-related drowning death and injury. This lack has not stopped local people in LMICs or high income countries (HICs) from wanting to do something to reduce or eliminate drowning deaths on coastal waterways, including the ocean, seas and major inland waterways.

The WHO *Global Report on Drowning* [2] has provided the world with a greater understanding of the drowning death problem across the world, including the needs of LMICs and also effective responses.

This chapter is focused on establishing a drowning prevention programme in a developing country (aka LMIC) with an emphasis on coastal settings and beach lifesaving.

Further, this chapter is based on the experience of the primary author, gained through a number of years working with and in LMICs in the Asia Pacific region aiding the establishment or improvement of beach lifesaving activities and services, in particular his work with Surf Life Saving Australia (SLSA) from 2007 to 2014.

METHODOLOGY

Getting started

ESTABLISHING THE NEED

At the outset in planning to introduce a beach lifesaving drowning prevention programme or service, it is important to establish the need.

The cost and effort required to establish a programme or service should be commensurate with the results that will be achieved. This consideration is especially important in LMICs where locals may see a drowning prevention intervention as reducing resources for other interventions (e.g. malaria and HIV/AIDS) that are seen as more important. This perception could exist despite the fact that any available funding is specifically earmarked for that particular project.

A successful and lasting programme will be one that has community 'buy-in', ownership. If the programme has been requested by the community, then the challenges of getting such buy-in will be smaller. However, if the programme is being implemented on the back of data or information not readily accessible to the community, then it is important that the need is clearly communicated to the local community and that the intervention is culturally and contextually appropriate.

A need must be based on evidence of a problem. There are often a range of challenges to establishing a good evidence base:

Available data. Drowning deaths in LMICs often go unreported due to:

1. Poor reporting systems.
   a. A lack of a standardized classification system means drowning deaths are often misclassified.
   b. Lack of a central recording database. Data are often collected and stored by multiple agencies (police, hospital, local healthcare facility, ambulance). A lack of a central database means records are often duplicated or inconsistent.
2. A body may not be taken to a health facility.
   a. Absence of transport or high transportation costs, particularly in rural areas and during a rainy season.
   b. Religious concerns may mean the body is buried or cremated soon after death.
   c. The body may never be found or identified.
3. Poor quality data collection, collation and analysis of data. There may be a lack of local skills or experience in the collection, collation and analysis of drowning data, leading to bias and error.

Even if a need has been established, the community may see the intervention as unneeded (or taking away from resources) if there are other problems that are considered more prominent.

In a local context, the need for a drowning prevention initiative such as a beach lifesaving service has arisen due to drowning death or injury, whether in a single or multiple incidents. Local communities want to act to reduce if not eliminate a future occurrence. This local response can

in part be explained in human needs similar to those outlined in Maslow's hierarchy of needs [3]. The safety and security response often feeds the desire for people to take immediate action rather than delaying action to learn more about the issue at hand. In the case of drowning in LMICs, experience has shown that local people and/or visitors want to take action to prevent further drowning, often without taking the time to learn more about any underpinning evidence.

START-UP TRIGGERS

Experience has shown there are numerous triggers that stimulate people and/or organizations to want to reduce drowning. The following are some of the more prevalent:

- A local community or organization recognizing drowning as a local problem.
- A LMIC government agency approaching an in-country HIC diplomatic post for assistance.
- An expatriate working and/or living in a LMIC community who wants to make a difference in reducing drowning.
- Tourists on vacation in a LMIC country who either witness, hear or read of a drowning event; are approached by a staff member at a holiday destination for assistance; or who are proactive and approach a senior manager at a holiday destination offering support.

Whatever the trigger, there is frequently someone or an organization who is available to assist in some form. However, there are generally three key issues that are often overlooked at the outset:

1. Assistance needs and wants
   a. What is the assistance that is actually needed versus what is wanted or requested? These often can be quite different as the perception of what is needed may be gained from a TV show or a person on holiday; it may not necessarily reflect an understanding of the needs of the local community. An investigation or more specifically a risk assessment should be conducted in the community in need, the results of which inform a meaningful plan of action.

b. Is external assistance wanted by the community? The local community as a collective may not want any external assistance even if one person or a small number of the community understand the need.

c. Could external assistance cause problems in the local area? Cultural issues can be quite strong in some if not many communities and external assistance may not be accepted until a relationship has been developed with the local community and the need has been clearly communicated.

2. Fit for purpose: Is the assistance to be provided or being provided fit for purpose for the country, its people, culture and needs or is it simply a transplant of an HIC programme?

   a. Is the intervention being offered the best control measure, given the data? (For example, is the provision of a beach lifesaving service the answer, or would it be preferable to teach people how to swim?)

   b. Is the intervention culturally sensitive?

   c. Is the intervention contextually appropriate? (For example, are lifeguards being taught to shout/go for help when doing CPR, even if none is likely to be around?)

   Quite often, well-meaning lifesavers from an HIC visiting another country take their HIC lifesaving education, training, resources and equipment without an understanding of local issues, which are likely to be significantly different to those they are used to.

3. Sustainable: At the start, how can one ensure that the assistance being provided will result in a service, programme and/or resource that can continue once the assistance is no longer provided?

   a. There are numerous examples across the globe whereby well-meaning people and organizations travel to a community in need for a week, or a month or maybe a year, provide some assistance and when their resources or interest diminish they leave. Is what remains sustainable without ongoing assistance? If no, then was it worthwhile starting in the first place?

Maybe there were some lives saved for a short while, but the longer term benefit is in doubt.

   b. Is there an appropriate local organization set up for the task (e.g. capacity)? There are a number of key factors in determining whether a programme and/or organization will be sustainable including governance, collaboration, finances, corruption, systems and monitoring and evaluation.

Multiple approaches to addressing drowning prevention

PUBLIC HEALTH APPROACH TO DROWNING PREVENTION

Over the past two decades the public health approach to drowning prevention has gained widespread support as the positive impacts achieved through the process have been demonstrated through rigorous research, in particular in Bangladesh [4,5].

The public health approach has four key stages [6] that are underpinned by an evidence base. The following sections outline the public health approach in a drowning prevention context.

Stage 1: Define the problem (surveillance). Before drowning can be effectively addressed it is important to understand the extent of drowning, where it occurs, who it impacts: i.e. to understand the *who, what, when, where, why* and *how*. This involves collecting and analyzing data such as the number of drowning-related deaths and injuries, the frequency of events, where drownings occur, trends and other relevant data. The data can often be obtained from a range of sources such as police reports, coroner's reports, hospital records and population-based surveys.

Stage 2: Identify risk and protective factors. It is also important to understand the risk factors that lead to drowning death and injury and what interventions may protect people from drowning. Since the 1990s, there have been advances in risk management processes and procedures that provide a systematic approach to understanding the risk and what risk mitigation strategies work better for any given situation.

Stage 3: Develop and test prevention strategies. The development and testing of drowning prevention strategies (aka risk mitigation strategies) are to reduce if not eliminate risk factors or to introduce interventions that may protect people from drowning. These strategies and intervention programmes are designed and developed using research data, risk assessment results and often the adaptation of strategies and programmes that have been shown to be effective in other countries. The strategies and programmes need to be continuously monitored and evaluated to ensure effectiveness.

Stage 4: Implement, evaluate and share. The drowning prevention plan is now implemented on a broad scale through community engagement, training, education, technical advice and encouragement. Periodic evaluation will ensure that the plan is fit for purpose and effective – e.g. continuous improvement. Scaled-up interventions will be most effective through a collaborative effort.

However, and contrary to modern public health principles and actions, establishing a drowning prevention programme in a developing country is not linear in a majority of cases. There are numerous entry points into a programme, which from the primary author's experience is triggered by a number of factors including the following:

- Initiation by expatriate living in-country
- Developer initiation
- In-country government requests to a diplomatic post or an emerging in-country organization with a humanitarian mission
- Diplomatic post of an alien government
- Intervention of a knowledgeable person while travelling

In an ideal world, the public health convention outlined above would be followed.

Where there is an entry point later in the public health approach steps, for example developing and testing prevention strategies such as introducing a lifeguard service, the local community should be encouraged to collect drowning-related data to better understand the drowning problem in the local community and whether or not the intervention strategy is effective.

It could be argued that in the year 2015 (and years beyond) the level of government recognition and/or support from private philanthropy will be less or even absent without a rigorous public health approach being taken. For example, the Bloomberg Philanthropies, which has in recent years funded drowning prevention projects in Bangladesh, has

six components to its distinctive approach [7]. One of these components is harnessing the power of data to assess opportunities, measure progress, evaluate impact and improve performance.

RISK MANAGEMENT APPROACH

As mentioned previously, over the past 20 years the adoption of a risk management approach to drowning prevention has been adopted by a number of lifesaving organizations in a number of HICs and also by the International Life Saving Federation (ILS) [8].

The release in 2009 of the international standard ISO 31000.2009 *Risk management – Principle and guidelines* [9] has provided an international framework which coastal managers and lifesaving organizations can use to identify hazards and risks and to introduce effective risk mitigation strategies.

Interestingly, these risk management processes, guidelines and standards that have emerged in the developed world over the past two decades are largely unknown in the developing world of LMICs. Experience has shown that to attempt to impose risk management in developing countries is largely futile. However, a gentle education of some of the basic principles of hazard identification, rudimentary risk assessment and some risk mitigation strategies such as provision of lifeguards has shown to be understandable and helpful in a range of coastal communities.

ILS TOTAL SERVICE PLAN AND DROWNING CAUSE AND RESPONSE DIAGRAM

The ILS is continually reviewing drowning prevention strategies to ensure effectiveness. In the second edition of 'Drowning Prevention Strategies, A framework to reduce drowning deaths in the aquatic environment for nations/regions engaged in lifesaving' [10], ILS acknowledges that its framework has been developed from the perspective of developed nations and regions with well-developed lifesaving practices. Further, for nations and regions without an established drowning prevention or lifesaving organization, the framework identifies the factors that cause people to drown and provides evidence-based measures to prevent and treat.

The document breaks out the causes and the broad responses that can be made for each cause. To help establish an in-country drowning prevention strategy, there are lists of responses presented that have been used in other nations or regions to deal with each cause. Further, the document notes that it is helpful to understand the drowning problem and at-risk populations. Research will assist in determining the target and prevention strategies that would be most effective.

The drowning cause and response diagram shown in Figure 18.1, which was originally developed by Surf Life Saving New Zealand and adopted by ILS, provides helpful guidance on the primary causes behind drowning and broad responses to each, all of which are underpinned by a risk management approach.

This drowning cause and response diagram is helpful in Step 3 of the public health approach, i.e. developing and testing prevention strategies.

SUGGESTED KEY STEPS TO ESTABLISHING AN EFFECTIVE LIFESAVING SERVICE

With the above image in mind, the following steps are provided as a guide to setting up an effective

lifesaving service, which is much more than just employing and training lifeguards.

1. Determine the area which requires lifeguard coverage. For a Greenfield site, this is often where most people are currently swimming or bathing. Unfortunately, quite often this is also where the land manager or local residents have developed car parking and change facilities with little regard for the hazards for those unaware of water safety matters. This is where risk assessment is vital.

2. Conduct a risk assessment to identify the hazards and use of the area by locals and visitors, and importantly the actions required to be taken to remove, reduce or manage those risks.

3. The person responsible for the lifesaving service should carefully select the location for a swimming/bathing zone taking into account the recommendations of the risk assessment.

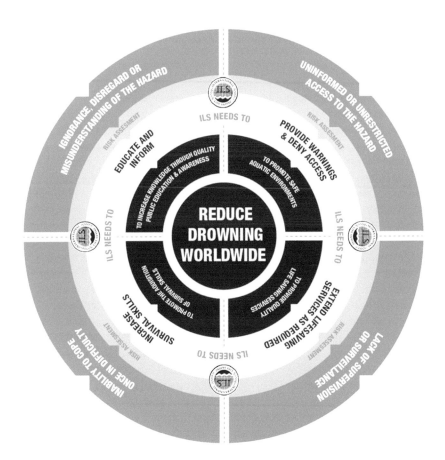

Figure 18.1 Drowning cause and response diagram. (Courtesy of International Life Saving Federation, Leuven, Belgium.)

The location should provide minimal risks to both the swimmers/bathers and the lifeguards, be situated such that it is easy to observe people in the water, have ready access and egress for users and emergency services, have good communication coverage and many others.

4. Prepare standard operating procedures (SOPs), inclusive of relevant emergency action plans (EAPs). The SOPs outline the information and processes required to manage the location from a public safety perspective, usually conforming to relevant international standards, guidelines and best practices. The EAPs provide guidance on the actions in the case of specific emergencies should they occur. The SOPs will ensure that all lifesaving service personnel know how the chosen location operates, that they follow the common procedures and that emergencies are dealt with effectively.

5. Lifesaving service management and communication systems need to be implemented to ensure that the number of beaches and operating times are continually managed effectively prior to, during and after the operating times each day.

6. Purchase of requisite equipment (training and operational) to ensure the service is able to be provided in accordance with the SOPs and also to manage and mitigate the risks identified in the risk assessment.

7. Recruitment and training of the required number of lifeguards ensuring that sufficient numbers are available to suitably supervise the number of locations and the duty periods, taking into account the turnover of staff and also the unavailability of some staff for sickness or family reasons.

8. Commencement of the service
   a. Deploy the service (equipment and personnel) in accordance with the SOPs.
   b. Communication: Inform the local community, potential tourists and relevant emergency services of the location and operating times of the service.

9. Regular monitoring and evaluation of the service is required to ensure the service is being provided to relevant standards and that the lifeguards are on duty at the required locations and at the most appropriate times to satisfy the needs of the venue users. SOPs will need to be periodically reviewed and updated.

10. Continual improvement should also be considered such as upgrading or introducing new equipment as it becomes available and/or affordable. This could include all-terrain-rescue vehicles, rescue watercraft, closed circuit television and the like.

INTERNATIONAL STANDARDS AND GUIDELINES

There are a number of international standards and guidelines that can guide the implementation and operation of effective beach lifesaving, including the risk management standard ISO 31000.2009 highlighted above in the section 'Risk management approach' and also the ILS drowning cause and response process depicted in Figure 18.1.

Another international standard that has proven to be effective is ISO 20712 (in three parts) *Water Safety Signs and Beach Safety Flags* [11], which was in part developed from the ILS *Lifesaving Position Statement on Beach Safety and Information Flags* [12]. However, simply having a standard is insufficient to be effective especially in LMICs and where there is not an established lifesaving organization to promote the standards. An example of this is in Vietnam where traditionally the red and yellow beach safety flags have indicated a private beach area and not an area that is generally a safer place to swim or under the surveillance of trained lifeguards. Figure 18.2 depicts the inappropriate use of red and yellow flags by a resort in Vietnam to cordon off its restaurant area. This is not helpful in promoting beach safety. Safety standards and guidelines must be used as intended.

SPORT FOR DEVELOPMENT AND PEACE

Another methodology that has proven to be effective in drowning reduction in a LMIC context is Sport for Development and Peace (SDP) [13] or more specifically the adaption of its principles.

The Sport for Development and Peace founder and special adviser to the UN secretary-general on Sport for Development and Peace, Wilfried Lemke has remarked that 'sport has a crucial role to play in the efforts to improve the lives of people around the world. Sport builds bridges between individuals and across communities'. The United Nations (UN) has been using sport as a tool in development cooperation and humanitarian aid efforts for decades.

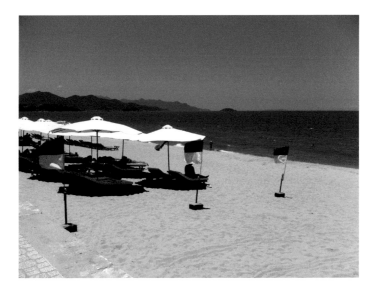

Figure 18.2 Incorrect use of beach safety flags. (Courtesy of N. Farmer. With permission.)

In India from 2009 to 2014, the SDP principles were adapted into a drowning prevention context by the Rashtriya Life Saving Society India (RLSSI) [14] in the Australian Sports Outreach Programme funded by the Australian Government and supported by SLSA. The programme goal was to enhance the capacity of the RLSSI to deliver high-quality (well-organized, regular, inclusive) pool-based swimming instruction, lifesaving and lifeguard training programs and facilitate increased participation in lifesaving sports, thereby contributing to the act of preventing accidental death and injury in India.

The outcomes achieved included significant increases in the participation of children and youth in the Swim and Survive program, primarily through capacity building activity for the trained swimming, lifesaving and lifeguard instructors and expanding the number of 'portable pools' in four states.

DEVELOPMENT EFFECTIVENESS: MONITORING AND EVALUATION

How do you know that your beach lifesaving service is effective? This is a question often posed by people from developed lifesaving organizations to people supporting the development and/ or improvements to beach lifesaving services in LMICs. The answers vary from 'I do not know' to 'we rescue people daily'.

Limited resources in the drowning prevention sector, especially in coastal settings, has limited and is currently limiting the level of monitoring and evaluation being undertaken. All available resources and funding are being applied to beach lifesaving programme set-up and running. This is not to say there is not a commitment to monitoring and evaluation.

In 2012, the ILS released a position statement titled 'Development Aid Effectiveness' [15], which provides guidance to ILS members and collaborating partners on what constitutes effective development aid. It describes how stakeholders can work within the frameworks of the Paris Declaration on Aid Effectiveness (2005), the Accra Agenda for Action (2008) and the Busan Partnership for Effective Development Cooperation (2011) to contribute to the achievement of ILS objectives across drowning prevention, lifesaving and lifesaving sport. At present, this body of work is largely unknown and unused and more promotional activity is required to take advantage of the guidance offered by this position statement.

DISCUSSION

This section provides information on a range of topics the primary author has encountered in his beach lifesaving development activities in LMICs.

Expertise of the service provider

The introduction of beach lifesaving services in LMICs is largely *ad hoc* and often provided by lifesaving people and organizations from HICs with limited resources and a low level of knowledge of the local needs in the LMIC community, but with a high level of humanitarian commitment.

The expertise of the individual lifesaving people in particular, who for the most part are providing support outside their traditional lifesaving organization, varies greatly from retired lifesavers to currently active and experienced lifeguards.

In many instances, the lifesavers and lifeguards have a good understanding of the well-developed high-quality lifesaving procedures, training, resources and equipment in use in their home location, for example the SLSA *Public Safety and Aquatic Rescue Manual* [16] but on occasion they do not. Very few will be familiar with the *International Beach Lifeguard* instructor and student manuals for use in areas where specialist equipment and facilities are unavailable. These publications were produced by the Royal National Lifeboat Institution (RNLI) and the International Drowning Research Centre – Bangladesh in 2012 [17]. This situation is further exacerbated by a limited knowledge of the needs, languages and cultures of the local community they wish to assist in establishing a beach lifesaving capability. However, this can be corrected with knowledge and guidance from those with experience.

Quite often one of the first responses is to say to the local community 'you need trained lifeguards and rescue boards'. However, in many cases there are very few people that can swim and those that can often cannot manage the distance which is expected of a lifesaver to international standards. In the case of a rescue board, the costs for which in 2015 vary from A$1,000 to A$1,500, the local community does not have sufficient funds to purchase such equipment. In a number of countries the primary author has assisted, the costs of a rescue board has been 12 months' wages for a local person.

In summary, not only does a travelling lifesaver wanting to assist a local community need up-to-date lifesaving skills and capabilities, they will also need a broad understanding of the local issues, needs, cultures, support systems and government requirements before starting any form of assistance.

Funding

The level of funding for international drowning prevention efforts is miniscule compared to funding for other public health causes.

However, while there is limited funding for beach lifesaving whether from governments, international philanthropy, lifesaving organizations, hotel and resort operators or from individuals wanting to help, there are still many developmental projects occurring across the developed world.

There are very few well-structured fundraising campaigns for drowning prevention in LMICs.

Government grants for drowning prevention vary from country to country but are largely nonexistent. Some government grants identified for broad developmental activities and often associated with the UN Millennium Development Goals [18] have been known to be adapted for use in a drowning prevention setting such as beach lifesaving.

The range of sources of funds for beach lifesaving vary greatly from an individual donating small amounts of money to purchase basic lifesaving equipment, to local fundraising events, to conducting training for hotels and resorts to raise money for programme delivery to the poor and to corporate sponsors supporting the provision of community lifeguard services.

Government support (intra- and inter-government)

There is no consistent method by which governments support or don't support beach lifesaving (safety) services.

On occasion, there have been instances where governments say they do not see lifeguards as a priority; if they do they spend a significant amount on facilities such as lifeguard towers, very little on labour to employ the lifeguards and even less on vital lifesaving equipment. The reasons behind these sources and application of government funds need further research, although anecdotal feedback indicates that political benefit is easier to gain through construction of fixed assets as opposed to the provision of people and equipment.

There is also the feeling that funding for labour and equipment is easily diverted where there is a culture of fraudulent or corrupt behaviours.

Fraud and corruption

As beach lifesaving organizations continue their developmental reach across international borders, it has become obvious that other cultures often view corruption and fraud differently. For example in the Asia Pacific region, there is a vast variation between countries where fraud and corruption are not tolerated and those where fraud and corruption is openly practised.

Similarly, there is variation on occasion between organizations across countries. For example, SLSA has a policy against fraud and corruption [19], which clearly states that its members representing surf lifesaving in Australia or internationally shall not engage in any corruption or fraud that will bring SLSA into disrepute. Discouraging corruption and fraud overseas also assists developing countries in bringing about a sustainable reduction in corrupt behaviour for the purpose of improving economic and social development.

There are a number of examples of corruption that have impacted beach lifesaving service, including equipment being impounded by customs officials while waiting for an *ex gratia* payment to certain officials before being released. Another example was donated rescue boards being used by lifeguards as a board rental service for the local community to use on payment. The situation was further exacerbated because the boards were not available for use in rescue while rented out.

A tool that can assist those organizations wanting to know more about corruption in particular countries is Transparency International's Corruption Perceptions Index (CPI) [20]. The CPI scores countries on how corrupt their public sectors are seen to be. Behind these numbers is the daily reality for people living in these countries. The index cannot capture the individual frustration of this reality, but it does capture the informed views of analysts, business people and experts in countries around the world.

Commercial enterprises versus safety

There are examples in the developing world in which government-backed welfare is not existent or very limited, where commercial imperatives outweigh any concern for safety.

One example is in a beach resort island in South Asia where beach safety flags have been taken down and lifeguards threatened for closing a beach in front of or near an on-beach restaurant and/or bar concession. The bar operator feared that people would not patronize the concession if the beach were closed or deemed dangerous.

The primary author is aware of an instance where a local government removed and relocated a restaurant concession to enhance beach safety and remove this threatening behaviour.

In addition, there is unfortunately evidence of some lifeguards having multiple jobs and leaving the beach unattended while they carry on other revenue-raising activities.

There are also a few instances where the local lifeguard has been working in the same stretch of beach for many years and has essentially become an institution. This fame and familiarity has had the result of diverting the lifeguard's attention from the task for which they are employed and in itself creating a safety hazard.

Expatriate communities

In a number of Asian communities, the expatriates (expats) who have taken up residence in a developing country, in many instances by marrying a local, have taken up the challenge to improve safety on the nearby beaches. On occasion, the expat may be a surfer or a past surf lifesaver with some knowledge of sea conditions and beach use observing the need for improved beach safety.

Quite often these expats provide valuable guidance on the local cultures, who are the important community, corporate and government contacts and importantly what are the correct channels and legal processes to be followed when wanting to introduce a beach lifesaving service.

As an example, in 1947 Mr Harry Nightingale [21], an expat Australian surf lifesaver from the Bondi Surf Bathers Life Saving Club who was appointed head coach of Ceylon Swimming, helped form the Life Saving Association of Sri Lanka (LSASL). The LSASL has in 2015 grown to an organization with more than 40 affiliated clubs, some of which provide a volunteer beach lifesaving service. The LSASL education and training is respected by a number of organizations including the Sri Lankan

Navy and the Sri Lankan Coast Guard, the latter also proving beach lifesaving services complementary to the LSASL.

Organizational capacity building

Organizational capacity building in the lifesaving sector is often focused on education and training; however, there are many more aspects to capacity building and development. For example, Wikipedia describes *community capacity building* as often referring to strengthening the skills, competencies and abilities of people and communities in developing societies so they can overcome the causes of their exclusion and suffering. Organizational capacity building is used by NGOs to guide their internal development and activities.

Often beach lifesaving organizations in LMICs have developed the practical lifesaving skills; however, there are numerous other skills and competencies that will define the effectiveness and sustainability of the organization and the services it provides. These can include the following:

- Leadership skills: for the organization's membership and for the cause
- Effective programme design and delivery: training and instruction skills
- Business development: how to ensure the organization can build the financial base to enable its services to grow
- Personal relationships: within the organization and external to business leaders and governments

There are numerous examples of effective organizational capacity building that have occurred in the Asia Pacific region in recent years including with the RLSS India and the Australian Sports Outreach Programme; LSASL and its support from SLSA and Life Saving Victoria; RLSS Australia and its work with the SwimSafe project in Thailand, Bangladesh and Vietnam; the RNLI and their Future Leaders programme; and also SLSA with the Nauru Surf Club.

Organizational capacity building cannot be achieved in the short term by 'flying experts in for a few weeks'. Successful programmes are those that are based on long-term relationships.

Collaboration

The potential for collaborative projects to deliver positive developments, social change, innovation and cost savings is undoubtable; however it is not always clear how to ensure that collaboration will be a success.

Quite often there are few international beach lifesaving development projects underpinned by effective collaboration. In our experience, there are numerous reasons for this, including the following:

- Recognition: The individual or organization wants to be recognized for their efforts, resource contributions and the like.
- Funding: The organization providing the highest level of funding wants the greatest recognition.
- 'It's too hard': It is difficult to work with a group with a range of interests, abilities, subject matter knowledge and resources or lack thereof.

There are examples of a collaborative effort at the planning stages; however very few follow through the implementation and onto the monitoring and evaluation stages. There are most likely many reasons for that, with each party having differing or non-aligned expectations and perceptions.

In 2012, the president and CEO of Living Cities, Ben Hecht [22], ???? across the United States there is a growing trend of leaders and organizations putting aside their self-interest to work together as private, public, philanthropic and not-for-profit collaborations. In doing so, they are acknowledging that 'even their best individual efforts cannot stack up against today's complex and interconnected problems'.

Hecht noted that the leaders in this trend are from business and philanthropy. After many years of seriously investing in a large range of programs, these leaders realized that the scale of the problems they were facing could never be adequately responded to by any single organization or initiative.

However, while there are numerous barriers to collaboration, like Hecht, we believe the tide is turning. In the words of Hecht, 'large-scale social change is turning away from competitive practices – the single cell organization asserting it has the solution that needs to be scaled – towards collaborative ones – the coming together of traditional and also non-traditional partners who are willing to embrace new ways of working together'.

The recent release of the 2014 WHO *Global Report on Drowning* and its recommendations will hopefully foster greater collaborative effort.

There is also a growing trend in beach lifesaving towards exchange programs where organizations share their expertise by having volunteers and/or staff visit allied lifesaving organizations to share development and to learn from each other. Since 2007, SLSA and the RNLI have had effective personnel exchanges as have SLSA and the RLSS India.

CONCLUSION

Quite clearly there is a growing trend for introducing beach lifesaving services in LMICs, in particular in major coastal urban centres and also high coastal tourist hubs across Asia and the Pacific. Generally, these lifesaving services are established in an unstructured manner and by well-meaning people and organizations who want to make a difference.

There is an opportunity for developed lifesaving organizations and international bodies such as the ILS to provide support, through a supported collaborative effort, to emerging lifesaving organizations and local communities in LMICs in the establishment and operation of fit-for-purpose beach lifesaving services that consider all local issues and needs.

DEFINITIONS

The following definitions are used in the context of this particular chapter and as such there may be slight definitional variations based on context used by different authors.

Beach lifesaving: The provision of a dedicated service, usually including lifeguards, which is aimed at protecting beach users from the potential dangers of the aquatic environment at a particular beach venue.

Collaboration: The action of working with someone to produce something.

Drowning: The process of experiencing respiratory impairment from submersion/immersion in liquid.

Expatriate (expat): A person temporarily or permanently residing in a country other than that of their citizenship. The word comes from the Latin terms *ex* ('out of') and *patria* ('country, fatherland').

Lifeguard: An expert or strong swimmer trained in first aid and certified in water rescue using a variety of aids and equipment depending on requirements of their particular venue.

REFERENCES

1. Labous, J. A Vaccine Against Drowning— Lifeguards and Swimming Lessons Can Keep Africa's Children Afloat. 2013. Available at http://www.huffingtonpost. co.uk/jane-labous/drowning-african-children-swimming_b_2922121.html
2. World Health Organization. *Global Report on Drowning: Preventing a Leading Killer*. Geneva: WHO; 2014.
3. Maslow, A H. *Motivation and Personality*. New York: Harper and Row; 1954.
4. Cox, R., et al. SwimSafe: A community based water safety and swim-learning Programme suitable for developing countries. *World Water Safety Conference Paper*, Porto Portugal, 27–29 September 2007.
5. Shanks, E. *SwimSafe Da Nang Drowning Prevention Program—Independent Evaluation Report*. Ho Chi Minh City, Vietnam: Mandala Consulting; 2012.
6. Sethi, D. *The Role of Public Health in Injury Prevention*. WHO European Centre for Environment and Health, WHO Regional Office for Europe; 2007. Available at http://www.euro.who.int/_data/assets/ pdf_file/0010/98803/Policy_briefing_1. pdf?ua=1
7. Bloomberg Philanthropies. About. Available at http://www.bloomberg.org/about/ our-approach/
8. International Life Saving Federation. *Position Statement: ILS Risk Assessment Framework*. Leuven, Belgium: ILS; 2008.
9. International Standards Organisation. *ISO 31000.2009 Risk Management— Principles and Guidelines*. ISO; 2009. Available at http://www.iso.org/iso/ catalogue_detail?csnumber=43170.

10. International Life Saving Federation. *ILS Drowning Prevention Strategies— A Framework to Reduce Drowning Deaths in the Aquatic Environment for Nations/ Regions Engaged in Lifesaving.* Leuven, Belgium: ILS; 2011.
11. International Standards Organisation. ISO 20712.1.2008 Water Safety Signs and Beach Safety Flags. 2008. Available at http://www.iso.org/iso/catalogue_detail. htm?csnumber=39682
12. International Life Saving Federation. *Lifesaving Position Statement LPS-14: Beach Safety and Information Flags.* ILS; 2010. Available at http://www.ilsf.org/about/ position-statements
13. United Nations. Sport for Development and Peace. Available at http://www.un.org/wcm/ content/site/sport/ and also http://www. sportanddev.org/
14. Rashtriya Life Saving Society India. Available at http://www.sportanddev.org/en/connect/ organisation.cfm?org=432
15. International Life Saving Federation. *Development Aid Effectiveness, Lifesaving Position Statement-LPS 11.* Leuven, Belgium: International Life Saving Federation; 2012.
16. Surf Life Saving Australia. *Public Safety and Aquatic Rescue.* 34th ed. Sydney, Australia: Elsevier; 2014.
17. International Drowning Research Centre Bangladesh and Royal National Lifeboat Institution. International Beach Lifeguard Instructor Manual. Version 1. IDRC-Bangladesh and RNLI, UK. September 2012. Available at http:// rnli.org/SiteCollectionDocuments/ InstructorManual%20Version%201.pdf
18. United Nations. Millennium Development Goals. Available at http://www.un.org/ millenniumgoals/
19. Surf Life Saving Australia. *SLSA Policy 6.27 Anti-Corruption and Fraud.* SLSA; 2013. Available at http://sls.com.au/sites/ sls.com.au/files/downloads/SLSA%20 Governance/Current%20Policies/6.27%20 Anti-corruption%20and%20Fraud%20-%20 February%202013.pdf
20. Transparency International. Corruption Perceptions Index (CPI). Available at http:// www.transparency.org/research/cpi/overview
21. Bondi Surf Bathers Lifesaving Club. Hall of Fame Members. Available at http://bondisurfclub.com/history/ hall-of-fame-members
22. Harvard Business Review. *Collaboration Is the New Competition.* Ben Hecht CEO of Living Cities; 2012. Available at https:// hbr.org/2013/01/collaboration-is-the-new- compe/

PART 7

Future Thoughts

19

Emerging technologies in beach lifeguarding

IAN GREATBATCH AND DAVID LIVINGSTONE

INTRODUCTION

Writing a chapter on the future technological advances of any sector is fraught with danger, and engaging in this process is to some extent becoming a hostage to fortune. Examples of terribly inaccurate predictions of the future technology are well known and numerous. They can be classified either as predictions that never happened (for example, the prediction in 1955 that 'nuclear-powered vacuum cleaners will probably be a reality in 10 years' [1]) or as predictions that underestimated the advance in science (for example, that it would be possible to travel from New York to Liverpool in two days [2]) (Figure 19.1).

However, despite these clear warnings from history, the authors have agreed to contribute this chapter, looking at the challenges facing lifeguards today and at a number of emerging technologies that may be applied in the future to the role. We humbly accept that we have not thought of everything and that there may be some common tools available to lifeguards in 25 years' time that were not considered or some predictions that do not come to pass. Nevertheless, it is hoped that the reader takes these potential flaws in his or her stride and views the chapter in light of the compatibility of beach lifeguarding with technology. This chapter will be informative if the reader considers the following suggestions as signposts to technology rather than complete and finished articles. We hope you enjoy the ride.

DEFINING THE LIFEGUARDED BEACH ENVIRONMENT

The previous chapters dealt with a number of ways of defining, structuring and understanding the beach environment. This chapter is primarily concerned with technologies and sectors *other* than lifeguarding and necessitates a different set of definitions and typologies in order to help apply technological solutions to lifeguarding challenges.

The beach lifeguarded environment can be regarded as a *community*, or rather a series of overlapping and interacting communities. These communities operate at a variety of scales and timescales using and interacting with the elements of the beach in a number of ways.

From a technological standpoint, these interactions are similar (in some cases identical) to interactions that take place in other environments and in other circumstances. This chapter looks at technologies emerging in a number of fields, many entirely unrelated to lifeguarding, and considers how they could be employed to make our beaches safer and better managed in the future.

THE LADIES' HOME JOURNAL

WHAT MAY HAPPEN IN THE NEXT HUNDRED YEARS

By JOHN ELFRETH WATKINS, JR.

Figure 19.1 What may happen in the next 100 years. (From Watkins JE. *The Ladies Home Journal*. 1900.)

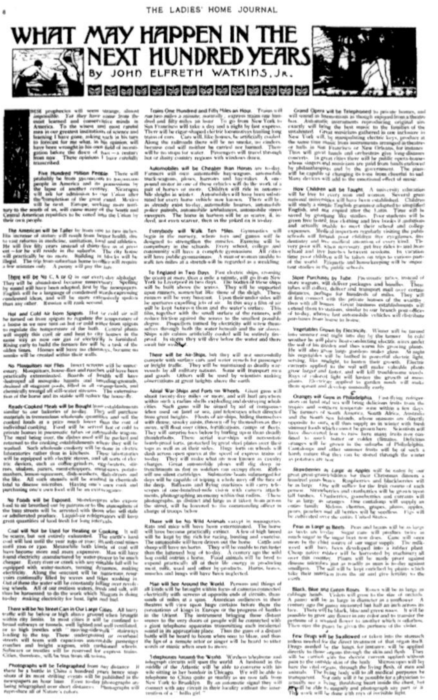

Communities that interact with the beach lifeguarded environment fall under the influence of its constituent factors. There may be many ways of typifying these factors; however, this chapter considers the influence exerted by *four* essential elements (Table 19.1).

These elements spell the acronym 'HOPE', which is appropriate considering the role of the lifeguard on our beaches, and they provide practical challenges to lifeguards operating in the beach environment. These challenges can be influenced by technologies employed in both allied and non-allied disciplines and that in future could be seen on our beaches. Again there are many ways in which one can attempt to typify technological factors that exert an influence on a chosen environment. Four particular technological application types (Table 19.2) are considered as having particular importance over the elements of the beach lifeguarding environment. Each of these applications is in turn considered with regard to the practical lifeguarding challenges faced today and probably those in the future.

These two conceptual axes allow us to treat each element in the subject individually to some extent, although there is some understandable overlap across themes.

Table 19.1 Four essential elements comprising the beach lifeguarded environment

Human environment	The ways in which people interact with and use the beach environment. The people in question can be visitors, staff, lifeguards or people carrying out business or industry or committing a crime – any person who is within the environs of the beach locale and has an impact, or is impacted by it.
Objects	The items within the beach environs that can be considered part of the beach environment at large. These can include pieces of rescue equipment, vehicles, buildings and the possessions of beach visitors. Any object which has been brought to or built upon the beach environment.
Physical environment	The natural features that create the beach environment. Typically these would be the sea, its tides and currents, animals on land and sea, cliffs, rocks or surrounding landscape, the beach, any vegetation on or around the beach and any freshwater objects such as rivers, lakes or pools.
Events	Activities that occur on the beach – legal, illegal, planned or unplanned, short or long duration, regular or irregular. They could include religious festivals, a rescue, a surf competition or a family picnic.

Table 19.2 Four technical applications of particular importance to the beach lifeguarded environment

Monitoring	Technology concerned with observing and recording any of the elements above
Communication	Technology allowing information to be passed between any of the four elements
Visualization	The application of technology to understanding, visualizing or portraying information, location or status of any of the four elements
Logistics	Technology applied to the running or organization of beach safety practices that impinge upon any of the four elements

THE HUMAN ENVIRONMENT

Monitoring

One way of regarding risk is that it consists of hazard plus people. It follows from this logic that a beach in itself is neither dangerous nor requires lifeguarding in the absence of people visiting it. In fact it is self-evident that a beach does not require lifeguarding if there is nobody using the beach or the water offshore, and from this it can be deduced that the human factor of beach use is foremost for any technological application that can assist. This observation is dramatically illustrated by the Mawgan Porth beach tragedy [3], where two people were killed while attempting to rescue other beach users during a period when there were no lifeguard patrols.

The nature and activities of the visitor population is the biggest single concern requiring the response of a beach lifeguard team. One of the traditional and key current roles of the lifeguard is that of surveillance and monitoring, observing numbers, behaviours and the constitution of the beach population. While this will continue to be a critical role, in the late twentieth and early twenty-first centuries there has been a massive growth in the scope and ubiquity of surveillance technologies which, albeit with legislative, social and personal considerations, have the potential to improve the efficiency, nuances, speed and scope of beach monitoring.

Surveillance and monitoring technologies can operate at a variety of spatial and temporal scales to build up a picture of the human environment at different levels of granularity. Intelligent transport systems use off-board and on-board surveillance techniques such as CCTV cameras, active street furniture (for example, streetlamps or bollards with sensors fitted on them), mobile phone signals and satellite navigation systems to monitor traffic movements at local, regional and national scales [4]. In turn CCTV, mobile phone and wireless signals are used to monitor the behaviour and movements of individuals in public spaces [5–7]. Positioning devices in mobile phones, wireless devices and GPS allow individuals to monitor their own locations and activities as well as those of their friends, family and even pets. Bio-monitoring devices such as heart monitors and accelerometers log information about health and fitness for personal use or for sharing with medical or social networks. Combined with affective computing techniques, they can be used to assess personal emotions and stress [8]. Location-aware and bio-monitoring devices integrated into 'always on' and 'always connected' computing devices form an extension to the notion of ubiquitous computing and move into a realm of pervasive computing devices that are embedded in a network space [5]. These devices provide both the information delivery and contextual information-gathering aspects of real-time mobile applications. At the time of writing, Google Glass [9,10] is perhaps the most extreme embodiment of vision, driving ubiquitous and pervasive computing devices, and thus they raise many technological, privacy and aspirational issues surrounding these devices [11,12]. As such Google Glass is the perfect technology to speculate about in a chapter such as this! All of the technologies briefly mentioned could play an increasingly important role in building up a picture of the state of the beach lifeguarding community, and some of the potential lifeguarding applications for monitoring the human environment are explained below.

The first and most basic requirement is to monitor the number of people that are expected at, and are currently on, the beach. Both car counting and footfall constitute important people-counting technologies used in applications such as intelligent transport systems, retail and urban planning and event management [12]. Adnan et al. [13] use the term *real-time geo-demographics*, which can be regarded as a means to provide services to communities of people derived from the knowledge of where they are or will be, rather than traditional geo-demographics, which are primarily concerned with where people live [14]. The raw number of people on the beach (in relation to the overall size of the beach) is a key factor in determining the requisite number and levels of specialism of the lifeguarding staff. Calculating the size of crowds accurately by eye is difficult; however, there are a variety of technologies that have emerged to address this problem. There are automated packages, in use in airports, sports stadia and other publicly accessible places that can do this routinely [15]. By definition, a mobile phone network needs to know the location of people within that network in order to route calls to that phone [7]. CCTV is used in conjunction with video surveillance to analyze traffic movements and to count the number of people in crowds [6] and their trajectories through spaces [5]. This technology has been used to some effect in the Australian CoastalCOMS project, using a combination of video and lifeguard observations to monitor beaches [16]. The world is increasingly immersed in a sea of electromagnetic radiation that interacts with and identifies the people and devices that move throughout it. Applied to the beach lifeguarded community, there is the potential to track their movements from city to surf and to react appropriately with the provision of lifeguarding resources.

However, that is not the only application of this technology. With recent threats from terrorism and insurgency, there have been developments in the automatic recognition of unusual behaviours within crowds [5,17] – exactly what a good lifeguard does already, but automated, on a wide scale and unlikely to be distracted. This technology can be adapted to detect either a swimmer who is beyond their abilities in the water, a crowd of visitors who are acting in an aggressive or threatening manner, areas of overpopulation that could make the beach unsafe or even those potentially about to commit or already committing a crime or an act of terror.

Technology allied to 'affective computing' [18], whereby computers can determine observed humans' emotional state from their stance, could be used to spot those acting unnaturally or those who are injured, drunk, affected by drugs or – most importantly – drowning or in difficulty. Simpler technology, already in use within swimming pools, alerts lifeguards to a swimmer who is motionless and directs the guard to a specific quadrant, shown on a wall display to speed up rescue and recovery. This technology, combined with improved ability to penetrate turbid seawater, could be applied to beach lifeguarding in order to identify and recover near-drowning victims quickly and turning fatal [19].

Other than being the objects of concern, communities that occupy beach environments can be the providers of information, either from their own pervasive devices or via crowd sourcing technologies, whereby online activity can be employed to understand the beach visitor population. Using location-aware applications on mobile phones, pads or smartwatches (in fact any smart device), the visitors to a beach can contribute intelligence on the composition and activities themselves. This may sound slightly sinister at first, and it is true to say that many people would be uncomfortable consciously supplying information to a monitoring system [12]. However, a fair trade can be accomplished, using rewards and trade-offs that will make cooperation more palatable.

For example, the beach management could offer visitors the opportunity to buy in to an information service, entertainment service or rewards service operating on the beach. This could achieve a number of operational aims. There could be competitions, whereby children have to identify beach dangers (see below section 'Visualization'); rewards systems where discounts or gifts are offered at beach outlets; or information, perhaps concerning upcoming events, the weather or tidal conditions. By signing up for this service, customers allow the beach management system to monitor their position and movements on the beach and also to have a communication channel to people to serve important messages. This system could also be used for missing child alerts, tsunami warnings or other safety messages; it could even be used to alert lifeguards or other trained responders to the location of an incident, without relying on visitors being able to describe their location [20].

The public are not the only human population at the beach, with lifeguards and other employees, such as cleaners, maintenance workers, shop or restaurant workers and other emergency services present on larger beaches. Using ubiquitous computing – smart devices with location awareness and computing power, but worn on the body – lifeguards can contribute to a wider intelligence picture of the beach, collecting data that can be compiled centrally, such as temperature, pollution levels, water temperature, rip locations, crowd numbers and so on. By combining this technology with biometric monitoring systems, the beach management could have real-time insight into the physical condition of lifeguards – breathing rates, speed over ground or through water. This technology could be employed to offset the requirement for regular physical tests, with the lifeguard effectively passing a physical test every working day. It could also be used to spot injuries or illnesses early and prolong lifeguards' working effectiveness.

However, the most useful and simple use of this technology would be to have a real-time picture of lifeguard locations, with the ability to match provision and position to requirements. The value of this as a tactical intelligence source would be invaluable, allowing managers at the tactical and strategic level to understand the distribution of resources in a truly spatial way.

Communications

COMMUNICATIONS WITHIN THE LIFEGUARD TEAM

Communication in a response emergency service is always critical. In order for a lifeguard to respond appropriately and in time to an incident, certain information is required, and for effective information passing, there must be good, effective communication. Effective communication can be considered to consist of two contrasting elements – technology and practice. This chapter will deal with the technological aspects, but it is worth considering that good communication is much more than the sum of the technical component parts. Good communication is a common understanding of terminology and concepts, as well as clear, unambiguous and appropriate descriptions

of the scene. In the absence of clear and appropriate communication, any technological advance is worthless. This is something that should be considered as a priority in training development.

Communications within the beach emergency and management community, that of lifeguards, ambulances, coastguard, lifeboat and fire service, who may co-respond to an incident is undeniably a critical component of the beach management infrastructure. There is a tradition of 'Tower Zero' or a 'Lifeguard Operations Centre', a central hub for handling radio traffic, dispatch and tactical structure of all lifeguards at larger beaches (such as Huntington Beach, CA, USA).

Traditionally, the greatest challenge has been the nature of the beach environment with regard to UHF or VHF radios. Rugged headlands, dune structures and bays have resulted in dead zones within the operating area, and subsequent operational inefficiencies. Mobile (or static) repeater units have been employed to some degree of success, but the system has always had some problems.

Recent advances in digital radio communications allow for not only improved direct communications, with crisper and clearer voice messaging, but also allows for some useful additional functionality. One of the main advantages of digital communication is the ability to work within 'talk groups' rather than frequency channels. In the past, if a UHF/VHF channel was in use, it effectively barred any other user (unless they had a more powerful transmitter). Talkgroups allow synchronous multiple messages to be transmitted, more akin to a conference call than a traditional radio call. Talk groups can be created so that routine messages are only passed between those who need to hear them, rather than everyone monitoring a channel – giving greater privacy and less redundancy.

Furthermore, digital radios can incorporate a GPS chip, transmitting the position of the handset at all times. This information can be transmitted to Tower Zero as a matter of course, allowing the tactical planning of the beach to truly understand the distribution of the lifeguard personnel at any given moment.

COMMUNICATIONS TO THE PUBLIC

One of the biggest challenges to a beach lifeguard organization is that of effectively communicating risk, hazards or safety information to beach visitors. This perennial problem, if addressed, has an enormous impact on the effectiveness of lifeguard operations. Through the effective communication of basic safety information, the lifeguard management can reduce the need for rescues, numbers of guards on duty and overall expenditure, while carrying out its primary function of reducing death or injury on beaches. However, it is accepted within the lifeguard community that visitors to the beach, while on vacation, are less aware of hazards, less open to safety messages and so focussed upon relaxing that safety messages are routinely ignored.

Recent technology in augmented reality (AR) [21,22], virtual reality (VR) [23,24] and location-based services [25] allow users to visualize and interact with their environment, via an information network that could have applications in this sector. For example, using a smartphone or pad with a large screen, the visitors could 'see' features of the beach that may normally escape them. These features could be locations of rip currents, real-time location of lifeguards or safe swimming flags. A reward system or game environment could be used, whereby points are won by correctly identifying features of either safety or danger, or perhaps acknowledging new dangers or events as they arise.

This usage can be thought of as effectively a hi-tech version of traditional beach safety colouring worksheets (see Figure 19.2)

By correctly identifying features, acknowledging updates and generally positively engaging with the beach safety management, the visitor could earn virtual tokens of some sort. These could be taken no further than the in-game environment,

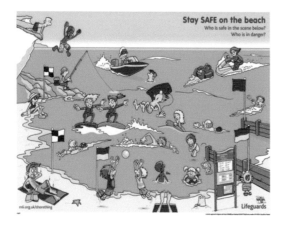

Figure 19.2 Classic beach safety worksheet. (Courtesy of Royal National Lifeboat Institution, Dorset, UK.)

or they could be used in a multiplayer online game setting – competing against other beach users. The tokens could actually be transferred into the real world, by either being exchangeable for products such as refreshments or gifts in beach stores, or for some other type of collectables, such as lifeguard-branded wristbands or beach toys.

Visualization

It is well accepted that the type of beach in question governs the provision and constitution of lifeguarding. However 'type' can mean a number of things; it could mean the physical characteristics of the sea, the beach or surrounding areas, or it could mean the make-up of the human population, the activities and demographic profiles of the visitors to the beach. The physical environment is dealt with in a later section, so this section will consider visualization of the human population of the beach.

Techniques can be adapted from human geography or the retail sector in the discipline of geo-demographics, a technique for segmenting populations into types based on their social, economic or behaviour characteristics, taking into account where they live. These techniques can be brought into beach lifeguarding directly, by considering what geo-demographic types visit the beach at what times and for what activities. In fact, a scheme developed by the Keep Britain Tidy campaign did just that in 2007, although it is now no longer in use [26]. This kind of scheme could be further advanced by using similar techniques to create a demographic clustering within the beach environment itself – using surveys or data collected by buy-in to some of the other participatory schemes on the beach – and running a clustering algorithm on the data to better understand the motivations and behaviours of the visitor population. As Adnan et al. [13] postulate a real-time demographic profile can also be created wherein the transient beach population is considered based on their current location, rather than home address.

Trends or fashions in beach use are hard to predict, as are all popular movements – for example, the invention of the Flyboard water jet pack was hard to predict. Human populations on beaches are equally as dynamic, changeable and difficult to predict as elements of the physical environment, arguably more so. However, generating or sourcing appropriate data and borrowing from disciplines that deal with understanding human populations enable the creation of models and visualization of the beach as a society.

Logistics

A perennial human issue facing lifeguards is that of lost children [27]. The beach is almost entirely perceived as a recreational space by visitors, and as such children tend to explore and parents relax, which results in the typically daily occurrence of lost children. Recent schemes with paper bands have been employed around the world, in which families register at the beginning of the day, possibly for a nominal fee. If a child turns up at a lifeguard station, using the contact information on the band, the family can be easily identified and contacted. Existing technology could take this further. By utilizing cheap, waterproof housings for technology, it is possible to create a location-aware smart band that can inform parents of the location of the child at all times, thereby allowing them to monitor their explorations, or even vibrate when a child is required to return to the family group or leaves a pre-designated area.

The usage of the bands could be expanded to encompass adults or incorporated into some other sort of wearable, ubiquitous computing technology. This technology could be hired out by the beach authorities or be used in conjunction with existing technology owned by the visitor. It would allow adults to not only know where they are on the beach but also would allow for information about events to be pushed to them as they entered designated areas on the beach or as events arose.

OBJECTS IN THE BEACH ENVIRONMENT

Communications

Radio communications were dealt with in the previous section, and still remain – as objects on the beach – the most critical and most common element of beach communications. However, there is no reason that objects themselves cannot communicate, or be communicated to, without human intervention. Embedded computing systems give the ability for pieces of equipment – personal watercraft, rescue boards, lifeguard huts,

whatever – to report their location and status. This would mean that in a central (or remote) location, an operator would be able to visualize the state of readiness of all of the equipment on the beach. The growth of the Internet of Things, whereby everyday objects can be permanently interconnected [28], provides the basis for infrastructure [29] that can integrate the animate with the inanimate. This has implications for both visualizing the current state of affairs and coordinating planning and logistical response to situations.

Visualization

There is a tendency for lifeguards to visualize and understand objects on the beach in terms of their inherent risk. In other words, grouping objects into 'things that may hurt us' or 'things that may save us', for obvious reasons. However, the nature and properties of beach objects is far richer than that, and by visualizing them, it is possible to make the management of beach safety easier and more effective.

Within an object-oriented model of the beach, the things that everyone uses, or interacts with on the beach, can all report any number of properties. Using techniques recently developed in Human Computer Interaction (HCI), or Data Visualization, a 'Tower Zero' would be able to see the beach as a programmer or systems analyst views a system: with interacting objects, reporting and co-interacting; a view of the mechanics of the beach that is totally different from a traditional lifeguard management perspective. It would probably be more akin to visualizations of the internet, or maps of space, but with the added functionality of being able to group or interrogate classes of objects. Protocols such as XMPP [30] can be used or extended to automate elements of inventorying and standard reporting, or alerts for safety of failure of an object.

Logistics

Having accepted throughout this chapter (and book) that the beach environment's key property is that of dynamism, it can be taken as read that this also applies to an object-oriented view of the beach. Objects, such as flags, move throughout the day, in response to the environment or changes in activity on the beach. Rescue equipment is moved closer to where it is needed, as are vehicles. Towers and Huts remain static, but properties within them change, such as the number of staff, the training or experience of those staff, and this too can be reported. As the human environment changes – in terms of activity, density or constitution, objects can change their properties or location in response.

THE PHYSICAL BEACH ENVIRONMENT

This section has dealt with considering the beach as a space filled with interacting objects up to this point. However, it can also be a space of non-interactive objects, which can simply improve their performance, with the addition of emerging technology. Considering a set of existing and familiar beach objects – rescue boards, jet skis, huts etc. – it is reasonable to assume that as technology improves and normal battery life increases, power outputs increase. As such we might then expect to see an increase in potential for any device that launches or throws something, such as rescue line launchers. Easily operated, maintained and deployed, line launchers could pass a rescue line or float to a casualty from the beach, harking back to the now-defunct rocket lines of the nineteenth century. The jet ski is now a common sight on lifeguarded beaches, but smaller powered craft, such as a form of powered rescue board, are evolving. It could combine increased speed and power, the ability to use hands to operate some other equipment or grab a casualty instead of paddling the board, with the lightness and proximity to water surface of a traditional surfboard.

Improvements in remote control signal transmission and reliability, as well as the creative combination of a number of existing technologies have resulted in rescue 'robots' such as EMILY [31] that allow aid to be 'driven' to casualties quickly and in all conditions, allowing the casualty valuable time before a fuller rescue effort reaches them. Robots are not limited to the water, and with the future of wider search and rescue very likely to involve heavy drone use, it would seem likely that some form of rescue device will emerge built on unmanned airborne technology.

Existing technologies for navigation could have a place, albeit in a modified form. The beach can be crowded, but with people moving around, leaving, arriving and so on throughout the day. As such, landmarks can be difficult to find and navigating throughout the beach environs can be difficult. A form of 'beach satnav' could use existing GPS technology to create an updated geography of beach objects and structure for visitors and staff alike.

Routine form filling and data collection is already being carried out using electronic devices, and that trend looks set to continue, albeit with smarter and more wearable devices. Patient reporting forms are well established in pre-hospital medicine, for example [32].

It may well be that the development with the greatest short-term impact will be in materials science. The major barrier to bringing mainstream technology onto the beach (or out to sea, into a fire, collapsed building etc.) is the issue of a lack of ruggedness. Sand, salt, water and electronic devices or devices with moving parts have always had a troubled relationship. The ability to take existing, widely adopted technology and *ruggedize* it for the marine environment and demanding rescue usage may well be a key step.

Monitoring

There are a number of long-standing and well-established sub-disciplines of geography that deal with the physical beach environment – from oceanography, studying the formation and impacts of waves, to beach geomorphology, coastal environmental management to geology and earth processes affecting beaches. This section will primarily deal with subjects allied to *physical geography*, specifically beach geomorphology and oceanography dealing with the littoral, eulittoral, sublittoral and supralittoral zones on the beach.

Monitoring and recording in order to understand the *process* behind geomorphological forms [33] is a key part of geomorphological research and as such has elements that are transferable to beach management [34,35]. For example, research into the formation of rip currents [36] has undergone recent advances with the employment of drones with remote sensing capabilities and 'smart buoys' to record wave strength and character. This technology gives the geomorphologist a greater insight into the processes behind rip current formation, but could be used to create a simple heat map of the beach, giving lifeguards a visualization of the areas most at risk from rips.

Future developments in micro-robots or nanorobotics may allow for a shoal of robots to live in the water off the beach, monitoring all aspects of the beach, from pollution and salinity levels of the water, to seabed profile (bathymetry), to wave surge strength/wave height/rips or undertows. Laser scanning is already well established and becoming cheaper and (perhaps in combination with drones) can scan beaches at low tide to allow us to predict the behaviours of the water at flood.

Robot fish, robot insects, and other unmanned, intelligent and self-navigating devices can take part in routine monitoring of all elements of the beach [37]. All of these technologies would build upon work started in the 1960s to automate and improve understanding of coastal process using technology (projects such as the US Army's DELILAH, Super Duck, DUCK94 and SandyDuck [38]).

General advances in technology supporting monitoring of ocean and atmospheric conditions and events, allied with improvements in computer-based modelling, will allow us to predict more accurately and earlier events that impact on the lifeguarded beach.

Harada et al. [39] demonstrated that lifeguards themselves can be used to monitor the physical beach environment [16]. By simply recording the location, state of tide and intensity of rip currents, a form of empirical data is generated that can contribute to a wider scientific body of knowledge and coastal systems.

It would seem likely that drones will play a major role in search and rescue, emergency response in general and law enforcement, as well as continuing the trend of use within military operations that started in the early 2000s. Numerous trials are already underway in the fields of Search and Rescue (SAR) in general, firefighting and lifeguarding. It would seem almost impossible to conceive that drones will not play a major part in beach lifeguard operations in the near future.

Communications

Automated reporting from smart buoys, nanobots or drones can piggyback on extant communications technology to contribute to an enhanced tactical picture of the working beach. The communication of information concerning the physical beach environment is intrinsically linked to the dissemination of information about the state of the beach, climate or water. Earlier in this chapter, the concept of geographical messaging or communication of information concerning the beach (especially incorporating ubiquitous computing technology) was covered. The same techniques and issues occur when disseminating physical geographic information on the whole.

Visualization

Advances in 3D or holographic projection, as well as existing 2D visualization techniques, can be employed to share and analyze this new information concerning the physical beach processes.

Innovative use of new technologies to allow a change of perspective will allow the physical beach to be viewed in a more effective manner, allowing data, changes and additional information to be seen as well as standard, visual observations. This could involve real-time drone footage, or the use of amphibious vehicles to create an 'island tower' looking at the beach from the sea. This could result in a more enhanced understanding of the physical construction of the beach, but could also result in faster rescues.

Wearable computing such as Google Glass allows the user to interact with services through an optical head-mounted display and natural language instructions. If such technology were ruggedized, it could be teamed with AR technology for lifeguards to see hazards and landmarks and pass on information. It has already been tested in the firefighting sector [40], and transferring the technology and utility of the technology to lifeguarding would be straightforward.

As this technology becomes more popular, products can be offered to beach visitors, enabling them to also see hazards, safe locations, lifeguard huts or beach amenities.

Logistics

One of the logistical issues facing lifeguards in a rescue or recovery scenario is water turbidity, wherein particles suspended in the water and potentially agitated by tidal action absorb or refract light, making the water unclear. Advances in water-penetrating scanning devices, allied to existing technology for detecting casualties on the floor of pools (such as the Poseidon system [19]), mitigate against this issue and allow scanning and detection to take place even in turbid water. Once this technology evolves sufficiently, real-time monitoring of the subsea environment will be possible.

EVENTS IN THE BEACH ENVIRONMENT

The final section in the chapter deals with technologies for understanding and handling events on the beach. The most obvious set of events affecting the beach are tidal or environmental events – the changes and extremes of water extent and height or of wave action. However, beach communities are also places of recreation, commerce and industry, so 'events' of many kinds are commonplace in the beach environment. Beaches are considered spiritual to many in either an informal or formal sense and so can hold a far higher significance for some individuals or communities. These can range from large-scale massive participation events such as parties, concerts or festivals, to individual activities such as surfing or jogging to traditional sunbathing and family recreation activities.

Monitoring

There are few social events, formal or otherwise, that do not have a presence on social media. Effective monitoring and engagement with social media will allow managing agencies to understand and prepare for events, even illegal or unauthorized events. The community in a virtual sense will change to accommodate the new event and this will in turn result in changes to the profile of the community. This can be as simple as an increase in traffic or chatter concerning an event. Although there are issues of privacy and legitimate concerns about the 'monitoring' of a beach community, it could be argued that a lifeguarding agency should be a part of the wider online (beach) community. As a result, any monitoring could be considered a passive and responsible part of good practice, rather than an active attempt to gather intelligence [41].

Communications

Large-scale events can stretch communication systems and will often require a communications network of their own. Digital radio systems (as discussed earlier) would allow specific talk groups

to operate solely concerned with the event, while lifeguarding operations could continue as normal.

Advances in communications technology (the ability to push and message geographically, for example) would also allow managing agencies to alert or inform visitors of upcoming events. In the case of emergencies – fire, tsunami or other events requiring evacuation or an elevated response – this functionality could be used to manage an evacuation, using targeted geographical messaging to distribute crowd numbers evenly across multiple escape points.

The beach and beach culture could be shared across virtual communities, using a number of emergent technologies. Real-time, multi-platform communications allow users or visitors to interact with management, reducing conflict and improving relations (as is being done already in many public spaces) [42]. If managed correctly, this ability will result in a better-managed beach. It is also possible to project the beach and its values beyond the traditional, geographically connected groups, which could be done for a number of activities from beach safety messaging to commercial activities.

Visualization

In the case of large public events (see Figure 19.3a&b), techniques mentioned previously in this chapter such as crowd density and behaviour allow a lifeguard management system to understand the nature, possible intentions and risk from a crowd at an event. With enough prior intelligence or data concerning the event, a VR or AR visualization could be used to prepare for the event, with lifeguards able to 'see' the structures or crowds in place to practise and plan before the event. If 'types' of beach days are created through statistical modelling of past events, preparation and training for types of days can be carried out, using VR/AR technology [21–24].

Visualization techniques could enable those not able to attend an event physically to experience it, democratizing and widening access to the beach. A combination of communications and visualization technologies would allow remote participants for events, increasing the reach of the beach.

Logistics

Taking as read that there are a catalogue of different types of beach days associated with the events that occur on those days, it makes sense to suggest

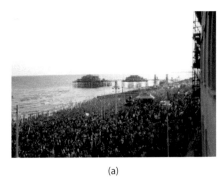 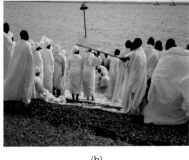

(a)   (b)

Figure 19.3 **(a)** Fatboy Slim at Brighton Beach, UK, in 2001 and **(b)** a North African Christian service in Southend-on-Sea, UK.

that this typology would be used to tailor the life-guarding response and setup for that day. Modular lifeguard units allowing different combinations of equipment and technology could be created, where only that equipment most useful or most likely to be used on that *kind* of day would be in the forward units.

CONCLUSIONS

Lifeguarding, although new as a subject in its own right, draws from a number of well-established disciplines – medical, geographical, technological, sociological and engineering-based – as can be seen in other chapters of this book. This chapter has tried to build on their good work and that of other experts in numerous disciplines to gather a set of suggestions for technological advances in the theoretical stage, or in early development in other fields.

This chapter has also viewed the technological challenges and opportunities within beach life-guarding as being fundamentally concerned with communities. It has considered that the beach and all of the interactions taking place on or around the beach form a kind of nexus of associations with either the environment, objects on the beach or the people that operate there.

Emerging technology is both changing and adapting to communities (as technology has always done), and as a result this wider beach community has itself been changed into a net-worked, real-time, communicating and reacting organism that can be understood, modelled and managed.

Technologies described in this chapter have the potential to become ubiquitous in the wider world (to the point of disdain) or to become a cul-de-sac in the tree of life of technological advance. Therein lies the danger of a chapter such as this. The nature of technology also needs to be considered in terms of its relationship to the whole range of human natures. Clearly the authors have taken a utopian view of technology – viewing technologies in terms of their inherent usefulness in lifeguarding. It should be considered that there is almost always a counter-view, and clearly there are dangers relating to privacy or civil liberties that are broached upon as soon as any organization attempts to monitor or understand a community, even for the most benign of reasons. The propensity for technology to be used for war, terrorism or crime is also a factor that has been overlooked in this chapter. Clearly any development that allows us to understand a phenomenon better allows us to exploit it better – not necessarily with good intentions.

That said, the authors hope that regardless of the fates of the individual technologies cited here, the principles of defining elements of the beach community and applying current emerging trends to those elements is not limited to a particular time or set of technologies. Ultimately, the purpose of technology is to promote society's wider aims – to prosper, preserve or prolong life and aid communities to work more effectively. These aims are clearly interchangeable with lifeguarding, and it is hoped that as a lifeguarding community we can embrace appropriate future technologies to keep ourselves and our communities safe on the beach.

ACKNOWLEDGEMENTS

We thank Matt Horton, senior lifeguard manager (Royal National Lifeboat Institution), and the lifeguards of Bournemouth, Boscombe and Poole Bay beaches for their input and time.

REFERENCES

1. New York Times. Vacuum cleaners eyeing the atom. *New York Times*, 11 June 1955, p. 13.
2. Watkins JE. What may happen in the next hundred years. *The Ladies Home Journal*, 1900; 8(1): 8.
3. BBC News. Mawgan Porth surf deaths tragedy was "unprecedented". Available at http://www.bbc.co.uk/news/uk-england-cornwall-29801594 (accessed 23 December 2014).
4. Khoudour L, Aubert D, Velastin S, Leung V. Video-based detection of specific events in public transport networks.
5. Makris D, Ellis T. Learning semantic scene models from observing activity in visual surveillance. *IEEE Trans Syst Man Cybern B Cybern*. 2005; 35(3): 397–408.
6. Fehr D, Sivalingam R, Morellas V, Papanikolopoulos N, Lotfallah O, Park Y. Counting people in groups. *2009 AVSS '09. Sixth IEEE International Conference on Advanced Video and Signal Based Surveillance*. September 2009, pp. 152–7.
7. Technology—Path Intelligence. Available at http://www.pathintelligence.com/technology/ (accessed 23 December 2014).
8. Greatbatch I, Kleinsmith A. Motion-capture technology for USAR: Only a matter of time. Industrial Fire Journal—Fire & Rescue—Hemming Group Ltd. Available at http://www.hemmingfire.com/news/fullstory.php/aid/2315/Motion-capture_technology_for_USAR:_only_a_matter_of_time.html (accessed 23 December 2014).
9. Rosenberger R. Google glass and highway safety—Messy choices. *IEEE Technol Soc Mag*. 2014; 33: 23–5.
10. Avsec R. Google Glass: 4 Good uses in firefighting. Available at http://www.firerescue1.com/fire-products/technology/articles/1461482-Google-Glass-4-good-uses-in-firefighting (accessed 23 December 2014).
11. Moncrieff S, Venkatesh S, West GAW. Dynamic privacy in public surveillance. *Computer*. 2009; 42(9): 22–8.
12. Norman BD. The paradox of wearable technologies. *Technology Review*, 2011; 116(5): 101–4.
13. Adnan M, Longley PA, Singleton AD, Brunsdon C. Towards real-time geodemographics: Clustering algorithm performance for large multidimensional spatial databases. *Trans GIS*. 2010; 14(3): 283–97.
14. Furness P. Real time geodemographics: New services and business opportunities (and risks) from analysing people in time and space. *J Direct Data Digit Mark Pract*. 2008; 10(2): 104–15.
15. Adey P. Airports, mobility and the calculative architecture of affective control. *Geoforum*. 2008; 39(1): 438–51.
16. Dusek G, Seim H. Rip current intensity estimates from lifeguard observations. *J Coast Res*. 2013; 288: 505–18.
17. Santofimia MJ, Martinez-del-Rincon J, Nebel J-C. Episodic reasoning for vision-based human action recognition. *Scientific World Journal*. 2014; 270171.
18. Picard RW, Healey J, and Vyzas E. Toward Machine Emotional Intelligence Analysis of Affective Physiological State. *IEEE Transactions on Pattern Analysis and Machine Intelligence*, 2001; 23(10): 1175–191.
19. Computer-aided drowning detection: An overview of the Poseidon System for architects and engineers. Available at http://www.poseidonsaveslives.com/Portals/0/Poseidon – Overview for Architects and Engineers 9.2.09.pdf (accessed 4 November 2014).
20. Cardiac Arrest App Crowdsources Good Samaritans. Available at http://www.emergencymgmt.com/health/Cardiac-Arrest-App-Crowdsources-Good-Samaritans.html (accessed 6 January 2015).
21. Siu T, Herskovic V. Mobile augmented reality and context-awareness for firefighters. *IEEE Lat Am Trans*. 2014; 12(1): 42–7.
22. Tsai M-K, Yau N-J. Improving information access for emergency response in disasters. *Nat Hazards*. 2012; 66(2): 343–54.
23. Cha M, Han S, Lee J, Choi B. A virtual reality based fire training simulator integrated with fire dynamics data. *Fire Saf J*. 2012; 50: 12–24.

24. Xu Z, Lu XZ, Guan H, Chen C, Ren AZ. A virtual reality based fire training simulator with smoke hazard assessment capacity. *Adv Eng Softw.* 2014; 68: 1–8.

25. Maglogiannis I, Hadjiefthymiades S. EmerLoc: Location-based services for emergency medical incidents. *Int J Med Inform.* 2007; 76(10): 747–59.

26. Mole MA, Mortlock TRC, Turner IL, Goodwin ID, Splinter KD, Short AD. Capitalizing on the surfcam phenomenon: A pilot study in regional-scale shoreline and inshore wave monitoring utilizing existing camera infrastructure. *J Coast Res.* 2013; 65: 1433–8.

27. Morgan D, Ozanne-Smith J. Surf lifeguard rescues. *Wilderness Environ Med.* 2013; 24(3): 285–90.

28. Xia F, Yang LT, Wang L, Vinel A. Internet of things. *Int J Commun Syst.* 2012; 25(9): 1101–2.

29. Ning H, Hu S. Technology classification, industry, and education for future Internet of things. *Int J Commun Syst.* 2012; 25(9): 1230–41.

30. Che X, Maag S. Testing protocols in Internet of things by a formal passive technique. *Sci China Inf Sci.* 2014; 57(3): 1–13.

31. Emily E.R.S. Available at http://emilyrobot.com/ (accessed 6 January 2015).

32. E-Health Insider. Ortivus wins £10m ambulance contract. Available at http://www.ehi.co.uk/news/EHI/9211/ortivus-wins-%C2%A310m-ambulance-contract (accessed 6 January 2015).

33. Raper J, Livingstone D, Bristow C, Horn D. Developing process-response models for spits. In Kraus D. (Ed.), *Proceedings of the Coastal Sediments 1999*, Long Island, NY; pp. 1755–69.

34. French JR, Burningham H. Coastal geomorphology. *Prog Phys Geogr.* 2011; 35(4): 535–45.

35. Thorpe A, Miles J, Masselink G, Russell P, Scott T, Austin M. Suspended sediment transport in rip currents on a Macrotidal Beach. *J Coast Res.* 2013; 65: 1880–5.

36. Dusek G, Seim H. A probabilistic rip current forecast model. *J Coast Res.* 2013; 289: 909–25.

37. Koprowski R, Wróbel Z, Kleszcz A, Wilczyński S, Woźnica A, Łozowski B, Pilarczyk M, Karczewski J, Migula P. Mobile sailing robot for automatic estimation of fish density and monitoring water quality. *Biomed Eng Online.* 2013; 12: 60.

38. Gunawardena Y, Ilic S, Pinkerton H, Romanowicz R. Nonlinear transfer function modelling of beach morphology at Duck, North Carolina. *Coast Eng.* 2009; 56(1): 46–58.

39. Harada SY, Goto RS, Nathanson AT. Analysis of lifeguard-recorded data at Hanauma Bay, Hawaii. *Wilderness Environ Med.* 2011; 22(1): 72–6.

40. Avsec R. Google Glass: 4 Good uses in firefighting. Available at http://www.firerescue1.com/fire-products/technology/articles/1461482-Google-Glass-4-good-uses-in-firefighting (accessed 23 December 2014).

41. Greatbatch I. The use of twitter as an early warning system for terrestrial search and rescue. *J Search Rescue.* 2014; 1(3): 47–50.

42. Botero, C-M, Williams AT, Cabrera JA. Advances in beach management in Latin America: Overview from certification schemes. In Finkl CW & Makowski C (eds.). *Environmental Management and Governance: Advances in Coastal and Marine Resources.* Springer, pp. 40.

20

Future additions and further research

ADAM WOOLER AND MIKE TIPTON

INTRODUCTION

As per the title of this book, *The Science of Beach Lifeguarding*, we have attempted to ensure that what is presented is underpinned by a scientific evidence base wherever possible. This evidence base is not always complete and sometimes we have had to make a judgement on what to include and what to leave out. Since the time this book was conceived and many of the chapters written, naturally more research has been conducted, and so this final chapter seeks to bring the reader up to date with important topics that didn't make this edition, and to suggest further research that is required to underpin many aspects of the practice of beach lifeguarding that have hitherto not been addressed.

To do this, a gap analysis was undertaken between this book, the recently published second edition compendium of papers entitled *Drowning: Prevention, Rescue, Treatment* [1] and the abstracts from the World Conference on Drowning Prevention 2015 [2]. Brief summaries of each topic that may warrant inclusion in a future edition of this book are presented here.

PUBLIC RESCUE EQUIPMENT, BEACH SAFETY SIGNS AND FLAGS

A number of organisations have conducted studies on the most appropriate and effective type of public rescue equipment (PRE) [3], and a comprehensive guidance document is available from the RNLI [4]. Irish Water Safety (IWS) has successfully introduced a small ring buoy supported by a public education and training programme in schools [5]. Further research into the effectiveness of similar national public education programmes and what equipment is appropriate for different locations is still required, though. For example, the IWS study suggested PRE should be deployed into rip currents to drift out to swimmers in distress, but this contradicts the RNLI guidance document which suggests that no PRE is suitable for shallow shelving beaches, where rip currents are often prevalent.

Following original work conducted by SLSA and the RNLI, ILS has helped with the establishment of an International Standards Organisation (ISO) standard for water safety signs and symbols [6,7]. The ISO 20712 document provides a standardised system for giving aquatic safety information that doesn't rely on the use of words to be understood. The standard consists of three parts:

- **ISO 20712-1:2008,** *Water safety signs and beach safety flags – specifications for water safety signs used in workplaces and public areas.* Intended for use by owners and operators of aquatic environments and by manufacturers of signs and equipment.
- **ISO 20712-2:2007,** *Water safety signs and beach safety flags – specifications for beach safety flags – Colour, shape, meaning and performance.* Specifies requirements for the shape and colour of beach safety flags for the management of activities on coastal and inland beaches.
- **ISO 20712-3,** *Water safety signs and beach safety flags – guidance for use.* Reflects good practice in the use of water safety signs and beach safety flags with examples.

These safety signs and symbols have been incorporated into standardised beach safety signs, many of which have been produced using sophisticated design principles to ensure ease of readability [8] and which are gaining universal acceptance (Figure 20.1). However, further research is required

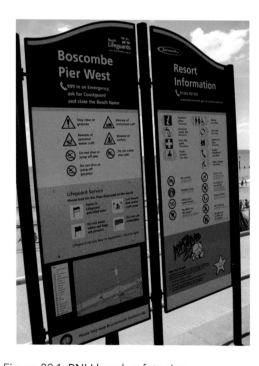

Figure 20.1 RNLI beach safety sign, Bournemouth, UK.

to ascertain whether they are an effective way of reducing risk. Do people read them, do they understand them, do they remember the information they have seen and do they act upon it? As these questions are addressed, we hope a chapter on the use of PRE, beach safety signs and flags will be included in a future edition of this book.

THE TECHNIQUES AND EQUIPMENT USED FOR RESCUE

A simple review of the lifesaving equipment currently being used on an international basis has been produced by Thompson and Wooler [9]. However, while numerous technical training manuals exist that demonstrate how to use this equipment [10], and its historical development has largely been documented [11], very little research has been conducted to determine whether the design is optimal for the tasks it is being used for [9]. A notable exception is the use of rescue fins, which have been looked at using sound scientific research principles [12]. It would be nice to see such scientific rigour applied to the design of the other equipment that beach lifeguards use, including: rescue tubes, rescue buoys, rescue malibu boards, rescue surf boards, inflatable rescue boats, rescue water craft and perhaps some of the beach-based equipment, including binoculars, sunglasses, observation towers, vehicles, first aid kits and even flagpoles. Just because certain things have always been used, this does not mean that with the application of some modern design principles and solid experimental research, new or better-designed equipment cannot be produced. It is hoped that a chapter on the techniques and equipment used for rescue will be able to be included in a future edition of this book.

TRAINING, EDUCATION AND LEADERSHIP DEVELOPMENT

In recent years, a number of countries have introduced competency frameworks that have modernized the approach to the training of beach lifeguards, often using a modular approach integrated into an existing national competency framework. In 2011, International Life Saving Europe (ILSE) helped create a cross-nation project to align the education of lifeguards across Europe as part of the European Qualifications Framework (EQF) under the guidance of the European Union.

This resulted in the first international qualification framework for lifeguards [13,14,15]. Building upon successful higher education programmes for lifeguards already running in Spain, Greece and Portugal [16], ILSE has created a qualification framework for levels 5 to 8 (lifeguard management, bachelor degree, masters degree and doctoral degree) [17]. There are now a number of higher education institutions across Europe looking to participate in this programme, including Cornwall College in the UK, which has developed a foundation degree in coastal safety management [18].

Although some countries have had a mature leadership development programme for many years [19], the advent of recent programmes such as the RNLI Future Leaders in Lifesaving programme is now seen as one of the keys to the success of international lifesaving development [20]. A chapter on the training, education and leadership development of beach lifeguards would therefore be a worthy addition to a future edition of this book.

MANAGEMENT FRAMEWORKS

Through a necessity to comply with both modern legislation and current best business practice, a series of reviews into the corporate governance of Surf Life Saving Australia [21], Surf Life Saving New Zealand [22] and Surf Life Saving GB [23] have taken place over recent years which have led to changes in the way that these organisations are structured and governed. In 2002, Surf Life Saving Victoria and the Royal Life Saving Australia, Victoria Branch merged to form Life Saving Victoria. The transition and subsequent management model and organisation role with the state emergency services framework is currently the subject of a doctoral research thesis (Taylor, N., personal communication, November 2015). Such studies provide an opportunity for established lifeguarding organisations to learn and if applicable, emulate. For those countries looking to establish a new lifeguard organisation, often a requirement as part of an international development programme, this type of review also provides a useful comparative starting point. A chapter dedicated to the management of a lifeguard service itself, and the organisation that supports it, would therefore be another useful addition to future editions of this book.

DROWNING

There are a wide range of studies that will benefit the understanding and thereby prevention and treatment of drowning [24]. For example, studies that will result in a better understanding of the mechanisms of cold shock in children, time to cold-induced physical incapacitation in different situations and the physiological substrates, and psychological fear of drowning may all contribute to prevention of drowning where these mechanisms play a role. A better understanding of the physiological mechanisms of deep tissue cooling and rewarming as well as water aspiration, and which drowning victims may or may not benefit from extracorporeal membrane oxygenation, would be beneficial. Greater insight into hypoxic cardiac arrest that results from drowning and the neurophysiology of central nervous system damage resulting from drowning should contribute to better treatment options, outcome and decisions on when to allow individuals to return home. Research on the physiological responses of breath holding, the diving response, upper airway reflexes, autonomic conflict, aspiration and swallowing, temperature, electrolytes and anoxia in drowning settings can be used to produce drowning-specific models which will allow greater understanding of drowning and the interactions among the responses that act as precursors to drowning.

OTHER RESEARCH RECOMMENDATIONS

There are a series of chapters entitled 'Future Research Questions' in the recent publication *Drowning: Prevention, Rescue, Treatment* [1], many of which are applicable to the beach lifeguarding environment. In addition, the United States Lifeguard Standards Coalition [25] has produced a series of research questions. Many of these have been addressed in this book and many are being addressed through various collaborative projects between academia and lifeguard practiners; a few of these seem to be a priority.

Evaluating and understanding the effectiveness of beach safety education programmes, the core of the prevention role that underpins a beach lifeguard's attempt to break the drowning chain early on, should arguably top the list. Although it is touched upon in Chapters 16 and 17 of this book, until we understand what the most effective measures are that the beach lifeguarding community can take to change people's behaviour, we may be wasting our efforts and deploying our resources inefficiently.

There is still no consensus on the definition of a rescue within the drowning prevention content [26]. It seems worthy of a debate and agreement in much the same way as there has been for the definition of drowning [27]. This would then help with the task of collecting appropriate data, without which we lack the evidence to underpin our research efforts. A universal agreement on rescue terminology, what beach lifeguard incident data we collect, both fatal and nonfatal, what format it is collected in and an international effort to share these data will help produce a much more credible evidence base on which future recommendations to increase the effectiveness of beach lifeguards can be made.

CONCLUDING REMARKS

In the World Health Organisation's recently published Global Report on Drowning, drowning was found to be the third leading cause of unintentional injury death worldwide [28]. The book has therefore become even more relevant and an important part of the global effort to reduce this global drowning burden. The scientific research techniques exist and the level of experience and expertise within the beach lifeguard community has never been so high. Surely there is now a collective responsibility on the worlds of academia and beach lifeguarding to collaborate in order to enhance our understanding of beach lifeguarding, to optimise its function and thereby to save even more lives.

REFERENCES

1. Bierens J (ed.). *Drowning: Prevention, Rescue, Treatment*. Berlin, Heidelberg: Springer-Verlag; 2015.
2. World Conference on Drowning Prevention 2015, Penang, Malaysia.
3. Nelson C, Wills S. Public rescue equipment. In Bierens J (ed.). *Drowning, Prevention, Rescue, Treatment*. Berlin, Heidelberg: Springer-Verlag; 2015.
4. RNLI. A guide to coastal public rescue equipment, p. 49. Available at http://rnli.org/aboutus/lifeguardsandbeaches/Documents/guidetopre.pdf (accessed 16 November 2015).
5. O'Sullivan M. *Public rescue equipment and the chain of survival*. World Conference on Drowning Prevention 2015, Penang, Malaysia.
6. Wills S, George P. Water safety signs and flags. In Bierens J (ed.). *Drowning, Prevention, Rescue, Treatment*. Berlin, Heidelberg: Springer-Verlag; 2015.
7. RNLI. Guide to beach safety signs, flags and symbols, p. 65. Available at http://rnli.org/aboutus/lifeguardsandbeaches/Documents/guidetobeachsafetysigns.pdf (accessed 16 November 2015).
8. Dyer B. RNLI Lifeguard signage design project. University of Bournemouth, UK; 2003.
9. Thompson M, Wooler A. Rescue techniques in pools and beaches with equipment. In Bierens J (ed.). *Drowning, Prevention, Rescue, Treatment*. Berlin, Heidelberg: Springer-Verlag; 2015.
10. Brewster C. *Open Water Lifesaving: The United States Lifesaving Association Manual*. Atlanta, GA: Pearson; 2003.
11. Brewster C. The history of beach lifeguarding (Chapter 1, this volume).
12. Stallman R, Abraldes A, Soares S. Direct body contact swimming. In Bierens J (ed.). *Drowning, Prevention, Rescue, Treatment*. Berlin, Heidelberg: Springer-Verlag; 2015.
13. Wilkens K, Brons R. European qualification framework for the lifeguard profession. In Bierens J (ed.). *Drowning, Prevention, Rescue, Treatment*. Berlin, Heidelberg: Springer-Verlag; 2015.
14. Bissinger D, Stoehr H. *EQF – A cross-national approach to harmonize lifesaving and lifeguarding education in European federations*. World Conference on Drowning Prevention 2015, Penang, Malaysia.
15. Mohr D. *Safer Europe by higher qualified lifeguards and water safety managers – Two projects for the European Qualification framework*. World Conference on Drowning Prevention 2015, Penang, Malaysia.

16. Queiroga AC, Abraldes A, Avramidis S. Higher academic education in lifesaving (EQF levels above 4). In Bierens J (ed.). *Drowning, Prevention, Rescue, Treatment*. Berlin, Heidelberg: Springer-Verlag; 2015.

17. Martin J. EQF2 – *Developing a European Qualification framework for water safety management for delivery in higher education institutions by working in partnerships*. World Conference on Drowning Prevention 2015, Penang, Malaysia.

18. FDA Coastal Safety Management. https://www.cornwall.ac.uk/courses/fda-coastal-safety-management (accessed 16 November 2015).

19. Fitzgerald J. *Leadership development within a water safety organisation*. World Conference on Drowning Prevention 2009, Porto, Portgual.

20. Farmer N, Mecrow T. Establishing beach safety and lifesaving programmes in a developing country (Chapter 18, this volume).

21. Barrington Consulting. *SLSA Organisational Effectiveness Review*. Perth, Western Australia: Barrington Consulting; 2009, 55 pp.

22. Research New Zealand. *Surf Life Saving New Zealand Organisational Development Project*. Wellington, NZ: Research New Zealand; 2008, 143 pp.

23. Conduco Consulting. *Saving Lives Together: Report on the Strategy and Governance of Surf Life Saving Great Britain*. Higher Denham, UK: Conduco Consulting; 2010, 44 pp.

24. Bierens J, Philippe Lunetta P, Tipton M, Warner D. Physiology of drowning: A review. *Physiology* (in press).

25. Wernicki P, Espino M. Evidence-based standards in lifesaving: The conclusions of the United States Lifeguard Standards Coalition. In Bierens J (ed.). *Drowning, Prevention, Rescue, Treatment*. Berlin, Heidelberg: Springer-Verlag; 2015.

26. Moran K. Towards a definition of aquatic rescue. In Bierens J (ed.). *Drowning, Prevention, Rescue, Treatment*. Berlin, Heidelberg: Springer-Verlag; 2015.

27. Beeck Ev, Branch C. Definition of drowning: A progress report. In Bierens, J (ed.). *Drowning, Prevention, Rescue, Treatment*. Berlin, Heidelberg: Springer-Verlag; 2015.

28. World Health Organization. *Global Report on Drowning: Preventing a Leading Killer*. Geneva: WHO; 2014.

Index